"Your skin is the largest organ of your body, and one of its most important. It is vital, then, to keep it healthy. *Smart Medicine for Your Skin* is loaded with information for keeping your skin youthful, as well as remedies and treatments for skin ailments, such as herbs, aromatherapy, homeopathy, supplements, and much more. I highly recommend that all women (and men) who wish to attain radiant skin read this valuable resource, as looking healthy is a major step on your way to a long and healthy life."

PHYLLIS BALCH, CNC, author of the bestselling
Prescription for Nutritional Healing

Smart Medicine for Your Skin

A Comprehensive

Guide to Understanding

Conventional and

Alternative Therapies

to Heal Common

Skin Problems

Jeanette Jacknin, M.D.

AVERY
a member of Penguin Putnam Inc.
New York

Most Avery books are available at special quantity discounts for bulk purchase for sales promotions, premiums, fund-raising, and educational needs. Special books or book excerpts also can be created to fit specific needs. For details, write Putnam Special Markets, 375 Hudson Street, New York, NY 10014.

AVERY

a member of
Penguin Putnam Inc.
375 Hudson Street
New York, NY 10014
www.penguinputnam.com

Library of Congress Cataloging-in-Publication Data

Jacknin, Jeanette.
    Smart medicine for your skin : a comprehensive guide to understanding conventional
and alternative therapies to heal common skin problems / by Jeanette Jacknin.
        p.   cm.
    Includes bibliographical references and index.
    ISBN 1-58333-098-4
    1. Skin—Diseases—Popular works.   2. Skin—Care and hygiene—Popular works.
    I. Title.
    RL85 .J33   2001   2001022741
    616.5—dc21

Printed in the United States of America
10 9 8 7 6 5 4 3 2 1

Book design by Tanya Maiboroda

To Ben, my angel in Heaven,
and Lauren, my angel here on Earth.
Because of Ben I started this book,
and because of Lauren, I finished it.

Acknowledgments

I would like to thank my family, especially my father, for his inspiration, and my mother, Charlotte, and my three brothers Sam, David, and Larry, for their encouragement in writing this book. I especially want to thank my daughter Lauren for being herself.

I would also like to thank the faculty of the Department of Dermatology at the Medical College of Virginia in Richmond, Virginia, for all they taught me about conventional approaches to clearing skin problems. Special thanks to Dr. Algin Garett and Dr. Jerome Parsons, who remembered and believed in me long after my residency was completed.

A warm thank-you to Michael Traub, N.D., for his valuable work on compiling a naturopathic approach to dermatologic diagnosis and natural therapeutics. Also, thank you to Dr. John O.A. Pagano, for his important contributions to natural therapies for psoriasis.

Additionally, I appreciate that the conventional medical dermatology community is now becoming more open and accepting of integrating a traditional and alternative approach to healing skin problems. This is evidenced by the American Academy of Dermatology's recent assignation of a task force to evaluate nutrition and alternative medicine in dermatology, and by the greatly increased number of articles pertaining to natural therapies in recent issues of highly respected and widely read professional dermatology journals.

A special thanks to Mr. Rudy Shur, my first publisher, who inspired me to discover and write more, and to Laura Shepherd, Carol Rosenberg, and Amy Tecklenburg at Avery/Penguin Putnam, who helped bring my work to fruition.

Contents

Part Three

SKIN-CARE TREATMENTS AND TECHNIQUES

APPENDIX

Preface

Our skin is extremely important to our everyday lives. How often have you heard the expressions "Beauty is only skin deep" or "He has thin skin"? Expressions like these show that the skin is more than a physical interface between our internal and external environments . . . it is also a psychological interface and mirror.

If a person's skin is flawed, it is one of the first things that others notice. It leaves a lasting impression. Think of the mythology surrounding "werewolves" with rare skin disorders, witches with facial warts and moles, and pirates with facial scars. These images have been with us in popular literature for centuries.

Today, with increased demand for age-defying cosmetics, creams, lasers, and surgical techniques, the public is even more interested in their own skin. They are more aware of the dangers of too much sun leading to skin cancer, and of the importance of using sunscreen.

With the advent of managed care and HMOs, people have less access to and less time with the doctor or dermatologist of their choice. Your health care has become more dependent upon your own education and research. With so much information readily available on the Internet and a surge in health-related books being written for the lay audience, people are beginning to learn about their skin problems before they see the doctor, to become more self-educated, and to take more responsibility for their own health care. Alternative medical philosophies are also based on the idea that patients are responsible for helping themselves to get better, and that they should not be just passive recipients of the healer's arsenal of drugs.

Over the last decade, I too became increasingly interested in what alternative therapies could add to the dermatologist's armamentarium in helping to heal skin problems. In looking through the consumers' guides to healthy skin, I found that most books dealt only with beauty issues. A few discussed conventional dermatologic approaches to common skin diseases. Rarely, a book discussed how a particular skin problem could be approached using only alternative medical therapies. Compendiums of alternative medical therapies only touched on the field of dermatology. I wanted to write a book that made sense of the increasing array of alternative medical therapies, describing them and ferreting out the most consistently helpful and scientifically substantiated treatments. I also wanted to integrate the conventional approach to treating skin problems and touch on a range of techniques to keep skin healthy and beautiful. I feel that only by understanding the nature of your skin, the newer alternative therapies gaining widespread acceptance, and the preventive and therapeutic options in both the conventional and alternative fields of dermatology can you really practice smart medicine for your skin.

This book is meant to be an easy-to-use, comprehensive guide to understanding conventional and alternative therapies for the skin and helping to heal common skin problems. There are many preventive and treatment modalities described in the book that you can use on your own to supplement your doctor's care. This book is designed to be used in conjunction with treatment by a dermatologist and other health-care practitioners. Its purpose is to add to their care and help give you control over the care of your own skin, so that it will be the healthiest it can be.

How to Use This Book

This is an in-home guide that will help you care for your skin through a unique approach that combines the best of conventional medicine, diet, nutritional supplements, herbs, aromatherapy, homeopathy, acupuncture, stress reduction, and mind/body medicine. Written by a board-certified, experienced dermatologist, it offers advice and explanations of the full spectrum of options available to treat the most common and threatening disorders of the skin.

This book was written to help you make informed decisions regarding the care of your skin on both a daily and occasional basis. The information and suggestions presented here are meant to be used together with the services of a well-trained dermatologist or other qualified health-care professional. This book is not a replacement for consultation with a skilled professional. If you have a troublesome problem with your skin, I strongly suggest that you visit your skin doctor for a thorough physical examination and treatment advice that is personalized to your situation.

The subjects in this book have been divided into three parts. Part One, The Elements of Health Care for Your Skin, discusses the basics for understanding the science of the skin, hair, and nails. The first section summarizes what techniques and therapies are commonly helpful in conventional dermatology. Included is a chart of the pharmaceuticals commonly prescribed for skin disorders, including their desired effects and also potential unwanted side effects. Further along in Part One, the basic history, theories, and practices of dietary therapies, nutritional supplements, herbal medicine, aromatherapy, homeopathy, acupuncture, and acupressure are described, with special emphasis on their application to skin problems. Other therapies important to the healing of the skin include stress reduction, relaxation therapy, meditation, mind-body medicine, emotional work, cognitive-behavioral techniques, spirituality and prayer, hypnosis, biofeedback, and neurolinguistic programming. These are described at the end of Part One.

Part Two, Common Skin Problems, contains an alphabetic listing and discussion of the problems that commonly affect the skin. Each of thirty-six common skin disorders is discussed, with information on causes, associations, signs, and symptoms. First conventional and then alternative treatment options are discussed at length, followed by general recommendations and preventive measures. The conventional therapy information is up to date and based on the standard of care you would expect from a medical doctor who is a board-certified dermatologist. Specific dietary measures, nutritional supplementation, herbs, aromatherapy, homeopathy, acupuncture, stress reduction, mind-body medicine, electrotherapy, light therapy, and music therapy are described for each common skin problem for which they have been found to be helpful. Part Two also contains a troubleshooting guide consisting of a list of symptoms and the conditions that may be causing them.

Part Three, Skin-Care Treatments and Techniques, explains in detail a number of the preventive and treatment procedures mentioned in Part Two. The locations of acupoints are illustrated, and guided imagery techniques are expanded upon. Relaxation techniques, meditation, yoga, therapeutic touch, massage, and bodywork are discussed in depth. Physical therapies, including light therapy, and sound and music therapy, are explained. Tips for daily skin, hair, and nail care are given, as are detailed instructions for performing a monthly skin self-examination for cancerous-looking lesions. The procedures for preparing different herbal treatments are also clearly described. Some of these techniques you are encouraged to do on your own, while others should be done in conjunction with an expert in that field.

Finally, in the Appendix are a glossary of some of the terms used in this book, a suggested reading list with detailed references, and a list of resource organizations that can provide additional assistance.

It is my hope that this book will be very helpful to you in maintaining the health and beauty of your skin through smart prevention and medicine.

PART ONE

The Elements of Health Care for Your Skin

Introduction

You may take for granted what a big job your skin does for you every day. It looks so good that you hardly realize it is working hard to protect your body from the effects of sunlight, water, pollutants, and attacking microorganisms. The skin is also important in temperature regulation, vitamin-D synthesis, and sensory perception, and as a storage site for calories, chemicals, and drugs. We are all very aware of the tremendous psychological effect the appearance of our skin, hair, and nails has on us as well.

The purpose of this book is to help you become informed about your skin in health and in illness. I want to give you a good understanding of what conventional and alternative methods you can use for skin care and for the prevention and treatment of any skin problems that may arise. In order to understand skin problems, you first need to know what normal skin, hair, sweat gland, and nail structure and function are on the microscopic level. In Part One, you will learn about the normal structure and physiology of your skin, the range of possible skin lesions (infected, diseased, or otherwise abnormal patches of skin), and all that both conventional and alternative dermatology have to offer you.

I first describe what the conventional medical approach to assessing and treating a skin problem would be. There are many time-tested and new treatments that conventional dermatology can offer to help with individual skin problems. A medical history and physical examination are always important in determining your type of skin problem. Laboratory tests and a skin biopsy may also be necessary to make a correct diagnosis. Conventional skin therapies involve pharmaceuticals, destruction of offending lesions, laser therapy, chemical peels, dermabrasion, and hair transplantation. Ultraviolet light therapy, photophoresis, and TENS or electrical therapy are other techniques that can play roles in conventional dermatology. These traditional dermatologic techniques are discussed in depth so that you will know what conventional dermatology can offer you to help you with any skin problems you may develop.

Sound nutrition is a core requirement for health. A balanced lifestyle—with plentiful exercise, rest, and sleep—and emotional tranquility are other prerequisites for good health. An integrated approach to skin health and healing considers these elements as well. A balanced, unprocessed, whole-foods diet is crucial to your skin's health. Drinking a sufficient amount of pure water is necessary to keep your skin well hydrated and healthy. Adequate intake of vitamins A, C, E, and K; the B vitamins (especially biotin); and beta-carotene are especially important in keeping your skin healthy. The minerals chromium, copper, and zinc are also necessary for the normal functioning of your skin. Taking nutritional supplements such as bioflavonoids and quercetin, coenzyme Q_{10}, dehydroepiandrosterone (DHEA), essential fatty acids, and selenium can often be very helpful for keeping skin healthy or restoring it to health. Helpful information about all of these nutritional factors is discussed in the section on diet and nutrition. It will help you to take control of your diet and nutrition as part of the self-care of your skin.

The field of dermatology is also very well suited to the acceptance and integration of alternative treatments. Alternative medicine uses a variety of substances and techniques that gradually restore proper functioning of the body to normal health. In Part One, alternative approaches such as herbal medicine, aromatherapy, homeopathy, acupuncture, and acupressure are detailed, with special emphasis on considerations for your skin's health. In most forms of alternative medicine, the mental and emotional aspects of illness are considered inseparable from its physical manifestations, so your individual physical and emotional situation is considered in addition to any localized physical symptoms and signs. Alternative medicine also incorporates methods of detoxifying the body to increase the efficiency of the body's organs and systems. Finally, in alternative medicine you are encouraged to take control of your own personal skin care and health. The success of alternative care depends on your being an informed, responsible patient and choosing to follow the advice and care of knowledgeable health practitioners.

It is important to know not only what alternative medical approaches are available to help you with your specific skin problem, but also to discover which approaches you would feel comfortable using. It is key that you believe in the alternative methods you have chosen to use. The positive effect of a therapy will be magnified if you understand how it works and if you are informed about studies and stories describing how it has helped other people.

In Part One, the alternative health-care approaches of herbal medicine, aromatherapy, homeopathy, acupuncture, and acupressure are each detailed, with special emphasis on considerations for your skin's health. You are encouraged to use many of the alternative methods described in this book at home for your preventive and therapeutic skin care. Other, more involved treatments have to be done in conjunction with a dermatologist and/or a qualified alternative health-care practitioner.

The section on herbal medicine should give you a better understanding of how plants and their parts can be used for medicinal purposes, especially for skin problems. First, I discuss the basics of herbal medicine, then turn to an exploration of individual herbal traditions from China, India, and Europe. Next, the rise of American herbalism is discussed. I look at the actions of various Western herbs, as well as the various forms in which the herbs can be used. Following this, common herbs used in dermatology are described in some detail. The last part of the section deals with possible side effects and drug interactions to be wary of when using herbal treatments.

Aromatherapy is a specific branch of herbal therapy that makes use of the pharmacological properties of certain plants' essential oils. Essential oils are highly concentrated aromatic essences distilled from various parts of certain plants. Like herbal therapy, aromatherapy can be very helpful for some dermatologic problems. This therapy is also well suited to self-care at home. In the section on aromatherapy, I discuss its history, studies of skin conditions helped with aromatherapy, how it works, and the various ways it is used. The characteristics of the essential oils most important in dermatology are outlined. Lastly, possible side effects of essential oils are discussed. After reading this chapter, you should better understand how to incorporate aromatherapy into good preventive and simple therapeutic self-care for your skin.

Homeopathy is an approach to health care that aims to stimulate the body's natural healing response. To do this, it makes use of remedies that are dilutions of natural substances derived from plants, minerals, and animals. In this section, the fundamentals of homeopathy are explained, followed by a brief history of homeopathy and a look at the extent to which homeopathy is used in the world today. Lastly, I will discuss the homeopathic remedies most commonly used in dermatology at the present time. This should give you an informed basis on which to choose some homeopathic remedies for simple home care, as well as an understanding of how an experienced homeopath (a professional practitioner of homeopathy) will treat you if you seek his or her help for a more difficult problem with your skin.

The next section reviews the healing arts of acupuncture and acupressure, with special emphasis on how they can help you with skin problems. I will discuss the fundamentals of the practice of acupuncture, the professional literature on acupuncture, the history of acupuncture in China and the United States, and the specific applications of acupuncture in treating skin problems. The last part of the section outlines certain cautionary notes to keep in mind with acupuncture. After reading this chapter, you should have a good understanding of how acupuncture may be able to help you with specific skin problems.

The last section of Part One explores other alternative approaches for the treatment of skin problems. These include stress reduction, relaxation therapy, meditation, mind-body medicine, emotional work, cognitive-behavioral techniques, spirituality and prayer, hypnosis, and biofeedback. All of these make use of the fact that there is a huge psychological component and an important mind-body connection in many skin disorders.

It is my hope that Part One will give you a good idea of what you can do for your skin at home, as well as what you can do, with the help of your traditional and alternative health-care practitioners, to prevent and treat skin disorders. You will be able to draw on your knowledge of the structure and function of your skin in health and disease, and integrate what both conventional and alternative dermatology can offer you and your family.

Understanding Your Skin, Hair, and Nails

I'd like to introduce you to several parts of your body that you see and feel all the time, but yet may still be a mystery to you—your skin, hair, and nails. You are covered in a wonderful, very large organ: the skin. You are continually grooming your skin's appendages, your hair and nails, to create a certain impression. As each of us knows, the skin is very important in social and sexual functioning. People with hyperpigmented skins, hypopigmented skins, and major facial blemishes often have their sense of well-being and self-worth lowered. Even the normal skin changes that come with aging—male pattern baldness, increased facial hairiness in women, and wrinkling—can cause us much anxiety. People also decorate their skin, hair, and nails with such items as nail polish, false fingernails, skin piercings, earrings, and tattoos to gain social acceptance and attention. It is impossible to overemphasize just how important the skin is to our whole way of interacting with others and our view of ourselves.

So hang on. You are about to start a fascinating trip into the world of your own skin. This section is not meant to be a technical medical synopsis of the anatomy and physiology of the human skin. However, it is intended to give you at least a general understanding of how the skin, hair, sweat glands, and nails are put together and how they work. That way you will have some background knowledge with which to make intelligent decisions about skin disorders and treatments. We will start with some basic skin anatomy. Then the basic types of skin lesions and the terms that skin doctors, or dermatologists, use are described. Finally, we explore hair, sweat gland, and nail anatomy.

STRUCTURE OF THE SKIN

Your skin is made up of three major layers: the epidermis, the dermis, and the subcutaneous tissue. The thick dermis contains hair shafts, sebaceous (oil) glands, sweat gland ducts, nerves, and blood vessels. The subcutaneous layer is full of fat, blood vessels, nerves, and the base of sweat glands. (See Figure 1.1.)

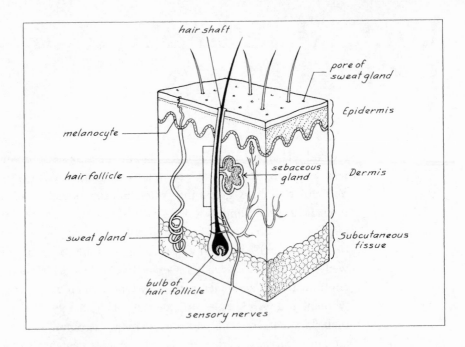

Figure 1.1 Basic Anatomy of the Skin

The epidermis is the outermost layer of the skin. It makes proteins for skin-cell growth, and also makes melanin and keratin, which protect the body from harmful substances in the environment. Keratin is a compact protein that provides a waterproof barrier to protect the body from environmental pollutants such as cigarette smoke. Melanin is a pigment in the epidermis that protects the skin and body from sunlight.

The cells of the epidermis multiply constantly, and they replace themselves approximately once every twenty-eight days. Basal cells from the bottom of the epidermis travel upward and turn into more mature, flatter squamous cells, replacing squamous cells at the top of the epidermis as they die and flake off. Cell turnover time gets longer with age and dramatically shorter in disorders such as psoriasis.

The dermis, the layer below the epidermis, is a complex network of collagen and elastic fibers, blood vessels, lymphatic vessels, nerve fibers, sweat glands, sebaceous glands, and hair follicles. Collagen and elastic fibers give flexibility, strength, and a nice tone to the skin. Sun exposure and aging cause these fibers to become damaged or reduced in number, and wrinkling and sagging of the skin becomes noticeable. Blood vessels supply blood to nourish the dermis and epidermis, remove toxins, and help to regulate body temperature. Age or cigarette smoking leads to reduced blood flow to the skin, and the skin becomes pale and sallow. Increased local blood flow to the skin, on the other hand, makes the complexion appear rosy and fresh. Lymphatic vessels in the dermis (as well as throughout the body) make, store, and carry inflammation- and infection-fighting white blood cells to points where they are needed.

Nerve fibers in the dermis convey our sense of touch, both pleasurable and painful. Sweat glands work with the blood vessels in the dermis to help control body temperature by producing perspiration, which is secreted onto the outer layer of the epidermis. There it evaporates, cooling the skin. Sebaceous glands produce sebum (oil), which keeps the skin moist and smooth. Too much sebum can lead to acne, while insufficient sebum production, common with aging, contributes to dry skin and fine wrinkles. Hair follicles produce hair and provide a channel to allow sebum and sweat to exit from their respective glands to the skin's surface.

Several important biochemical reactions take place in the skin, the most well known being the role of the skin in vitamin-D synthesis. The skin is also involved in the metabolism of androgen, a type of steroid hormone, and it has receptors for other steroid hormones as well, including estrogen, progesterone, and glucocorticoids, as well as for vitamin A.

The skin is an important site of immunological activity, with many specialized cells in both the epidermis and the dermis. A variety of cells and chemical messengers are very important in starting and increasing the body's responses to immunological threats.

Under the dermis is the subcutaneous tissue, which is made up mostly of fat used for insulation and storage of calorie (energy) reserves. Importantly, subcutaneous tissue also acts as a storage site for chemicals, drugs, and nutrients.

SKIN LESIONS

In disease, some component or components of the epidermis, dermis, or subcutaneous tissue may be affected by thickening (or too much of that component), thinning (or too little of that component), or disruption of that component. Doctors describe skin lesions according to what part of the epidermis or dermis they affect, and in what way, and what the lesions look like to the human eye and under the microscope.

Primary lesions—early, uncomplicated skin changes—are described by dermatologists as macules, papules, plaques, nodules, wheals, vesicles, bullae, and pustules, depending on their size and other characteristics. A lesion that has undergone some type of natural evolution from its early stage or that is artifically altered in some way (scratched or picked at, for example) is considered a *secondary lesion.* These include crusts, scales, erosions, ulcers, fissures, atrophy, and scars, and they form after the primary lesions. Other types of lesions, classified as *special skin lesions,* include excoriations, comedones, milia, cysts, burrows, lichenification, telangiectasia, petechiae, and purpurae. For descriptions of the characteristics of these various types of lesions, see Table 1.1.

Skin lesions can be arranged in different ways. The individual lesions can be arranged in lines, circles, gyrating patterns, groups, or not show any particular arrangement. The presence of several or many lesions can be characteristic of a particular skin problem.

HAIR AND HAIR FOLLICLES

There are three types of human hairs: *lanugo, vellus,* and *terminal.* Lanugo is a type of soft hair that covers the body of the human fetus. Vellus hairs are fine and cover most of the bodies of children and adults. The long, coarse, pigmented hairs of the scalp, beard, eyebrows, eyelashes, underarms, and, in adults, pubes are terminal hairs. Terminal hairs differ in structure from lanugo and vellus hairs in that they have a central core, or *medulla.*

During its lifetime, an individual hair follicle may produce different types of hair. Genetic and hormonal influences determine the increase in hairiness around puberty and throughout adult life, as well as the loss of terminal hairs on the scalp with age that is commonly known as male pattern baldness.

Each part of the body has its own genetically determined pattern of hair growth, with individual hairs growing for a set period of time. This period is much longer for scalp hairs, which can grow for longer than three years and reach the mid-back. Pubic and eyebrow hair grows actively for only a few months. This active growing phase is called the *anagen phase.* After the anagen phase comes the resting phase, or *catagen phase.* Finally, during the *telogen phase,* the resting hair is shed. A new hair then normally develops from the same hair follicle and the process repeats itself. Figure 1.2 illustrates how a hair develops, with separate layers with specialized cells.

TABLE 1.1 TYPES OF SKIN LESIONS

Lesion	Description	Examples
PRIMARY SKIN LESIONS		
Bulla	Larger blister, greater than ½ centimeter (about ⅜ inch) in size.	A bad second- or third-degree sunburn or burn will produce bullae.
Macule	Flat spot ranging from red to white to purple to black in color.	Freckles, age spots. Vitiligo is made up of macules without pigment.
Nodule	Large bump, greater than ½ centimeter (about ⅜ inch) in diameter caused by the three-dimensional growth of a papule (see below). Color can range from red to white to purple to black.	Skin cancers such as basal cell and squamous cell carcinomas and melanoma are often nodules.
Papule	Small bump, up to ½ centimeter (about ⅜ inch) in diameter, ranging in color from red to white to purple to black.	Warts and moles are papules. Insect bites and acne also form papules. Basal cell carcinomas, a type of skin cancer, are often papules.
Plaque	Papules that have grown together in a horizontal direction, forming a plateau greater than ½ centimeter (about ⅜ inch) in diameter. Plaques can secondarily scale and crust and be of different colors.	Psoriasis, eczema, and mycosis fungoides (an uncommon form of lymphoma that affects the skin) can be made up of plaques.
Pustule	Vesicle (see below) or small papule less than ½ centimeter (about ⅜ inch) in size filled with pus, or dead white blood cells.	Acne pustules are a common example.
Vesicle	Small papule filled with clear fluid, less than ½ centimeter (about ⅜ inch in diameter).	Shingles are made up of vesicles.
Wheal	A temporary firm elevation of the skin with irregular borders, a red exterior, and pale interior. The dermis is being filled with fluid.	Hives and insect bites are examples of wheals.
SECONDARY SKIN LESIONS		
Atrophy	A depression in the skin resulting from thinning of the epidermis or dermis.	Discoid lupus erythematosus and stretch marks often show atrophy.
Crust	A collection of fluid and cellular debris that reaches the skin's disrupted surface and dries there.	Scabs are the most common crusts. Crusts can form from cold sores, eczema, and bacterial infections of the skin.

TABLE 1.1 TYPES OF SKIN LESIONS (continued)

Lesion	Description	Examples
SECONDARY SKIN LESIONS		
Erosion	A limited, distinct area where there is a loss of epidermis only. Erosions heal without scarring.	Fungal infections and eczema often form erosions.
Fissure	A crack—a linear loss of epidermis and dermis with sharply defined, nearly vertical walls.	Chapped hands and fingertip eczema often form fissures.
Scales	Dry, whitish thickenings of the outermost layer of dead epidermal cells.	Psoriasis, dry skin, seborrheic dermatitis, and althete's foot often form scales.
Scar	The visible change in the appearance of the skin following the healing of an injury or disorder that damages the dermis.	Acne and deep burns can often heal with scarring. Scars usually start out thick and pink and become whiter and thinner with time.
Ulcer	A hole in the epidermis and part or all of the dermis. Ulcers heal with scars.	Bedsores often rapidly develop into ulcers. Canker sores in the mouth and changes due to poor circulation in the legs form ulcers as well.
SPECIAL SKIN LESIONS		
Burrow	A narrow, elevated, tortuous channel made by a parasite.	Scabies form burrows.
Comedone	A plug of sebaceous (oily) and keratinous (protein) material lodged in the opening of a hair follicle.	Blackheads and whiteheads. Blackheads form in open hair follicles, whiteheads in closed or narrowed follicular openings.
Cyst	A limited, distinct lesion with a wall and a central open area filled with liquid or semisolid materials.	Acne cysts and abscesses are two examples of cysts.
Excoriation	An erosion (see above) caused by scratching.	Poison ivy is often excoriated.
Lichenification	An area of thickened epidermis caused by scratching.	Scratching of eczema often forms areas of lichenification.
Milia	A small, superficial keratin cyst with no visible opening.	Milia are common in acne.
Petechia	A spot of blood less than ½ centimeter (about ⅜ inch) in diameter.	Trauma to the skin can form petechiae.

Purpura	A spot of blood greater than ½ centimeter (about ⅜ inch) in diameter.	Trauma to the skin can form purpura.
Telangiectasis	A dilated superficial (surface) blood vessel that is big enough to be visible to the naked eye.	Telangiectasia over the nose and cheeks are very common in rosacea. Basal cell carcinomas and lupus erythematosus lesions often contain telangiectasia. Vascular spiders occur with age and pregnancy.

The hair follicles are set into the dermis at an angle, with the end, or bulb, setting deep down, just above or in the subcutaneous fat. The hair bulb contains a group of cells that divide and diversify to produce the early hair shaft. The hair bulb also contain *melanocytes,* which produce pigment. The hair shaft, as it grows toward the mouth of the hair follicle, consists of several tubular layers. The medulla is the central core, present only in terminal hairs. The *cortex* surrounds the medulla, and keratinization (deposition of a layer of keratin, a tough protein) takes place here. The *cuticle,* a layer of overlapping keratinized plates, lies outside the cortex. The *inner root sheath* and the *outer root sheath* lie in concentric layers outside the cuticle.

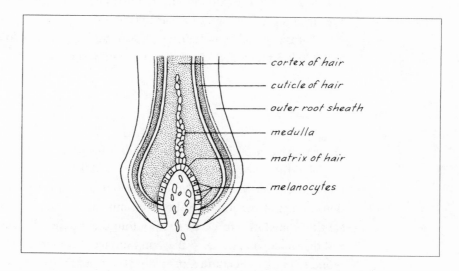

Figure 1.2 Cross-Section of a Hair Follicle

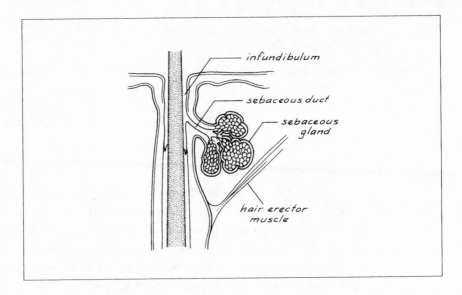

Figure 1.3 Sebaceous Gland Joint to a Hair Follicle

Partway up the hair follicle, a duct delivers sebum, or lipid (oil), from the attached sebaceous gland onto the surface of the hair. Thus, the hair's surface and then the skin's surface is lubricated with lipid. Figure 1.3 depicts a sebaceous gland joined to a hair follicle.

Hair is generally cosmetically pleasing and has a lot to do with our self-image, self-esteem, and attraction of the opposite sex.

SWEAT GLANDS

Humans have two kinds of sweat glands: eccrine and apocrine.

The true sweat gland is the eccrine gland. About 3 million of these are present from birth. Sweat glands are present almost everywhere on human skin, except at the junctions between mucous membranes and skin. They are tiny coiled structures, ascending from the junction between the dermis and the subcutaneous fat to the skin's surface. Most of the sweat glands respond to body temperature, increasing their output of salty water when the body becomes hot, and functioning to dispel heat from the body. The eccrine glands on the palms of the hands, the soles of the feet, the underarms,

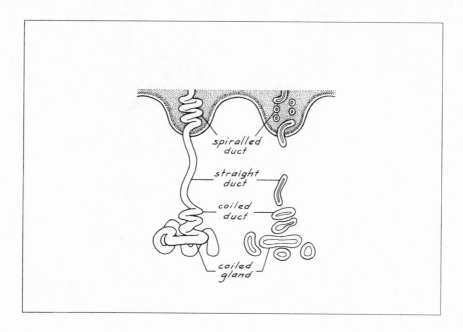

Figure 1.4 Eccrine Sweat Gland

and the forehead also respond to emotional stimuli, such as pain, fear, or anger. Figure 1.4 is an illustration of how a typical eccrine sweat gland appears in the skin.

Apocrine sweat glands are also coiled structures with a duct, but they open into associated hair follicles, just like sebaceous glands do. They are mostly found under the arms, on the scalp, around the nipples, near the navel, and in the outer ears, eyelids, and perineum, or genital area. At puberty, these glands begin to secrete a milky substance that forms when portions of the apocrine cells' cytoplasm (the semiliquid substance that makes up the living matter of cells) separate out, enter the duct, and go through it up to the skin surface. Apocrine glands have a nerve supply, and also depend on the presence of male hormones, or androgens, to trigger secretion of their milky substance. At this time, we know of no function for the apocrine glands in people, although it is known that they serve as a source of sexual scent hormones, or pheromones, in other mammals. Figure 1.5 shows how an apocrine sweat gland looks in your skin.

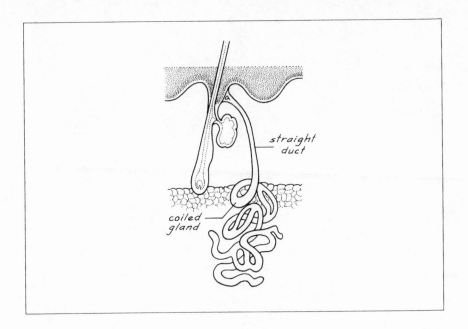

Figure 1.5 Apocrine Sweat Gland

NAILS

The nail unit consists of the nail plate and the tissues around and under it. The area of skin that surrounds the cuticle is known as the *nail fold* (that at the bottom of the nail is the *proximal nail fold;* that on the sides is the *lateral nail fold*). The *cuticle* arises from the cornified, or hardened, layer of the proximal nail fold and extends a few millimeters onto the surface of the nail, known to dermatologists as the *nail plate.* The proximal nail fold covers the white part, or *lunula,* of the nail. The lunula is most visible on the thumbnails. Figure 1.6 depicts the anatomy of a nail.

The nail plate rests upon the tissues of the nail bed. It is made up mostly of keratin, a protein rich in sulfur-containing amino acids, which gives the nail its strength and hardness. Contrary to common belief, calcium is present only in tiny amounts in the nail plate and does not contribute to the hardness of nails. Fingernails grow by about 0.1 millimeter—less than a hair's breadth—a day. This means it takes about six months for a fingernail

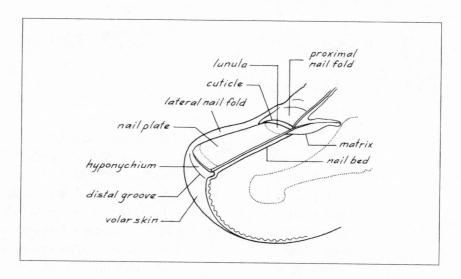

Figure 1.6 Anatomy of a Nail Unit

to grow back completely if it is removed. Toenails grow at about one-third this rate.

The *nail bed,* the tissue under the nail plate, is made up of *epithelium* (the type of tissue that makes up the surface of most of the body) overlying a dermis very richly supplied with tiny blood vessels and resting on top of the bone. The dermis contains a huge network of sensory nerves. The *nail matrix,* which produces the nail, is continuous with the nail bed and extends beneath the proximal nail fold for about three-eighths inch. The cells of the nail matrix gradually move upward to form the nail plate, becoming keratinized—that is, toughened—as they do so.

Nails have several important functions. They protect the ends of the fingers and toes in a cosmetically pleasing way. The multiple sensory nerves in the dermis of the nail bed allow us to feel fine touch and pain, which is a protective mechanism. Nails are also important tools with which we can scratch and grasp and enhance other fine motor skills of the fingers and toes.

Now that we have examined how the skin, hair, and nails are put together and how they work, let us turn to the various ways in which these wonderful structures can be cared for and, should they develop problems or disorders, treated.

Conventional Approaches
to Skin Care

Let's take a look at what conventional dermatology can offer you and your family if a skin problem arises. After all, modern Western medicine has helped hundreds of thousands of people with their skin disorders and has been extensively studied. First, let's look at a typical visit to a dermatologist. Next, let's see how he or she will approach helping you with your skin problem. Then you will know exactly what to expect during your visit to the doctor. We will take a look at the questions he or she will ask, what type of exam you can expect, and what sorts of tests your dermatologist may perform. After reviewing the most common medications used for various skin disorders, you won't be surprised by what your dermatologist may prescribe. After reading this chapter, you will also be familiar with the various surgical and other specialized treatments your doctor may use to help you. So, hang on, and let's take a trip to your dermatologist's office!

A VISIT TO THE DERMATOLOGIST

A dermatologist is a skin-care professional very well versed in conventional Western medical therapies. A dermatologist is a medical doctor who has not only completed four years of medical school, but also spent at least a year of internship in internal medicine or surgery and three years of dermatology residency at a teaching hospital. That is a lot of studying and working with patients with skin problems! Dermatologists are well versed in dealing with the common problems of acne, warts, psoriasis, eczema, sunburns, poison ivy, and skin cancer, as well as recognizing and treating the hundreds of other more unusual skin problems. Because of his or her comprehensive medical background, a dermatologist is also an expert at interpreting signs of internal medical problems that show up in the skin.

When you are choosing a dermatologist, I recommend going to one who is board-certified in the specialty of dermatology. This means that after training for at least eight years in medical school and residency programs, he or she has passed a very difficult test administered by the professional dermatological association.

Other medical doctors also practice dermatology as part of what they do. Family-practice doctors, internists, and pediatricians have all had some training in dermatology and treat the more common skin problems. They usually refer more difficult dermatologic problems to a board-certified dermatologist.

Conventional dermatology has helped many people with their skin problems through the years. However, possible side effects from the long-term use of corticosteroid preparations and other more potent drugs in the dermatologist's arsenal can be a problem. Also, like other forms of conventional medicine, conventional dermatology is often most helpful for the treatment of acute problems and is less successful with chronic, recurring problems that are not life threatening but are bothersome. For many skin problems, there are also many alternative therapies that can be tried first at home. With a knowledgeable integration of both alternative and conventional dermatology, you can take more responsibility for the health of your own skin before turning to a skilled dermatologist and/or other professional if that becomes necessary.

Let's look first at what you can expect from a visit to your dermatologist and what techniques and procedures dermatologists are experts in.

Medical History

The conventional approach to assessing and treating an individual with skin disease starts with taking a history. Questions such as "What brings you here today?" "Where is your skin problem?" "How long have you had it?" "How does it bother you?" "How have you treated it already?" will be asked about the current skin problem. The dermatologist will inquire about your history of skin diseases, allergies, and general medical disorders. You will be asked about whether family members and close contacts have any skin diseases or allergies. The dermatologist will inquire into your occupation and hobbies, paying careful attention to any history of exposure to irritating or allergenic materials at work or at home. Also important to the dermatologist is detailed information about which treatments, both conventional and alternative, you have already tried, and whether or not these treatments helped or worsened the skin problem. It is also important for the doctor to know which other creams and cosmetics you routinely apply to your skin.

Skin Examination

Next, the dermatologist will physically examine your skin. Problem areas are examined first, then the doctor looks at the other sites he or she anticipates may be involved. The skin lesions need to be felt as well as looked at. Often lesions are measured and drawn or photographed for the doctor's medical records. Dermatologists are trained to look for and categorize the appearance of individual skin lesions, the arrangement of these lesions, their distribution over your body's surface, and their color, in order to make the correct diagnosis and prescribe helpful treatments.

Skin lesions can involve just the scalp, mouth, palms of the hands, soles of the feet, nails, face, groin, arms, legs, trunk, or any combination of these. Particular diseases or skin problems tend to affect characteristic areas. Also, if the disease starts in one area and then spreads, that will give your dermatologist clues as to the cause and type of the condition. The color of the skin and skin lesions gives the trained physician further clues as to problems of the skin or underlying internal organs. It is always a good practice for the dermatologist to examine the whole skin the first time he or she sees a patient. This is to make sure no dangerous lesions are present that the individual may be unaware of.

Laboratory Testing

In some cases, laboratory tests are done to help determine the diagnosis and to rule out possible associated problems. Blood, urine, and x-ray studies are sometimes helpful in diagnosing people thought to have a disease involving other organs, such as systemic lupus erythematosus, that affects other organs as well as the skin.

The skin itself can be more closely examined using a magnifying glass or a special light, known as a Wood's light, that aids in detecting the presence of some bacteria and yeast. Cell specimens removed from the very top layer of the skin with a scalpel may be examined under a microscope to look for fungi, yeast, bacteria, herpes virus, scabies, and lice. Cell specimens may also be cultured to identify specific offending bacteria, mycobacteria, fungi, or viruses. This can be very helpful in determining effective treatment.

Patch tests are used to investigate the causes of allergic contact dermatitis. In this test, materials that are suspected of causing allergic or irritant rashes are deliberately applied to the skin and then covered with tape.

The doctor examines the patches of skin where suspected allergens were placed after forty-eight hours, and then again after ninety-six hours, to see if there is redness, hardness, and itchiness of the skin. If there is, this is an indicator of the type and degree of irritant or allergic dermatitis.

A skin biopsy examines all the layers of the skin, from the epidermis to the subcutaneous tissue. In this procedure, local anesthesia is administered and a small piece of skin is removed. The incision is closed with a stitch or stitches, and the tissue sample is sent to a specialist known as a dermatopathologist (a dermatologist with an additional year's training in studying skin cells under the microscope) for processing and examination under a light microscope. An expert's opinion of what the skin sample or biopsy looks like under the light microscope is often very helpful in defining a difficult diagnosis, as each specific skin problem typically looks quite different under the microscope. Further specialized examination and testing on the small piece of skin, using an electron microscope or bacterial, fungal, and viral culture of the tissue, can also be done.

Working Diagnosis

Next, the dermatologist creates a differential diagnosis of possible skin diseases that the individual may have. That is, he or she determines which disorders are capable of producing the symptoms, and then selects the most likely working diagnosis by ruling out as many of the candidates as possible. The working diagnosis is what the dermatologist thinks the patient is being bothered by, until proven otherwise.

CONVENTIONAL DERMATOLOGY TREATMENTS

Once a working diagnosis is arrived at, the dermatologist will recommend a course of treatment. Conventional dermatologists primarily use creams, lotions, shampoos, pills, shots, and soaks to help alleviate skin problems. They often also remove the skin lesions, whether by excision (cutting out), freezing off with liquid nitrogen, electrodesiccation (burning off with electric current), or laser removal. Other specialized dermatologic techniques include chemical peels and dermabrasion to diminish signs of aging or old acne scarring, sclerotherapy for unwanted leg veins, and hair transplantation. Ultraviolet light therapy is commonly used for problems such as pso-

riasis, eczema, mycosis fungoides, and vitiligo. The technique of photophoresis, a blood treatment utilizing ultraviolet light, is becoming much
more important in dermatology. Electrotherapy using the transcutaneous
electric nerve stimulation, or TENS, unit is a much less commonly used
but helpful tool for skin problems. Referrals to another medical specialist,
such as a psychiatrist, rheumatologist, plastic surgeon, internist, radiation
therapist, or oncologist, sometimes becomes necessary. Thus, conventional
dermatology has a lot of different treatment modalities to offer that have
worked well for many people.

Medications

Throughout the years, many pharmaceutical creams, ointments, and pills
have given people great relief from the signs and symptoms of various skin
disorders. Their value is not to be underestimated. However, some medications can produce irritating or dangerous side effects, and the potential risks
and benefits of various treatments must always be considered. Table 1.2 lists
many of the conventional medications most commonly prescribed for various skin problems.

Liquid Nitrogen Therapy

Liquid nitrogen sprayed from a special canister or applied with a cotton
swab is often used to freeze off benign lesions such as age spots (or *lentigos*),
warts, and sun spots (or *actinic keratoses*). Sometimes a very deep freeze is
used to treat basal cell carcinomas. A few minutes after the lesion has been
frozen, thawed, and refrozen, a hive forms. Later, a blister develops. This
peels off within a week, taking the unwanted lesion with it. The freezing is
painful for a few seconds, but usually does a nice job of removing these unwanted lesions.

Excision

Dermatologists are skilled in skin surgery, and they sometimes need to cut
out, or excise, a skin cancer, mole, or other lesion. Excised skin specimens
are then sent to a dermatopathologist, who confirms the diagnosis by
examining the sample under a microscope and lets your doctor know if he

TABLE 1.2 CONVENTIONAL MEDICINES
COMMONLY PRESCRIBED FOR SKIN PROBLEMS

Medication (Examples)	Beneficial Effects	Possible Side Effects/Cautions
TOPICAL PREPARATIONS		
Acyclovir (Zovirax)	Fights viral infection. Used for genital herpes.	Should avoid contact with the eyes.
Alpha hydroxy acids (many products by many different manufacturers)	Exfoliates and moisturizes skin to help make it appear younger. Used for acne, wrinkles.	Can be irritating to sensitive skin.
Anthralin (Drithocreme, Micanol)	Inhibits the proliferation of skin cells. Used for psoriasis.	Very strong—should not be applied to sensitive areas. Causes discoloration of skin and clothing.
Antifungals (ciclopirox [Loprox], clotrimazole [Lotrimin, Mycelex], econazole [Spectazole], ketoconazole [Nizoral], miconazole [Micatin, Monistat-Derm, and others], naftifine [Naftin], oxiconazole [Oxistat], terbinafine [Lamisil], tolnaftate [Aftate, Tinactin, and others], undecylenic acid [Cruex, Desenex, and others])	Fight fungal infection. Used for athlete's foot, candidiasis, ringworm, and yeast infection.	Topical treatment is usually not adequate if toenails, fingernails, or scalp is affected.
Antipruritics (oat protein [Aveeno], calamine lotion, menthol/phenol combination [Sarna and others])	Relieve itching. Used for dermatitis; hives; itching; poison ivy, oak, or sumac; psoriasis; seborrhea; sunburn.	If used for longer than a week or so, calamine lotion can harden and dry the skin. Menthol/phenol can be irritating for some individuals.
Azelaic acid (Azelex)	Kills bacteria and encourages skin cells to slough off. Used for acne.	May lighten the color of the treated skin.
Benzocaine (Americaine, Lagol)	Minimizes pain of rashes or aftermath of skin surgery. Used for shingles, any disorder necessitating skin surgery.	Unless directed by a health-care professional, should not be used on open wounds, burns, or broken or inflamed skin. Should be used with great care near the eyes.

Medication (Examples)	Beneficial Effects	Possible Side Effects/Cautions
TOPICAL PREPARATIONS		
Benzoyl peroxide (Benoxyl, Persagel, Clearasil Maximum Strength, Fostex, Oxy 10, and others)	Kills bacteria and breaks up contents of blackheads. Used for acne.	Alcohol-based creams and gels, especially 5% and 10% concentrations, may be drying and irritating. Can bleach skin and clothing. May inactivate retinoids if applied at the same time.
Calcipotriene (Dovonex)	Inhibits the proliferation of skin cells. Used for psoriasis.	Can cause skin irritation. May increase the risk of kidney stones. Expensive.
Capsaicin (Capzasin-P, Zostrix)	Increases local blood flow and relieves pain. Reduces redness and scaling in psoriasis. Also used for scleroderma, shingles.	Should not be applied to broken skin.
Clindamycin (Cleocin T)	Antibiotic that works against propionibacteria, the type of bacteria involved in acne. Used for acne.	Formulations usually contain alcohol, which may be drying and irritating. Should not be used in combination with retinoids.
Coal tar (Aquatar, Denorex, DHS Tar, Doak, Estar, Fototar, Ionil T, Lavatar, Medotar, Psorigel, Tegrin, Tersa-Tar, Zetar, and others)	Soothes itchy and inflamed skin, and helps to thin rough, thickened patches. Used for dermatitis, psoriasis.	Stains bedclothes. Has an unpleasant odor. Should not be used on infected, blistered, or oozing skin. Should be kept away from the eyes. In rare cases, can cause skin irritation. Treated areas should be protected from sunlight.
Corticosteroids (alclometasone [Aclovate], amcinonide [Cyclocort], betamethasone [Diprolene, Diprosone, and others], clobetasol [Temovate], desonide [DesOwen, Tridesilon], desoximetasone [Topicort], diflorasone [Florone, Psorcon, and others], fluocinolone [Fluocet, Fluonid, and others], fluocinonide [Fluocin, Licon,	Fight inflammation. Help relieve redness, swelling, itching, and discomfort. Used for most acute and chronic dermatoses, such as atopic dermatitis, insect bites, hives, lupus erythematosus, poison ivy, psoriasis, seborrheic dermatitis, sunburn.	High-potency topical corticosteroids can cause thinning of the skin if used for long periods of time, especially on the face, underarms, neck, and groin.

Lidex], fluticasone [Cutivate],
halcinonide [Halog],
hydrocortisone valerate
[Westcort], mometasone
[Elocon], triamcinolone
[Aristocort, Kenalog, and
others])

Diphenhydramine (Benadryl)	Helps relieve itching. Used for dermatitis, insect bites, itching, sunburn.	May sensitize skin, causing contact dermatitis.
Doxepin (Zonalon)	Helps relieve itching. Used for dermatitis, insect bites, itching, sunburn.	May sensitize skin, causing contact dermatitis. May cause drowsiness—should not be used while driving.
Erythromycin (A/T/S, Benzamycin, Emgel, Erycette, T-Stat, Theramycin, Erygel, Erymax, Erythra-Derm)	Antibiotic that works against propionibacteria, the type of bacteria involved in acne.	Formulations usually contain alcohol, which may be drying and irritating. Should not be used in combination with retinoids.
Fluocinolone (Derma-Smoothe/FS, Fluonid)	Helps loosen scales. Used for seborrhea of the scalp.	Oily. Has to be left on overnight.
5-Fluorouracil (Efudex, Fluoroplex)	Fights cancer by interfering with the growth of abnormal cells. Used for actinic keratoses (certain cancerous and precancerous lesions).	Area treated may become inflamed and red. Sun sensitivity increases. There may be a burning feeling upon application. Also can cause itching, oozing, soreness or tenderness of skin.
Gentamicin (Garamycin, Gentamar, G-Myticin)	Kills bacteria. Used for bacterial infection of the skin; body odor.	Can cause itching, redness, swelling, or other signs of irritation in some individuals.
Imiquimod (Aldara)	Aids the immune system to help protect the body from viruses that cause warts. Helps relieve and control wart production. Used for genital warts.	Can cause mild skin irritation.
Lidocaine (DermaFlex, Lidoderm, Xylocaine)	Minimizes pain of rash or skin surgery. Used for shingles, any disorder necessitating skin surgery.	Unless directed by a health-care professional, should not be used on open wounds, burns, or broken or inflamed skin. Should be used with great care near the eyes.

Medication (Examples)	Beneficial Effects	Possible Side Effects/Cautions
TOPICAL PREPARATIONS		
Nitrogen mustard (mechlorethamine)	Interferes with abnormal cell growth. Used for mycosis fungoides.	May cause hives, shortness of breath, skin rash or itching. May also cause dry skin and reversible darkening of the skin.
Mupirocin (Bactroban)	Kills bacteria. Used for abscesses, boils, and other *Staphylococcus* and *Streptococcus* infections of the skin. Also used for skin ulcers.	Should not make contact with the eyes.
Neomycin/polymyxin B/bacitracin combination (Neosporin, Polysporin)	Kills bacteria. Used for abscesses, boils, and other *Staphylococcus* and *Streptococcus* infections of the skin. Also used for skin ulcers.	Can be sensitizing and cause a rash.
Penciclovir (Denavir)	Fights viral infection. Used for cold sores.	Can cause mild pain, burning, or stinging; headache; altered sense of taste; decreased sensitivity of the skin; redness, skin rash. Should not be used in or near the eyes or inside the mouth or nose or on other internal parts of the body.
Podofilox (Condylox)	Destroys warts. Used for genital warts.	Can cause irritation and burning. Should not be used during pregnancy.
Podophyllin (Podocon-25, Podofin)	Causes destruction of wart tissue. Best for genital warts.	Must be used with care to avoid harming normal skin. Can cause burning, redness, irritation, skin rash, itching.
Pramoxine (Pramagel)	Helps relieve itching and inflammation. Used for dermatitis, eczema, insect bites, itching, sunburn.	Can cause burning, stinging, tenderness, skin rash, redness, itching, or hives.
Retinoids (tretinoin [Retin-A, Renova], adalapene [Differin])	Break up whiteheads and blackheads, and encourage sloughing off of skin cells. Used for acne, wrinkles. Retin-A may also be used for warts (best for flat warts).	Differin and Renova are less irritating than Retin-A, but all can cause dryness, redness, and sun sensitivity. All may worsen acne at first. Should not be used during pregnancy or by nursing mothers.

Salicylic acid (Calicylic, Clear Away, Clearasil Clearstick, Clearasil pads, Compound W, Duofilm, Freezone, Mediplast, Occlusal, Propa pH, Sal-Plant, Sebucare, Stri-Dex pads, Trans-Plantar, Trans-Ver-Sal, Wart-Off, and others)	Helps skin to slough off. Reduces seborrhea. Used for acne, seborrhea, warts.	Can be overly drying and irritating. Has an unpleasant odor.
Silver sulfadiazine (Silvadene, SSD, Thermazene)	Fights/prevents bacterial and fungal infection. Used for burns, surgical wounds.	Should not be used by those allergic to sulfa drugs.
Sodium sulfacetamide	Fights bacterial and fungal infection. Used for acne.	Should not be used by persons allergic to sulfur.
Tazarotene (Tazorac)	Vitamin-A derivative that keeps pores clear. Decreases redness and reduces the number and size of lesions in psoriasis. Used for acne, psoriasis.	Irritates skin; can cause burning, stinging, itching, dryness, peeling, redness, pain, or swelling. Should not be used during pregnancy or by nursing mothers.
Trichloroacetic acid	Causes skin to slough off; destroys warts.	Can cause burning, tenderness, pain.

ORAL MEDICATIONS

Acitretin (Soriatane)	Vitamin-A derivative that inhibits psoriasis and allows normal skin growth. Used for severe psoriasis, some other forms of dermatitis.	Can cause severe headache, nausea or vomiting, visual problems, chapped lips, abdominal pain, liver inflammation, stiff or painful muscles, bones, or joints. Causes severe birth defects—should not be used during pregnancy, and pregnancy should not be attempted for three years after stopping this drug. Alcohol should be avoided while taking this drug and for two months after stopping.
Acyclovir (Zovirax)	Fights viral infection. Used for cold sores, genital herpes, shingles.	Can cause skin changes, vision changes, difficulty breathing, dizziness, irregular heartbeat, muscle cramps or weakness, nausea or vomiting, mood changes. If kidney function is impaired, a lower dose should be used.

Medication (Examples)	Beneficial Effects	Possible Side Effects/Cautions
ORAL MEDICATIONS		
Amoxicillin (Amoxil, Polymox, Trimox, Wymox)	Fights bacterial infection. Used for abscesses, boils, cuts, wounds, and secondarily infected dermatitis.	Can cause stomach upset. Should not be used by anyone who is allergic to penicillin.
Antihistamines (astemizole [Hismanal], brompheniramine [Bromphen, Dimetane, and others], cetirizine [Zyrtec], chlorpheniramine [Chlor-Trimeton, Teldrin, and others], clemastine [Tavist], cyproheptadine [Periactin], diphenhydramine [Benadryl, Diphenhist, and others], fexofenadine [Allegra], hydroxyzine [Atarax, Hyzine-50, Vistaril], loratadine [Claritin], promethazine [Anergan, Phenergan, and others])	Help relieve itching. Used for dermatitis, eczema, hives, itching.	Most cause drowsiness; alcohol and driving should be avoided while using these medications. Astemizole, cetirizine, fexofenadine, loratadine do not cause drowsiness, but may worsen stomach ulcers.
Azathioprine (Imuran)	Suppresses the immune response, inhibits rheumatoid conditions such as lupus. Used for dermatomyositis, psoriasis, systemic lupus erythematosus.	Can lower blood counts. Should not be used during pregnancy.
Azithromycin (Zithromax)	Fights bacterial infection. Used for abscesses, boils.	Can cause stomach upset and nausea.
Cephalosporins (Cefaclor, Cefixime, Ceftriaxone, Cephalexin, and others)	Fight bacterial infection. Used for acne, boils.	May cause diarrhea in some individuals. Alcoholic beverages should be avoided while using these drugs.
Chloroquine (Aralen)	Suppresses rheumatoid conditions such as lupus. Used for systemic lupus erythematosus.	May cause flare-ups of psoriasis.

Cimetidine (Tagamet)	Helps to relieve itching of hives and is thought to change immunologic response in warts. Used for hives, warts.	Can cause abdominal pain, diarrhea, dry mouth, changes in vision, dizziness, irregular heartbeat, breathing changes, mood changes, increased sweating.
Cyclophosphamide (Cytoxan, Neosar)	Interferes with abnormal cell growth. Helpful for systemic lupus erythmatosus.	May lower blood counts or cause bleeding into bladder.
Cyclosporine (Neoral, Sandimmune, SangCya)	Suppresses the immune response, inhibits psoriasis. Used for severe atopic dermatitis, psoriasis.	Can cause kidney toxicity, liver toxicity, high blood pressure, birth defects.
Dapsone	Fights bacterial and fungal infection. Suppresses certain skin problems. Used for systemic lupus erythematosus.	Breaks down red blood cells. Can cause fatigue.
Dicloxacillin (Dynapen, Dycill, Pathocil)	Fights bacterial infection. Used for abscesses, boils, and other *Staphylococcus* and *Streptococcus* infections. Also used for bite wounds.	Can cause diarrhea. Should not be used by anyone who is allergic to penicillin.
Doxycycline (Doryx, Monodox, Vibramycin, Vibra-Tabs)	Fights bacterial infection. Used for acne, rosacea.	Can cause increased sun sensitivity, tooth discoloration.
Erythromycins (E-Mycin, ERYC, Erythrocin, Ilotycin, and others)	Fights bacterial infection. Used for acne, secondary infection.	Can cause stomach upset.
Etretinate (Tegison)	Inhibits psoriasis. Used for severe psoriasis.	Can cause elevated blood fats, bone changes, liver toxicity, headache, visual difficulties. Causes birth defects; should not be used during pregnancy.
Famciclovir (Famvir)	Fights viral infection. Used for cold sores, shingles.	Can cause headache, digestive disturbances, unusual tiredness or weakness. Expensive.
Fluconazole (Diflucan)	Fights fungal infection. Used for fungal infection.	Can cause liver damage.
Griseofulvin (Fulvicin, Grifulvin, Grisactin, Gris-PEG)	Kills fungi. Helps to clear fungal infection of the fingernails and toenails.	Can cause stomach upset, sun sensitivity. White blood cell count and liver enzymes should be monitored while taking this drug. Many fungi are resistant to treatment. It can take more than a year to clear toenails.

Medication (Examples)	Beneficial Effects	Possible Side Effects/Cautions
ORAL MEDICATIONS		
Hydroxychloroquine (Plaquenil)	Suppresses rheumatoid conditions such as systemic lupus erythematosus.	Can cause retinopathy, blood cell problems. Should not be used by anyone with liver disease.
Isotretinoin (Accutane)	Vitamin-A derivative that disrupts plug formation, shrinks the sebaceous (oil) glands, and reduces the amount of oil produced. Used for severe acne.	Raises blood fat levels. Can cause chapped lips, dry eyes, severe headache. Liver enzymes should be monitored while taking this drug. Causes birth defects; pregnancy should be avoided while taking this drug.
Itraconazole (Sporanox)	Kills fungi. Used for fungal infection of the nails.	Can cause hepatitis, which is usually reversible.
Ketoconazole (Nizoral)	Kills fungi. Used for fungal or yeast infection of the nails.	Can cause liver damage, which is usually reversible. Should not be used during pregnancy.
Methotrexate (Folex, Rheumatrex)	Interferes with the growth of abnormal cells. Used for mycosis fungoides, severe psoriasis.	Can cause fever, chills, reduction in blood cells, liver toxicity, stomach ulcers, diarrhea, lung inflammation, decreased kidney function. Interacts badly with many other drugs. Can cause birth defects; should be avoided during pregnancy.
Minocycline (Dynacin, Minocin)	Fights bacterial infection. Used for acne vulgaris, rosacea.	Can cause increased sun sensitivity, tooth discoloration.
Photosensitizers (Methoxsalen [8-MOP, Oxsoralen-Ultra], trioxsalen [Trisoralen])	Increases the skin's sensitivity to sunlight. Used in conjunction with ultraviolet light to treat mycosis fungoides, psoriasis, vitiligo.	Can cause itching, nausea, dizziness, headache, depression, nervousness, trouble sleeping. Strict sun-protection measures must be adhered to while using this drug.
Terbinafine (Lamisil)	Kills fungi. Used for fungal infection.	Can cause liver damage, a decrease in white blood cells.
Tetracycline (Achromycin V)	Fights bacterial infection. Used for acne, rosacea.	Can cause increased sun sensitivity, tooth discoloration.

Trimethoprim (Proloprim, Trimpex)	Fights bacterial infection. Used for acne.	Rarely, can cause severe drug reaction with loss of skin.
Valacyclovir (Valtrex)	Fights viral infection. Used for cold sores, shingles.	Can cause headache and stomach upset. Should not be used by people with depressed immune systems.

or she has removed the lesion in its entirety. Some dermatologists also do more complicated skin surgeries, including flaps, grafts, and specialized Mohs microsurgery, which is done with the aid of a microscope. Others refer these procedures on to a plastic surgeon whose work they like and respect.

Electrodesiccation

Electrodesiccation, or electrocautery, is a procedure in which a very fine electric needle is used to char or burn off an unwanted growth. For small benign lesions, such as telangiectasia on the face, a low setting is used and local anesthesia is not necessary. For deeper lesions, such as basal cell carcinomas, a higher setting is used, local anesthesia is administered, and the lesion is burned and then curetted, or scraped off, three times in a row. This treatment is referred to as *electrodesiccation and curettage times three.* Electrodesiccation has been very useful in dermatology for decades.

Sclerotherapy

Sclerotherapy has been used for many years to remove unattractive leg veins that tend to appear with time. Recently, laser therapy has also been used for this purpose, but some types of leg veins are still better suited for removal by sclerotherapy. Using a very fine needle, a dermatologist injects a liquid compound directly into the veins you want eliminated. This causes the blood vessels to shut down and their walls to be destroyed. Hypertonic salt, or saline, solution is most commonly used on the smaller spider veins. Sodium tetradecyl sulfate works much better on larger blood vessels. Uncommon side effects of sclerotherapy with sodium tetradecyl sulfate include local redness, bruising, light brown spots, small ulcers, and the appearance of very tiny new blood vessels around the treated sites.

Chemical Peels

Chemical peels are regaining popularity as newer, gentler variants are being developed. They are also increasingly being combined with laser treatments to eliminate signs of aging. In these procedures, a selected chemical compound is applied to the skin, left on for a specific length of time, and then removed. Chemical peels are classified as superficial, medium, and deep, depending on the degree to which they penetrate the skin. The deeper the penetration, the greater the results, but also the greater the possibility of unwanted side effects and the greater the time needed for recuperation.

Superficial chemical peels, or "lunchtime peels," are almost free of side effects, but the "healthy glow" they produce only lasts a few weeks or months. Salon-strength superficial peels are usually done using low concentrations of glycolic acid, an alpha-hydroxy acid, to gently exfoliate the skin. Prescription-strength superficial peels applied by dermatologists are usually made from concentrations of 30 to 70 percent glycolic acid, 20 to 30 percent salicylic acid, 10 percent trichloroacetic acid (TCA), or a chemical called Jessner's solution. If they are done repeatedly, they can reverse some of the irregular blotchiness, fine wrinkling, and brown spots of age, in addition to giving the skin a healthy glow. They are slightly uncomfortable, but do not require local anesthesia. Sometimes there is facial redness and peeling for several days. The main risk with these peels is the chance of irregular pigmentation resulting.

Medium-depth chemical peels generally last for up to a year, and are for people who want to improve moderate to severe sun damage. They are given with 20 to 40 per cent TCA, or by combining 10 percent TCA with Jessner's peel or high-strength glycolic acids. The popular Obagi Blue Peel is a medium-strength peel that uses a 30 percent TCA solution. It turns your skin blue as it works so that your doctor can gauge the depth of penetration of the peel. Oral sedation is given before medium-depth peels because they can be quite uncomfortable. The peeling can last from several days to two weeks. In uncommon cases, medium-depth peels can cause severe peeling, increased irregular pigmentation, and scarring.

Deep chemical, or phenol, peels are done to reverse the effects of severe sun damage and wrinkles, acne scars, and/or unwanted brown spots. They are comparable in strength to laser skin resurfacing with a superpulsed carbon dioxide laser (more about laser therapies later in this chapter). Accordingly, intravenous sedation or general anesthesia is used for pain, intravenous fluids are administered, and heart function is monitored. One has to be prepared for severe redness, peeling, and scabbing for several weeks. Potential unwanted side effects include scarring, long-lasting redness, and blotchiness. However, skilled dermatologists have used these peels for over thirty years, with many happy clients.

Dermabrasion

Microdermabrasion, the new "lunchtime peel" approved by the U.S. Food and Drug Administration (FDA) several years ago, has increased the popularity of dermabrasion, which has been used by dermatologists for years. Dermabrasion removes the sun-damaged top layers of skin so that newer, smoother skin can take its place. With microdermabrasion, age spots and fine lines are usually gone after several thirty-minute treatments. Most patients need no topical anesthetic, and the treatments are usually repeated six times, once every two weeks. There appears to be less risk of scarring and color loss than with chemical peels.

Dermabrasion is performed using a sterilized electric sanding device that removes the outer skin layer by layer, as deep as your doctor feels is necessary. Dermabrasion removes fine and deep wrinkling, acne scars, and blotchy pigmentation for years, but the patient needs to understand that his or her face will be painful, red, and raw-looking for several weeks immediately after the procedure. If a small area of dermabrasion is done, local anesthetic is used. Intravenous sedation is required for full-face dermabrasion. As with other skin-removal techniques, there is a risk of scarring and blotchy pigmentation.

Hair Transplantation

As with other forms of cosmetic dermatology, hair transplantation is becoming increasingly popular. In this technique, hairs from the sides of the scalp are grafted in small amounts to areas of the scalp where hair is sparse. There they grow and respond to hormones as if they are still on the sides of the scalp. Hair transplantation is a slow, painful process, though, requiring many treatments, local anesthesia, and some postsurgical scabbing and redness. Older men with lighter colored hair usually benefit most, as their hair loss has stabilized. Risks include scarring, temporary numbness of the scalp, infection, and the formation of small skin cysts. However, many men are happy to risk these side effects for the chance to look younger.

Laser Therapy

The term *laser* is an acronym that stands for *l*ight *a*mplification by *s*timulated *e*mission of *r*adiation. A laser beam is a uniform, one-directional beam of only one wavelength of light energy that is created when gases (such as carbon dioxide) or crystals (such as ruby) are stimulated with electricity. Many specialized lasers have become available in the last twenty years for use in dermatology, and in some cases are replacing other surgical techniques as the treatments of choice. In laser therapy, a dermatologist uses a particular laser, with unique light waves that target and destroy specific components of the skin, leaving surrounding skin components unharmed. Usually lasers are named after the element that is stimulated with electricity, such as ruby, alexandrite, erbium, or neodymium.

Laser therapy for the treatment of wrinkles and the natural signs of aging has become increasingly popular in our youth-oriented culture. The superpulsed carbon dioxide (CO_2), erbium:yttrium–aluminum–garnet (Er:YAG), and neodymium:yttrium–aluminum–garnet (Nd:YAG) lasers are currently the most popular lasers for removing wrinkles. They emit a single wavelength of light that destroys anything with water in it. Because the skin has water in it, these lasers vaporize and remove targeted wrinkled skin on contact. The Er:YAG laser is used to remove more superficial wrinkles, as it doesn't go as deep as the superpulsed CO_2 laser. Be aware that prolonged redness and scarring can occasionally occur with the CO_2 laser.

The pulsed dye, or vascular, laser gives off a single wavelength of yellow light that is toxic only to components of the blood. Thus, it travels harmlessly *through* the skin cells above and below the blood in the epidermis and dermis. This allows a dermatologist to treat any blood-filled spot, such as a broken blood vessel or telangiectasis (spider veins), and other unwanted red-colored spots on the skin using this pulsed dye laser. Occasionally, blotchy brown pigmentation may be an unwanted side effect.

The neodymium:yttrium–aluminum garnet (Nd:YAG), alexandrite, and ruby lasers are used to remove unwanted darkly pigmented spots, which they specifically target and destroy. Pigmentation that forms after a rash has healed, sun freckles, tattoos, and age spots can all be treated with these lasers. Care has to be taken, as occasionally the laser can remove too many pigmented cells in a brown spot, leaving it as a white spot. Because all skin, especially darker colored skin, has some degree of pigmentation, care has to be taken not to lighten normally pigmented skin. Unwanted hair also can be removed with these lasers because they target the pigment cells that are near the part of the hair where growth takes place.

Recently, "tuneable" dye lasers have been developed in which different types of lasers are combined in one unit. Thus, a dermatologist doesn't have to buy several big machines. Instead, he or she can set the machine for the specific colored wavelength needed to target the component of the skin the patient wants destroyed. This has been an important advance.

Low-intensity laser light therapy stimulates the natural healing process at the cellular level and has been very helpful for pain control and improving microcirculation. Laser light treatments have also increased collagen synthesis in the skin and the efficient production of neurotransmitters. With the rapid development of more advanced and more specialized lasers, we will see them play an increasingly important role in the treatment of many dermatologic problems.

Ultraviolet Light Therapy

Another common treatment is the *light box,* capable of producing high doses of ultraviolet-A (UVA) and/or ultraviolet-B (UVB) light for the treatment of eczema, psoriasis, vitiligo, and mycosis fungoides, a form of lymphoma that shows up in the skin. A person goes into a box-shaped machine at the doctor's office several times a week, depending on the severity and extent of the skin problem. The machine gives off UVA and/or UVB radiation in the precise doses and for the precise time that the dermatologist desires to treat the person's skin problem. Usually multiple treatments are given for several weeks or months.

Ultraviolet light therapy began in the 1890s, when the Danish "father of photobiology," Dr. Neils Finsen, used ultraviolet light to successfully treat skin tuberculosis. He later won the Nobel Prize for his work. Today, dermatologists routinely use UVA and UVB light therapies to treat patients with eczema, psoriasis, vitiligo, and other, rarer, diseases. Often patients are given psoralen, a drug that increases sensitivity to ultraviolet light, one to two hours before being exposed to UV light. This intensifies the therapy and produces results more quickly.

Photophoresis

Photophoresis, or *hemoirradiation,* is the term for a technique in which blood is removed from the body, irradiated with ultraviolet light, and then reinfused into the patient. Up to a pint of blood at a time can be treated in this manner. The absorbed light energy is thought to activate oxidation of the blood, kill bacteria, restore chemical balances, and reduce the effect of toxins in the blood. Photophoresis has been used successfully to treat several types of infections and some types of cancer, and holds greater promise for the future.

Electrotherapy

Using electrical current for healing purposes is becoming much more common and accepted. Transcutaneous electric nerve stimulation (TENS) therapy has been successfully used for a number of painful or itchy skin problems. It has also been helpful for skin problems involving the cutaneous nerves (the nerves in the skin) and the skin's blood supply. In dermatology, TENS has been used successfully for pain control during leg-vein sclerotherapy, cryosurgery, and debridement of ulcers. It has also been helpful for the discomfort of postherpetic neuralgia (a pain syndrome that sometimes occurs following a bout of shingles), itching, and diabetic neuropathy. Raynaud's phenomenon, scleroderma, wound healing, increased survival of skin flaps, keloid scars, tumors, and various kinds of skin ulcers have benefited from TENS therapy as well.

Electrotherapy was probably used by the ancient Egyptians, as evidenced by drawings of electric fish on their pottery, paintings, and walls. In Rome, in about the year 50, black torpedo fish were used to relieve gout pain. These fish, which produce electric currents similar to those used with TENS machines, were put under the feet of gout patients as the patients stood in water. Since the 1850s, the usefulness of local electrotherapy for anesthesia and for treating circulation problems has been discovered, forgotten about, and rediscovered. The modern era of TENS began in 1965.

Living tissues have the ability to form a small electrical charge at their surfaces. Thus, they have an electric and biochemical communication and control network. This plays an important role in normal wound healing, pain control, and dilation of microscopic blood vessels serving the skin. In 1983, it was demonstrated that there are biologically closed electrical circuits in our bodies that carry currents along blood vessels and through various organs. It is thought that in many diseases, such as scleroderma and dermatomyositis, there is an electrical derangement in the body's biologically closed circuits.

After tissue damage, an electropotential difference (a negative electrical current) forms across the top layer of the skin, the epidermis. This inherent type of "skin battery" helps to start the biological repair and healing in animals. The equivalent of a human "skin battery" thought to be capable of driving substantial currents into wounds was demonstrated in normal human volunteers' skin by researchers I.S. Foulds and A.T. Barker. They published their findings in the *British Journal of Dermatology* in 1983. If the above studies are accepted, then wound healing is mediated in part by electrical signals. Therefore, external electrical stimulation of wounds should change the healing process.

Electricity flows between negative and positive electrodes by the shortest route. The current from an externally applied source enters the body from the positive electrode, or anode, and streams toward the negative electrode, or cathode. Cells and ions with a net positive charge are repelled by a positive electrode and move away from it. Blood cells that have a negative charge, such as white blood cells, are driven away from a negatively charged cathode, and back up in tissues and blood vessels. Nerves also are polarized and depolarized by this applied electricity. Thus, a current flowing across cell membranes in turn causes biochemicals to be transmitted across synapses. Because it activates these various electrical and biochemical pathways, locally applied electricity is thought to have system-wide effects in the body.

Referrals to Other Specialists

Sometimes a dermatologist may need to refer a patient to another type of medical specialist. Occasionally a rheumatologist, allergist, oncologist, or internist is consulted for expertise in these areas that relate to the individual's skin problem. A psychologist may need to help the person address in more depth psychological factors contributing to or resulting from the skin problem, or aid in learning stress-reduction or mind-body techniques.

Conventional Psychiatric Counseling

Anecdotal reports as well as a recent controlled study suggest that psychological counseling can play an important role in increasing recurrence-free survival in people with malignant melanoma. A 1993 randomized, controlled study by F.I. Fawzy and colleagues at the University of California-Los Angeles Medical School found that in their test group of sixty-eight patients with malignant melanoma, those who participated in an intensive six-week psychiatric counseling group immediately after diagnosis and initial surgery had a much lower rate of recurrence and a significantly decreased rate of death from their skin cancer.

It is not too much of a stretch to surmise that if psychiatric or psychological intervention has a significant impact on the prognosis of people with melanoma, it may also be highly beneficial for people with other difficult or chronic dermatologic problems.

CONVENTIONAL DERMATOLOGY'S VIEW OF ALTERNATIVE THERAPIES

The field of dermatology is very well suited to the acceptance and integration of alternative therapies. Many creams and lotions are routinely compounded by pharmacists at dermatologists' requests. Doctors sometimes combine ingredients that they have discovered are helpful to the patient, but that are not commercially prepared in large quantities. Dermatologists are often open to using such preparations on a trial basis to see if they work, as often one topical treatment will help one patient with a given disease, while a different cream works better for another patient with the same disease. Dermatologists are used to viewing their craft as a cross between science and art, and use their experience and intuition about which treatment may work best for a particular patient based on the appearance of his or her skin problem. Because of its location, the skin itself can give the doctor immediate and obvious answers as to whether a specific therapy is effective. Thus, dermatologists can easily see if alternative therapies integrated into their practices work effectively and quickly, with few side effects.

The prestigious *Archives of Dermatology* recently devoted an entire issue to articles on alternative medicine in dermatology. Even the traditional American Academy of Dermatology has approved the formation of a task force of leading dermatologists to study nutrition and to evaluate alternative medical therapies in dermatology.

Many people with skin conditions—especially chronic, hard-to-cure ones—have turned to alternative medicine for help. In a 1989 German study of 71 patients with chronic skin diseases and allergies, 66 percent thought alternative medical treatments had been helpful. Likewise, in a 1990 study Norwegian study of 950 atopic dermatitis and psoriasis patients, 47 percent used one or more types of alternative medical treatment. A more recent 1993 study done at the Wake Forest University Department of Dermatology revealed that of 317 adults with chronic psoriasis who responded to a questionnaire, 51 percent used alternative therapies.

Therefore, physicians taking care of patients with skin diseases need to recognize that many of their patients, especially those with long-standing, difficult dermatologic problems, are using alternative therapies. They need to ask every patient about his or her use of alternative medical treatments. In this way, doctors can discover helpful information about results of complementary medical therapies as well as unwanted side effects. They can then work together with their patients to achieve the most beneficial results, using both traditional and alternative methods, depending on which therapies are most helpful for a particular individual. That is truly smart medicine, and that is the idea behind this book.

Diet and Nutrition

A healthy diet, with proper nutrition, is one of the crucial building blocks of your skin's good health. In this section, we will take a look at what a healthy diet really consists of. We also will look at certain foods and spices that can be very helpful for various diseases that affect the skin. The importance of drinking enough pure water every day cannot be stressed enough. Certain vitamins, minerals, and other food components are especially important for your skin's health, and will be discussed in detail in this chapter. Thus, after reading this chapter, you should have a good idea of how important your diet is for your general health as well as your skin's health, and what you should be putting into your mouth every day.

DIET

To maintain healthy skin, your diet must be rich in antioxidants, essential fatty acids, and the B and D vitamins. Antioxidants are nutrients that protect against oxidation, a chemical reaction that profoundly damages cells. Oxidation occurs when free radicals—electrically imbalanced molecules or fragments of molecules—"steal" electrons from components of cells to balance themselves energetically. In turn, this process generates even more damaging free radicals. Free radical damage has been shown to be an important factor in the aging process and in the development of cancer.

Omega-3 essential fatty acids (EFAs) are "good fats" found in fish oil and fatty fish. They are an important component of healthy cell membranes, including those of skin cells. Without sufficient omega-3 EFAs, the hair and skin become dry and brittle.

Also important is the concept of multiple marginal nutrient deficiencies. This means minor deficiencies in several nutrients, which together render the body less effective at fighting off disease and cancer. In this country, with the typical American diet, multiple marginal nutrient deficiencies are very common—much more so than deficiencies of single nutrients. These marginal nutrient deficiencies are very important, as they can lead to or cause flare-ups in infectious disease, carcinogenesis, and reduced immunity. Nutritional deficiencies are even more frequent in older adults, whose recommended daily intake of vitamins is actually higher than that of younger people, but whose diets tend to be even poorer.

Poor dietary habits and dietary nutrient deficiencies increase a person's susceptibility to skin disorders. This is largely due to the fact that skin-cell turnover time is so short. Skin cells are produced, die, and are replaced by new cells every few weeks. The condition of the skin is therefore a good mirror of a person's overall nutritional status. Also, many vitamins and minerals in a healthy diet help to maintain good circulation to the skin, increase the skin-cell levels of nutrients and oxygen, and remove the waste materials. Crash diets in particular can lead to brittle nails and hair loss.

A Healthy Preventive Diet

In general, a balanced diet of whole, unprocessed foods that is rich in whole grains, legumes, fruits, and vegetables will provide the necessary nutrients for healthy skin, hair, and nails. It is advisable to eat a variety of foods to reduce repeated exposure to food toxins, and to choose organic foods whenever possible. Wash all fresh food thoroughly before eating it.

Eating some form of fiber with every meal is a good idea, as this speeds the passage of toxins through the intestinal tract. Reduce your fat intake, especially your consumption of animal fats and saturated fats, as toxins concentrate in these fats. Avoid highly processed foods, which have high levels of additives but relatively little nutritive value, and may contain concentrated toxins. Instead, eat all natural foods whenever possible.

Avoid eating foods, especially (but not only) meats, that have been burned. Burning foods causes the formation of carcinogens, or cancer-causing substances. Alcohol, caffeine, sugar, and fried foods, which are sources of harmful free radicals, should be avoided also. Finally, if you have a problem such as acne, eczema, hives, or itching, it is wise to investigate the possibility of food allergies, which can cause or contribute to these problems.

Therapeutic Diets

Because certain foods are rich in one nutrient or another, specific foods are naturally helpful for certain disorders. For example, garlic is one of the strongest natural broad-spectrum antibacterial agents, and eating raw garlic cloves is a great boost to antibacterial activity. Onion is also a strong natural antibiotic and antiseptic, as are honey and wine. Still other foods have antiviral activity. Apples, blueberries, cranberries, grapes, grapefruit juice, mushrooms, peaches, plums, sage, tea, and red wine all have antiviral activity.

Other foods help to reduce inflammation. These include apples, black currants, fatty fish such as sardines and salmon, garlic, ginger, onion, pineapple, sage, and hot chili peppers. Garlic, shiitake mushrooms, and yogurt greatly stimulate the immune system. So do fruits, vegetables, nuts, grains, and shellfish that contain beta-carotene, vitamin C, vitamin E, and zinc.

Natural compounds found in many fruits and vegetables can interfere with some stages in the development of cancerous cells. Citrus fruits, tomatoes, broccoli, carrots, brown rice, oats, and soybeans are among the many foods that have natural anticancer activity.

Food can also change your mood by affecting the body's level of *serotonin,* a key brain neurotransmitter. Caffeine, ginger, honey, and sugar are all known to elevate mood. Carbohydrates, folic acid (found in green leafy vegetables), and selenium (in seafood, grains, and nuts) also work to heighten your mood. Caffeine, chili peppers, cloves, garlic, ginger, licorice, onion, peppermint, and sugar all have analgesic, or painkilling, activity.

PROPER HYDRATION WITH PURE WATER

It takes at least six to eight cups of pure water each day to keep the skin and body well hydrated. Good hydration is necessary for the skin to feel and look smooth. Hair looks and feels brittle and dry if you are not drinking enough water. Also, dehydration is often mistaken for hunger, and you may be tempted to overeat if you fail to realize that it is really water that your body craves.

Make sure your source of water is pure and filtered. Don't forget that drinks containing caffeine, such as coffee, tea, and some soft drinks, are actually diuretics and cause you to lose more water than you take in.

IMPORTANT NUTRIENTS AND NUTRITIONAL SUPPLEMENTS

It's best to get your essential nutrients through your daily diet, but sometimes this is not entirely possible. If you suspect that this may be the case, supplements can help. Begin by taking supplemental antioxidants—vitamins A, C, and E; beta-carotene, selenium, and zinc—as well as the fatty acids found in fish oil, the B vitamins, and vitamin D. These nutrients can be taken in capsule, pill, or liquid form. In the 1980s, patented spray forms of vitamins, minerals, and other nutrients were introduced. They are absorbed directly into the body though the tissues lining the mouth. Manufacturers claim that they provide an over 90 percent absorption rate within thirty seconds, nine times as fast as pills or capsules.

Today, an estimated 24 million Americans take dietary supplements, although fewer than 40 percent of them have discussed it with their doctors. It is a good idea to let your doctor know which supplements you are taking, as some can interact with certain drugs. Rarely, a nutritional supplement may can cause an unwanted side effect.

The Office of Dietary Supplements was established in 1994 at the National Institutes of Health (NIH). The NIH recently launched a new online database devoted entirely to dietary supplements that cites studies from more than 3,000 scientific journals. With the increasing popularity of alternative medicine and the emphasis on individuals assuming greater responsibility for their own health care, the over-the-counter supplement business has expanded rapidly in recent years. It promises to grow to even greater proportions in the years to come.

Let's look at some individual nutrients and what they do for the body, particularly for the skin, hair, and nails.

Vitamins

VITAMIN A

Vitamin A is very important for the health of the skin. It increases a person's immunity to infection, protects against damage from pollution, helps to block cancer formation, slows the aging process, and is essential for the maintenance and repair of normal skin tissue and mucous membranes. It is one of the very helpful antioxidants that neutralize damaging free radicals.

Great food sources of vitamin A include fish oils, animal livers, and green and yellow fruits and vegetables—specifically, apricots, asparagus, beets, broccoli, cantaloupe, carrots, garlic, kale, liver, mustard, papaya, parsley, peaches, pumpkin, red peppers, spinach, sweet potatoes, turnip greens, watercress, and yellow squash.

It is thought that, on average, people need 5,000 international units (IU) of vitamin A daily. Vitamin A should not be taken in large amounts by pregnant women, children, or people with liver disease. Overdosage can cause headaches, nausea, itchy skin, brittle nails, liver toxicity, bone pain, and birth defects.

Potent vitamin-A derivatives have been very useful in the treatment of severe acne, psoriasis, and other, less common, skin disorders. Isotretinoin (sold under the brand name Accutane) has helped many sufferers of severe acne, although great care needs to be taken not to become pregnant during therapy or for several months afterward, as this medication can cause birth defects. Etretinate (Tegison) has been very important in the treatment of difficult psoriasis cases. Most recently, a metabolite of etretinate, a retinoid also related to vitamin A, has been developed to treat severe erythrodermic psoriasis (an inflammatory form of the disorder characterized by widespread reddening of the skin, with fine scales that shed) and generalized pustular psoriasis (psoriasis with blisterlike lesions) that are unresponsive to other therapies. This is acitretin (Soriatane). Like the other vitamin-A derivatives, it causes birth defects, and is hazardous to the fetus if taken during pregnancy and for up to three years after the discontinuation of therapy.

The medications discussed in the preceding paragraph are taken orally. There are also several derivatives of vitamin A that can be applied topically for various purposes, among them the prevention and treatment of acne, psoriasis, and wrinkles and other signs of aging. Some are available by prescription only, while others are available over the counter. Retinol (ROC) is a nonprescription form of vitamin A useful for diminishing the dark spots and changes in the tone, texture, and moisture level of the skin that accompany aging.

Tretinoin, another vitamin-A derivative, is available in two prescription forms. Renova, or tretinoin emollient cream, is the only topical medication proven and approved for the treatment of wrinkles. It decreases the production of the pigment melanin in the skin, increases the rate of skin-cell turnover, and affects the growth and differentiation of skin cells, or keratinocytes. It is best used for the reduction of fine wrinkles, mottled increased skin pigmentation, and roughness of facial skin in people less than fifty years old. It is not effective for significant chronic sun exposure with deep wrinkling. It is thought to be an important addition to a comprehensive skin-care program for the early signs of aging from the sun. Retin-A, or tretinoin cream or gel, has been on the market for more than twenty years. It is officially approved only for the treatment of acne, although many people have used it in an unapproved manner to reduce facial wrinkling.

One of its main drawbacks has been the side effects of skin irritation, redness, and photosensitivity. Recently, a new formulation of Retin-A, Retin-A micro, or tretinoin gel microsphere, has been developed. It appears to be as effective as the original Retin-A, but with very little skin irritation. Like Retin-A, however, it is officially approved only for the treatment of acne, not wrinkles.

Another in the class of vitamin-A derivatives, or retinoids, is tazarotene (Tazorac). This is a topical gel that comes in two strengths. It is indicated for the treatment of stable plaque psoriasis that covers up to 20 percent of the body, and for mild to moderate facial acne.

Vitamin A and its derivatives have been very important in maintaining healthy skin and improving skin problems. Further research into the applications of vitamin-A derivatives in skin care appears very promising.

B VITAMINS

The B vitamins should always be taken together. They are coenzymes, or helpers needed by enzymes to carry out many functions. Vitamin B_1 (thiamine), vitamin B_2 (riboflavin), vitamin B_3 (niacin), and vitamin B_6 (pyridoxine) play an important role in energy production in the body, nerve-signal transmission, and the synthesis of hormones. Vitamin B_{12} (cobalamin) and folic acid are critical to the formation of red blood cells and the production of DNA, which is important for the health of skin, hair, and other cells. These two vitamins often work together synergistically to magnify each other's effects.

Biotin, another member of the B-complex family, is needed to process fats, carbohydrates, and proteins, and in the utilization of the other B vitamins. It is important for cell growth and for the formation and maintenance of strong nails and healthy skin. Taking supplemental biotin may help to prevent or reduce hair loss in some individuals. The body needs 300 micrograms of biotin a day, but deficiencies are rare. Most people normally get enough biotin in the foods they eat, and biotin can also be produced in the intestines from ingested foods. Good food sources of this vitamin include cooked egg yolk, saltwater fish, meat, milk, poultry, soybeans, peanuts, walnuts, corn, cauliflower, whole grains, and yeast.

Niacin is the B vitamin with the greatest potential to cause unwanted side effects, such as flushing and liver toxicity, if it is taken as a supplement. Side effects are most likely when niacin is taken in high doses and over long periods of time. Its ongoing use should therefore be closely monitored.

BETA-CAROTENE

Beta-carotene is one of a group of substances known as carotenes, which are yellow-orange pigments found in plants. When ingested, it is converted into vitamin A in the liver. Thought to be an even stronger antioxidant than vitamin A, beta-carotene aids in cancer prevention and slowing of the aging process. Actually, other carotenoids and disease-fighters, such as alpha-carotenes, lycopenes, lutein, and zeaxanthin, which are present with beta-carotene in foods, may be the best antioxidants, since taking pill forms of beta-carotene alone is much less helpful than is eating foods high in beta-carotene. These food sources include sweet potatoes, carrots, cantaloupe, spinach, winter squash, and dark-green leafy vegetables. The recommended daily dose of beta-carotene is between 8,000 and 25,000 international units (IU), or between 5 and 15 milligrams (mg), each day, depending on your age.

Although the skin can turn yellow-orange if you get very large amounts of beta-carotene, no overdose can occur, so it is relatively safe. However, people who have diabetes or underactive thyroids should not take beta-carotene supplements, as people with these conditions often have difficulty converting beta-carotene into vitamin A.

VITAMIN C

Vitamin C, or ascorbic acid, is an antioxidant essential for the manufacture of collagen, the protein that makes up cartilage, tendons, and other connective tissues of the body, including the skin. Vitamin C also aids in the absorption of iron and folic acid, and it is needed for the metabolism of these nutrients. In addition to maintaining healthy gums and tissues, it is important in reducing bruising and blood-clotting problems, strengthening blood-vessel walls, and healing wounds. Vitamin C protects cellular structures, including DNA, from damage. It protects against the harmful effects of pollution, increases immunity, aids in interferon and antistress-hormone production, and thereby helps to prevent cancer. By increasing immunity, it also helps to guard against infection. Taken orally, vitamin C helps to prevent cancer and speed the healing of skin ulcers and wounds.

There is evidence suggesting that vitamins C and E work synergistically, magnifying each other's effects and together greatly increasing antioxidant activity. Vitamin E scavenges for harmful oxygen radicals in the cell membranes, while vitamin C works in biologic fluids to attack free radicals.

Vitamin C is found naturally in green vegetables, berries, and citrus fruits. Asparagus, avocados, beet greens, broccoli, Brussels sprouts, cantaloupe, collards, currants, grapefruit, green peas, kale, lemons, mangos, mustard greens, onions, oranges, papayas, parsley, persimmons, pineapple, radishes, spinach, strawberries, sweet peppers, tomatoes, turnip greens, and watercress all contain an abundance of vitamin C.

Supplementation to increase vitamin-C levels is thought to help both preventively and therapeutically. The oral esterified polyascorbate form of vitamin C (such as Ester-C) is best to supplement the diet with, as it enters the bloodstream, tissues, and white blood cells four times as quickly as does the usual vitamin-C product. In this form, ascorbic acid is bound to calcium, magnesium, potassium, zinc, and/or sodium, with any one of these minerals allowing for more rapid absorption. High doses of vitamin C can cause diarrhea. Additionally, if you take large doses of vitamin C, your body gets used to these doses. Therefore, if you choose to reduce your intake, you have to taper off gradually to avoid a rebound vitamin-C deficiency.

Topically, the antioxidant vitamin C inhibits skin aging caused by ultraviolet light and increases the production of the proteins collagen and elastin, which are necessary to maintain firm skin that does not sag or wrinkle. Vitamin C also neutralizes free radicals, and promotes skin-cell renewal. Thus, it is very important in reducing the appearance of fine lines and wrinkles, returning and maintaining youthful skin resilience, and lightening and evening skin tones. It is available in many over-the-counter cosmetics, lotions, creams, eye-lift gels, and transdermal patches that are applied to the wrinkled areas and left on overnight. There is also a new patch out on the market that is applied for only forty-five minutes prior to an important event to reduce the appearance of wrinkling for up to six hours.

VITAMIN E

Vitamin E, or tocopherol, is an antioxidant that also helps to improve blood circulation, promote normal clotting, repair tissue, improve healing, and reduce scarring. It helps to maintain the integrity of cell membranes, and it is needed to synthesize DNA. Like vitamin C, it inhibits free radicals, thereby preventing cell damage, helping to prevent cancer, and retarding the signs of aging.

Cold-pressed vegetable oils, whole grains, dark-green leafy vegetables, nuts, seeds, and legumes are great sources of vitamin E. Additional sources include dry beans, sweet potatoes, brown rice, oatmeal, cornmeal, wheat germ, eggs, milk, and organ meats.

The body needs zinc in order to help maintain the correct blood levels of vitamin E. Vitamin E works better when taken with selenium. Iron supplements should not be taken at the same time as vitamin E.

Vitamin E applied topically is very soothing and moisturizing, and therefore has been very popular in skin care. It is available in stick, oil, and cream form for use on the face, lips, and body as a moisturizer and anti-aging cream, and to reduce the prominence of healing scars.

VITAMIN K

Vitamin K is needed for blood clotting, and is therefore useful in treating bruises. Vitamin K-rich foods include alfalfa, broccoli, dark green leafy vegetables, and soybeans.

Vitamin K is also available in cream form to help reduce the appearance of spider veins, or small, visible capillaries near the surface of the skin. These frequently develop on the legs with age. Accentuations of the capillaries also often develop on the cheeks or chest with rosacea or chronic overexposure to the sun.

Minerals

CHROMIUM

Chromium is involved in the metabolism of glucose (sugar) and is needed for energy and the synthesis of cholesterol, fats, and protein. It helps to maintain stable blood sugar levels. Chromium-rich foods include beer, yeast, brown rice, cheese, meat, whole grains, corn, mushrooms, potatoes, and dried beans. Many people do not get enough chromium through diet alone, as there is a lack of chromium in our water and soil, and because the typical American diet high in refined white sugar, flour, and junk foods is deficient in chromium. It often needs to be supplemented at a dose of 150 micrograms (mcg) per day.

COPPER

Copper aids in the formation of hemoglobin and red blood cells, and therefore is important for healthy circulation of blood to the skin. This mineral also works in balance with zinc and vitamin C to form elastin and collagen, the protein building blocks necessary for toned, supple skin. Thus, copper is also important for normal hair and skin coloring and health.

About 3 milligrams of copper is needed on a daily basis; over 35 milligrams a day is toxic. Copper is naturally found in most vegetables, nuts, and seafood. Most people do not need supplemental copper.

SELENIUM

Selenium is a vital antioxidant, especially when combined with vitamin E. It aids in the production of antibodies, protects the immune system, and helps prevent cancers, including skin cancer. Some feel that selenium depletion may be a trigger that allows harmful viruses, including HIV, to "turn on" and damage the body.

Plants get their selenium content directly from the soil in which they grow. Vegetables grown in selenium-rich soil, such as is found in Brazil, are higher in selenium than those grown in the eastern United States, where selenium stores in the soil have been depleted and are very low. Thus, depending on the soil content of the food's place of origin, selenium can be found in meat, vegetables, and grains. Good sources of selenium include Brazil nuts, yeast, broccoli, brown rice, chicken, dairy products, garlic, liver, onions, and seafood.

Our bodies need 70 micrograms of selenium a day; over 200 micrograms a day can be toxic. Early evidence of overdosage include a metallic taste in the mouth. Later signs include fragile or black nails and hair loss.

ZINC

Zinc is an essential mineral required for protein synthesis and collagen formation, promoting the healing of wounds. It is also important to help keep the immune system healthy and to maintain the proper concentrations of vitamin E in the blood.

Great sources of zinc include fish, legumes, meats, oysters and other seafood, poultry, and whole grains. A daily intake of approximately 15 milligrams of zinc is desirable. Interestingly, while consuming up to 100 milligrams of zinc daily enhances the body's immune response, taking in more than 100 milligrams a day actually depresses immunity. In too-large quantities, zinc can cause nausea, vomiting, diarrhea, and abdominal pain, and can deplete copper stores in the body.

Other Nutrients

BIOFLAVONOIDS AND QUERCETIN

Bioflavonoids, while not true vitamins, enhance absorption of vitamin C, and should be taken with it. They act together with vitamin C to preserve the structure of capillaries, or small blood vessels, and reduce symptoms of oral herpes (cold sores). Bioflavonoids also promote good blood circulation and have an antibacterial effect. Apricots, black currants, cherries, grape-fruit, grapes, lemons, oranges, peppers, and prunes are good dietary sources. Quercetin, one of the many different bioflavonoids, is found in blue-green algae, and is used for the treatment of allergies when taken in supplement form.

COENZYME Q$_{10}$

Coenzyme Q$_{10}$, or ubiquinone, is a vitaminlike substance similar to vitamin E, but even more powerful as an antioxidant. It is an essential part of the mitochondria, the energy-producing part of almost all of the cells in the body. It plays a key role in the effectiveness of the immune system and in delaying the aging process. It also fights the effects of histamine, the body chemical that triggers allergic reactions, so it is valuable in dealing with allergic skin problems and hives.

The amount of coenzyme Q$_{10}$ stored in a person's cells declines with age, so supplements are recommended. Mackerel, salmon, and sardines contain large amounts of coenzyme Q$_{10}$. At least 30 milligrams of coenzyme Q$_{10}$ a day should be added to the average American diet to maintain mitochondria that function effectively.

Coenzyme Q$_{10}$ is also available in topical form, added to various moisturizers and sunscreens. It is thought that this nutrient can be absorbed and act directly on the skin as an antioxidant, reducing the signs of aging and enhancing the skin's natural immunologic ability.

DHEA

DHEA, or dehydroepiandrosterone, is a potent steroid hormone produced by the adrenal gland. Recently it has been being promoted as an anti-aging, anticancer agent. The body's levels of DHEA peak at twenty to twenty-four years of age and fall by about 20 percent with each subsequent decade of life. Isolated studies have shown improvement in the symptoms of systemic lupus erythematosus and atopic eczema with DHEA supplementation. Possible side effects of DHEA include acne and increased growth of body hair in women. DHEA supplements must be treated with care as a potent drug.

ESSENTIAL FATTY ACIDS

Essential fatty acids (EFAs) are polyunsaturated fatty acids (building blocks of fat and oils) that cannot be made by the body and therefore must be supplied by the diet. There are several different families of EFAs. Of these, the most important are the group designated omega-3 essential fatty acids. The EFAs have anti-inflammatory effects and have been shown to help eczema and psoriasis in some (though not all) studies.

The daily requirement for EFAs is satisfied if they make up about 15 percent of total daily caloric intake. However, there aren't any known adverse effects to consuming larger amounts. Pure, cold-pressed, nonhydrogenated fortified flaxseed oil, primrose oil, black-currant seed oil, and other vegetable oils contain high amounts of linoleic acid, an important EFA. Evening primrose oil contains the highest amount of gamma-linolenic acid, another EFA, of any food substance, and is often used in the treatment of atopic dermatitis. Salmon, mackerel, herring, and sardines—fish that come from cold, deep-water environments—are great sources of fish oil because they have the highest fat content and provide more omega-3 factors than other fishes.

Whether you have a skin problem or not, you should eat a balanced, healthy diet to meet as many of your vitamin and mineral needs as possible. However, for some disorders, higher doses of certain nutrients can be beneficial. When I list recommended supplements in Part Two, Common Skin Problems, I am also suggesting that the diet be composed of foods high in these specific nutrients. It is preferable to consume nutrients in foods, as there are probably many as-yet-undiscovered valuable nutrients and synergistic relationships among various factors in our foods.

Herbal Medicine

In recent years, Americans have fallen increasingly in love with herbal therapies. More and more pharmaceutical and cosmetic companies are incorporating herbs in their formulations and actively marketing these herbal preparations. With all this hoopla, it's easy to forget that the use of herbs is actually the most ancient form of health care known to humankind. So let's see what all this fuss over herbs is about. In this chapter, we will take a look at the science, action, forms, and history of herbs from different cultures around the world. Then I will describe in more depth the herbs that have been found to be most helpful with skin problems. Herbs, although they come from plants, can still have unwanted side effects and drug interactions, and we will look at that, too. When you have finished this chapter, you will have gained a good understanding of herbs and how you can use them at home for self-care with your skin problems.

AN INTRODUCTION TO HERBAL MEDICINE

An herb, as used in herbal or botanical medicine, is a plant or part of a plant used to make medicine, spices, or aromatic oils for soaps and fragrances. Of the approximately 265,000 plants worldwide, only about 5,000 have been studied for their medicinal uses. Thus, there exists a very real possibility that cures to many different diseases may still exist in the 98 percent of the plants yet unstudied.

Recently, tremendous advances in screening processes have made it possible to do the initial screening of plants for useful components in just a few days, without using animals. (In the past it took an average of twelve years and up to $300 million to come up with a single new drug.) With this financial incentive, there has recently been a huge increase in the number of specialists in medicinal plants working for or with pharmaceutical companies. They scour the world's flora in search of plants that will benefit Western medicine. Often, they are in a race against other human activities, such as farming, logging and road-building, that are driving innumerable plant species to extinction before anyone is able to study them. Some people with vision offer cash-poor native peoples, particularly those in rainforest areas, where the diversity of plants is enormous, an alternative such as tourism to help them avoid selling off the forests to loggers. Botanical specialists are also in a race with time to learn the art of the traditional healers of the world before these individuals cease to exist, as various cultures abandon traditional healing practices for Western pills and creams.

Much of the earth's biodiversity is concentrated around the equator, and medicinal plants are sought in such far-flung places as Samoa, the South Pacific, Southeast Asia, South America, and East Africa. Some people randomly collect thousands of plant samples, while others believe it is more productive to interview and work with local native healers. The different herbal traditions of the world are richly varied, depending on cultural context, although their goals and effects are similar. There is much herbal healing knowledge in the Native American, European, Ayurvedic, and traditional Chinese medical cultures.

HERBAL TRADITIONS FROM CHINA, INDIA, AND EUROPE

Traditional Chinese herbal medicine is based on balancing two complementary forces, the yin and the yang. Five elements—fire, earth, metal, water, and wood—are thought to give rise to the five tastes, by which all herbs are traditionally evaluated. Each taste is thought to have a specific healing action. Therefore, in this view, fire gives rise to bitterness, and bitter-tasting herbs drain the body of excess fluid, internally or externally, and dry it out. Earth gives rise to sweetness, and sweet herbs tonify, or nurture the body, build vital energy, and also decrease pain. Metal is associated with acrid-tasting herbs, which disperse, or scatter, cells or fluids for medicinal purposes. Water gives rise to saltiness, and salty herbs nourish the kidneys. Wood gives rise to sourness, and sour-tasting herbs are astringent, having binding effect on mucous membranes and skin, thereby preventing unwanted loss of body fluids and energy. Herbs that are bland and have none of these tastes are thought to be diuretic, helping in the elimination of wastes through the kidneys. In the traditional Chinese medical view, different herbs are also associated with different target organs and different temperatures, as well as the five different elements, tastes, and healing actions described above.

Ayurvedic medicine, from India, also recognizes five different elements.

Fire, water, and earth are the same as in the Chinese view, but ether and air replace metal and wood. These five Ayurvedic elements are believed to manifest themselves in the body to form three basic humors: vata, pitta, and kapha. It is thought that in healing one tries to achieve a balance between vata (air or wind), pitta (fire or bile), and kapha (water or phlegm). Again, the different tastes of herbs are supposed to be indicative of the herbs' characteristics. For example, pungent, sour, and salty-tasting herbs are thought to cause heat and so increase fire, or pitta. Sweet, bitter, and astringent herbs are supposed to do the opposite—cool, and decrease pitta. Ayurvedic medicine categorizes all healing herbs according to this age-old system.

Herbal medicine is much more accepted in Europe, especially in Germany, than it is in the United States. Since 1933, all German doctors have studied herbal medicine in medical school and must pass a section of their board exams on these herbal remedies before becoming licensed physicians. European physicians and researchers have coordinated their efforts and have formed the European Scientific Cooperative for Phytotherapy (ESCOP). ESCOP publishes monographs on individual herbs, and soon will publish a definitive European Pharmacopoeia of herbal medicine.

HERBALISM IN AMERICA

Modern Western medicine is actually deeply founded in herbal medicine. Almost 25 percent of all prescription drugs are derived directly from chemicals that come from about 40 trees, shrubs, or herbs. Of 119 plant-derived pharmaceuticals, about 74 percent are used in modern medicine in ways similar to the ways that, according to folklore, native cultures used them.

However, for a number of reasons, modern American medicine typically hasn't used the pure herbs for medicinal purposes. First, herbs cannot be patented, so there is no economic incentive on the part of pharmaceutical companies to use pure herbs. The collection and preparation of herbs cannot easily be controlled, and this also makes profits less dependable. Most importantly, in the past, Americans have preferred to rely on synthetic, commercial drugs, which concentrate a single active ingredient to provide quicker relief, although the risk and severity of potential side effects can be greater. However, with the increasing disenchantment with modern health-care practices, the interest in herbal medicine is a growing American phenomenon.

In December 1994, a historic conference entitled "Botanicals: A Role in US Health Care?" was held in Washington, DC, sponsored by the Office of Alternative Medicines of the National Institutes of Health in cooperation with the U.S. Food and Drug Administration (FDA). The conference brought together for the first time regulators, researchers, practitioners, and herb manufacturers. All agreed that this was the beginning of a new era in herbal medicine in the United States. With the retail botanical market booming, it is estimated that the herbal market will increase from the $1.5-billion-a-year industry it is now to a greater-than-$5-billion-a-year industry over the next several years.

However, accurate education about the safe and effective use of herbs has lagged behind this heightened consumer demand. This is because much of the information available today is taken from herbal traditions in which herbs were used for the treatment of acute conditions that require aggressive treatment. However, the majority of our health problems today are chronic ones, in part arising from the effects of chronic stress, pollution, and poor nutrition. These chronic diseases require a new supportive, enhancing, and nourishing approach to the use of herbs. Herbs are not used in the same manner as conventional medications, where the most active and strongest remedy is used to stop a symptom. Therefore, many new techniques for herbal usage must be learned.

Because there is currently no licensing body for the practice of herbal medicine in the United States, one must beware of the qualifications and knowledge of herbal practitioners. Naturopathic doctors, who have completed a four-year training program after college, have a very good foundation in botanical medicine and are often reliable sources of herbal information.

Several established institutions, including Columbia University and Temple University, have set up educational programs to help meet the new consumer demand for herbal remedies and information. In response to the 74 percent of recently surveyed pharmacists who said they were interested in more information on herbal medicine, the American Botanic Council is planning to provide home-study training for pharmacists in the area of botanical medicine.

Herbal remedies have also been passed down for generations in the cultural melting pot that is America. Although these are often called "Grandma's cures" or "Great-Auntie's home remedies," some are in fact based on herbal medicine. I use the term herbal here in its full sense, defining herbs to include roots, leaves, fruits, flowers, seeds, and those plants generally used as spices.

These represent remedies that are mostly Western, as opposed to strictly Chinese, Indian, North American Indian, or other cultural remedies.

For cosmetic applications, many herbal treatments are extremely economical alternatives to expensive, highly advertised beauty aids. Also, the latest trend in chic cosmetics and skin-care products is to incorporate herbal ingredients into various formulas and promote them on the basis of their use of "natural" elements. These products can be good for those with multiple allergies to all the ingredients, preservatives, and fragrances crammed into many commercial products, and are recommended for those with chemical allergies.

TYPES OF HERBS IN WESTERN HERBALISM

Herbal medicines work according to their chemical makeup, similar to the way conventional pharmaceutical drugs work. However, their effects are usually weaker and slower than those of purified pharmaceutical drugs, which use more direct routes to the bloodstream and target organs. Therefore, one must be more patient when using botanical therapy. The positive aspect of this is that there is less danger of the severe side effects found in drug-based medicine. One still has to be wary of adverse effects, though, especially if an improper dose, a low-quality herb, or the wrong herb is used, or if herbs are used by pregnant or nursing women.

Herbs can be categorized in Western medicine according to the kinds of problems they can be used to treat. Their effects are due to the actions of specific chemicals in the herbs, or due to a complex interaction between different constituents of the plants. For skin problems, herbs classified as *alterative, anti-inflammatory, antimicrobial, bitter, hepatic, nervine, tonic,* and *vulnerary* are most commonly used.

Various types of alteratives gradually alter and correct a "polluted" bloodstream, and have been nicknamed "blood cleansers." Some work mostly on cleansing the liver, while others work on the kidneys. Herbs with a bitter taste trigger a response in the central nervous system leading to increased bile flow, liver detoxification, and intestinal self-repair. Hepatic herbs strengthen the liver, thereby helping to remove toxins from the body. These toxins are often one of the underlying causes for dermatologic diseases. Diuretics cleanse the urinary system. Alteratives frequently used in the treatment of skin problems include blue flag, cleavers, figwort, fumitory, goldenseal, nettle, Oregon grape root, red clover, sarsaparilla, sassafras, thuja, and yellow dock.

As the name suggests, anti-inflammatories decrease the inflammatory response of tissue. Antimicrobials usually aid the body's natural immunity and resistance to infective organisms, and occasionally contain chemicals that are poisonous to certain organisms. Antimicrobials commonly used for skin problems include chickweed, echinacea, garlic, marigold, myrrh, thuja, thyme, and wild indigo.

In August of 1987, Dr. A. Caceres and his colleagues at the Center for Mesoamerican Studies on Appropriate Technology at the University of San Carlos in Guatemala City, published an assessment of the antimicrobial activity of eighty-nine plants commonly used in Guatemala for the treatment of diseases of the skin and mucous membranes. In the laboratory, almost one-third of the plants at least partially inhibited the growth of the four most common bacteria and yeasts that cause skin and mucosal infections. Dr. Caceres published a further study in December 1993 showing that half of the fifty-two Guatemalan plants screened were active against different types of fungi that attack the skin. He also evaluated and confirmed the antifungal activity of seven American plants.

Drs. M.J. Plotkin and R.E. Schultes of Conservation International in Washington, DC, reported in 1990 that the resin of the plant virola showed very promising results for the treatment of deep fungal infections. Virola is traditionally used by many different Indian tribes for difficult deep fungal infections. The authors suggested further study and purification techniques be done immediately because this antifungal treatment had proved so successful.

In 1993 Dr. M. Kurokawa and colleagues at the Department of Virology at Toyama Medical and Pharmaceutical University in Japan tested the laboratory efficacy of traditional antiviral medicines used against herpes simplex virus 1 (HSV-1), polio, and measles. Out of 142 medicines traditionally used in China, Indonesia, and Japan, 32 showed activity against HSV-1, 55 worked against the polio virus, and 30 were effective against the measles virus. Additionally, 12 of the 32 extracts that showed anti-HSV-1 activity in the laboratory were also effective in limiting the development of cold sores in mice. Interestingly, these 12 medicines were currently being used in Asia for the treatment of things other than viral infections. Therefore, 12 new candidates for the use of traditional Asian medicines against herpes simplex virus 1 infections were discovered!

Nervines tone and strengthen the nervous system, some stimulating it and others relaxing it. Tonics are frequently used for preventive as well as for therapeutic treatments, as they nurture the body and build vital energy.

Vulneraries, which include astringents, help to heal external wounds and cuts. Astringents help to stop bleeding and condense tissue. They also help to dry up wound discharges. Vulneraries important in dermatology include aloe, chickweed, comfrey, elderberry, goldenseal, marigold, marshmallow root, slippery elm, and witch hazel.

Herbal medicine is most helpful for chronic, ongoing problems. When treating chronic skin problems, the entire body must be considered, and the therapy must include nutritional, tonic, digestive, eliminative, and restorative herbs. Chronic problems such as psoriasis and eczema can especially benefit from herbal therapies.

FORMS OF HERBS

Herbs now come in many forms: capsules, tablets, extracts, tinctures, essential oils, ointments, whole herbs, and teas. They are available in natural food stores, grocery stores, and drugstores, and through many mail-order catalogues, Internet sites, and multilevel marketing organizations. Therefore, it is wise to shop around and compare qualities, combinations, and prices, as they all vary tremendously.

Herbal Extracts and Tinctures

Extracts and tinctures are high concentrations of herbs in alcohol, which works as a solvent and as a preservative. They are rapidly assimilated and have a much quicker effect than tablets and capsules. Tinctures can contain up to 80 percent alcohol, and therefore these products have an almost indefinite shelf life.

Herbal Salves

Salves made from plants have been used for thousands of years. Today, vegetable oil or petroleum jelly is often made into a salve containing aloe, marigold, chamomile, or other herbs to treat skin irritations, wounds, and bites.

Essential Oils

Essential oils, used in aromatherapy, are essences of aromatic plants that are extremely concentrated and distilled, or, in the case of citrus fruits, squeezed directly from the peels. One or two drops is all that is generally needed. Eucalyptus and tea tree oils can be used directly on the skin, but most other oils have to be diluted in a carrier oil or water first before they can be used topically, as they are highly irritating if used by themselves. They will be discussed further in a subsequent section.

In addition to the forms discussed above, it is possible to buy whole herbs, which are plants or plant parts that are dried, and herbal teas, or infusions, which are one or more finely cut herbs designed to be steeped in water and drunk.

HERBS COMMONLY USED FOR SKIN PROBLEMS

Aloe Vera

Several controlled scientific studies have shown statistically significant antibacterial benefits of aloe vera. Other studies have shown statistically significant improvement in skin symptoms when aloe vera has been used in the treatment of radiation ulcers, burns, and frostbite injuries in animals.

In 1953, Drs. C.C. Lushbaugh and D.S. Hale found that treatment with aloe vera sped up the repair of skin ulcers caused by radiation in rabbits. It took less than half the time for the aloe-treated ulcers to heal as compared with the untreated group. Drs. S. Goff and I. Levenstein in 1964 found that aloe vera helps surgical wounds in mice to heal more quickly for the first two weeks after surgery. In a related study in 1994, Dr. F.M. Strickland and colleagues at the Department of Immunology of the University of Texas and the M.D. Anderson Cancer Center in Houston, Texas, found that aloe vera gel extract spread on the skin of mice exposed to ultraviolet (UV) radiation lessened the degree of UV-induced immune suppression.

In 1964, Dr. L.J. Lorenzetti and others found that aloe juice significantly inhibited the growth of four strains of virulent bacteria in the lab. Similarly, in 1982, Dr. M.C. Robson and others found that aloe vera extract killed two strains of clinically important bacteria.

In 1982, Dr. Robson and Dr. J.P. Heggers found that aloe vera increases the blood supply to the second layer of skin, the dermis. This speeds healing by bringing in vital nutrients and removing dangerous toxins. The researchers also found that aloe vera decreases tissue destruction after a burn, and that it can increase survival in white rabbits with frostbite injuries by a statistically significant amount. In seven independent studies done from 1968 to 1982, four pharmacologically active ingredients were identified in aloe vera that together reduce the pain, itching, and inflammation of a rash.

Thus, aloe vera has been proven to be an important antibacterial and anti-inflammatory agent that speeds the healing of all kinds of wounds, burns, and ulcers. Aloe vera gel is one of the most common botanical additions to first-aid creams, moisturizers, and shampoos.

Calaguala Fern and Pine Tar Products

Calaguala fern, known to the Mayan people since 350 BC for its use in dry, itchy skin and scalp problems, has been combined with pine tar, a European remedy with similar uses. Skin creams, bath products, soaps, shampoos, and conditioners have been made from this combination and are very helpful for dry, itchy skin and scalp problems.

Calendula

Calendula (or pot marigold), with its deep yellow and orange flowers, is one of the best all-around skin remedies, good for minor cuts and burns, insect bites, dry skin, and acne. Calendula blossoms have antibacterial and antiviral properties, soothe inflammation, and speed wound healing. Therefore, it is simultaneously potent and gentle, which makes it very useful for all skin types. Calendula tea can be used as an astringent facial rinse two or three times a day for acne. More convenient preparations are available over the counter as salves, creams, oils, and lotions.

Chamomile

Chamomile is an anti-inflammatory agent that soothes the skin when used topically and soothes the bowels when taken internally. It also has a gentle tranquilizing effect on the central nervous system, and soothes nervous tension and irritability. It is often used for eczema and psoriasis. Generally, it is best taken three times a day as a great-tasting apple-scented herbal tea made from its flowers. Or a clean cloth can be soaked in the chamomile tea and applied to the areas of inflamed skin for fifteen minutes four to six times a day. Chamomile also forms the base for many moisturizers, under-eye therapies for puffiness and dark circles, and many soap and shampoo combinations.

Comfrey

The leaves and roots of comfrey have been used for centuries to treat cuts, burns, and other wounds. Comfrey contains allantoin, a compound that is quickly absorbed through the skin to stimulate healthy cell growth. It also has astringent and soothing actions. Comfrey is a very common ingredient in over-the-counter and prescription skin-healing salves and ointments. Comfrey poultices, made from powdered comfrey root and hot water mixed to make a thin paste that is spread on a cloth, can be applied on a surface wound. If left on overnight, there is very fast healing by morning. However, since some of the alkaloid compounds comfrey contains can cause serious liver damage if the plant is ingested, comfrey should never be taken by mouth. Also, you should not use comfrey on deep wounds, as an abscess may form if surface healing occurs faster than the deep tissue healing.

Emu Oil

Advertisers are using the Internet to sing the praises of emu oil. Not only do they say that it's great for cuts, bites, burns, and the itch of poison ivy, but they also claim that it promotes hair growth by rejuvenating skin and hair cells. It has been combined with other ingredients to make cleansers, masques, shampoos, conditioners, shaving creams, body lotions, and lip balms.

Flaxseed

Flaxseed comes from the herb flax and contains those omega-3 essential fatty acids necessary for the proper synthesis of immune and anti-inflammatory compounds. It is useful in the management of skin disorders such as eczema and psoriasis, which are associated with inflammatory processes. One to two tablespoons of cold-pressed flaxseed oil should be taken daily, preferably with other foods.

Goldenseal

Goldenseal is obtained from the underground parts of a member of the buttercup family, *Hydrastis canadensis*. It was introduced to early European settlers in America by Cherokee natives, who used it as a wash for skin diseases. Goldenseal has astringent and antiseptic properties, and inhibits the growth of bacteria, yeast, and parasites. Goldenseal is best taken in capsule form, as it stains the hands and clothes easily and has a bitter taste. Pregnant women should not take goldenseal, as it stimulates uterine contractions. Neither should it be used by people with high blood pressure, as it can cause blood vessels to contract further, thus raising blood pressure.

Licorice

Taken internally, licorice can reduce inflammation. It helps the body to maintain its own healthy levels of cortisol, and so is very helpful for those who have had to use large amounts of cortisone ointments for a long time. To reduce internal inflammation and stabilize cortisol levels, you can drink a cup of licorice tea two to three times a day. Or you can take 2 to 4 milliliters of liquid extract, or 250 to 500 milligrams in capsule form, three times daily. However, you should not take licorice on an ongoing basis, as it can raise blood pressure in some people, and you should not take it if you already have high blood pressure.

Milk Thistle

Milk thistle is an anti-inflammatory agent. It is also a liver detoxifier and encourages the regeneration of new liver cells. It helps in chronic skin diseases that are related to food allergies and toxic bowels. It is best taken in tincture form, one dropperful four to six times daily, or 100 to 200 milligrams of concentrated extract in capsule form three times daily.

Oregon Grape Root

Oregon grape root is helpful for eczema, psoriasis, and acne, as it contains alkaloids that reduce inflammation and soothe mucous membranes. It also stimulates the secretion of bile by the liver, promoting detoxification, which is key for healthy skin. If you take this herb to enhance detoxification and decrease inflammation, look for a standardized extract containing at least 8 to 12 percent alkaloids and take 6 to 12 milliliters of tincture, 2 to 4 milliliters of liquid extract, or 250 to 500 milligrams in capsule form daily.

Tea Tree Oil

Tea tree oil is an essential oil distilled from the leaves of a plant called *Melaleuca alternifolia*. It has been shown to kill germs and decrease bacterial, fungal, and viral activity. This versatile botanical is sold in oil, soap, ointment, toothpaste, mouthwash, and lozenge form, and is included as an ingredient in many herbal combinations.

POSSIBLE SIDE EFFECTS OF HERBAL MEDICINES

There is a common misconception that herbs are harmless because they are natural products sold over the counter. This is not the case. Discovering the causes of some complications may be difficult, as many people, during a standard medical history, do not consider herbs worth mentioning along with the conventional medications they take. Some people may also be embarrassed to admit to a doctor that they are taking herbs instead of more conventional medicines. Doctors should remember to inquire about this, as it can be important.

There are references to skin problems associated with exposure to certain plants from as far back as the first century AD. Pedianos Dioscorides was a Greek botanist who wrote a text on 600 medicinal plants. In it he first described plant irritants. Poison ivy was first mentioned in 1609 in the diary of Captain John Smith, written during his settlement of Jamestown, Virginia. Chinese primrose became a useful material for contact dermatitis research in the late 1800s. By the beginning of the 1900s, the study of dermatitis due to plant exposure in the West had merged completely with the research of contact dermatitis in general.

In the recent professional literature, contact with the following herbs has been mentioned as causing sensitivity reactions in some cases:

- Burdock (*Arctium lappa*).
- Chamomile (*Chamaemelum nobile*).
- Elecampane (*Inula helenium*) extract.

- Nettle (*Urtica dioica*).
- Slippery elm (*Ulmus fulva*).
- Spurge (*Euphorbia bougheii*).
- Tea tree (*Melaleuca alternifolia*) oil.

A very small number of diverse side effects due to the use of herbal preparations have been reported in the professional medical literature over the past fifteen years. In a number of studies between 1987 and 1992, it was well documented that traditional Chinese herbal medicine could, in very rare cases, cause liver damage. In her 1994 study, Dr. M.P. Sheehan of the Department of Dermatology at the Hospital for Sick Children in London, England, refers to two cases previously reported by others in which two children contracted hepatitis after receiving traditional Chinese medicine treatment for atopic dermatitis. There has been a single case reported of abdominal pain due to taking a Chinese herbal medicine with clamshell powder that contained lead, and another isolated case of reversible weakening of the heart after a two-week treatment with traditional Chinese herbal medicine. The number of people who have experienced unwanted side effects from traditional Chinese herbal preparations appears to be very, very tiny, but you should remember that side effects are still possible.

Dr. C.P. Siegers and colleagues at the Institute of Toxicology, Medical University of Lübeck, Germany, concluded from their studies that laxative abuse with aloe, cascara, senna, frangula, or rheum may cause a 2.5-fold increased risk for colorectal cancer. This does not mean that these natural laxatives pose an increased risk for colorectal cancer when taken as directed, only if they are overused and abused. In general, herbal preparations are most likely to cause problems if taken in too-high doses, too frequently, and/or for too long a period of time.

Aromatherapy

Like herbal therapy, aromatherapy has become quite popular in the United States. Aromatherapy diffusers and essential oils are now sold in drugstores and department stores, not just in specialty stores. Aromatherapy is the specific branch of herbal therapy that makes use of the medicinal properties of the essential oils of plants. The essential oil is the volatile part of the plant's oil, its essence, which is extracted from its other parts. Because essential oils are rapidly absorbed by the skin, they are an ideal addition for baths, compresses, and massage oils to aid damaged skin or enhance healthy skin. Unlike some other treatments, using them can be fun and enjoyable as well. So let's learn more about them, so you too can enjoy the many benefits of essential oils.

AN INTRODUCTION TO AROMATHERAPY

The essential oils of plants have been used therapeutically since ancient times in many countries, including China, India, Egypt, and Italy. The modern-day science of aromatherapy for the treatment of common medical problems began with the French chemist and perfumer René-Maurice Gattefossé in 1937. He began to research the curative powers of essential oils when he found that pure lavender oil was very helpful in treating a burn he received while working in his family's perfume laboratory. It was he who coined the term "aromatherapy," which has stuck until this day.

Today, essential oils are still widely used in most of the rest of the world, including Europe. In France, a system of medical aromatherapy is already well established, and French physicians routinely prescribe aromatherapy preparations that can be purchased in neighborhood pharmacies. There, it is routine for doctors to send culture samples to the pharmacist for testing and identification of the relevant aromatherapy for the patient's condition.

In England, aromatherapy is used by hospital nurses to give essential-oil massages for stress reduction, pain relief, and insomnia. English hospitals also diffuse essential oils such as lemon, lavender, and lemongrass into the air to help fight the transmission of airborne infections.

With an increasing demand here in the United States for less toxic alternative therapies for mild and chronic conditions, the popularity of aromatherapy has grown rapidly over the last ten years. Aromatherapy has an increasingly promising future as more Americans come to accept its use and effectiveness.

Aromatherapy is very helpful for bacterial infections, viral infections, and immune deficiency. Because the oils work in a different way than antibiotics do, they do not have the same side effects and do not destroy necessary intestinal bacteria. The oils tend to stimulate the immune system rather than depress it, as more conventional treatments do. Essential oils can also be used to promote the excretion of urine, widen or narrow blood vessels, act on the glands, and facilitate digestion. The oils interact immediately and strongly with all branches of the nervous system, harmonizing moods and emotions, and are very effective for stress management.

Numerous skin disorders can be improved with the use of aromatherapy. Isabelle Hay and colleagues at the Department of Dermatology, Aberdeen Royal Infirmary in Foresterhill, Scotland, recently reported in the *Archives of Dermatology* that aromatherapy was found to be a safe and effective treatment for alopecia areata, an autoimmune condition characterized by severe hair loss. In a randomized, double-blind, controlled trial of seven months' duration, researchers treated forty-three alopecia areata patients with a daily scalp massage of essential oils of thyme, rosemary, lavender, and cedarwood in carrier oils. The control group unknowingly used only the carrier oils for their daily scalp massage. Three times as many patients in the active group showed improvement in their hair growth compared with the control group.

HOW AROMATHERAPY WORKS

Aromatherapy works because of the pharmacological properties of essential oils, as well as their small molecular size. When small aromatic molecules enter a person's nasal cavity, they easily penetrate body tissues. They are rapidly changed by various biological processes before traveling to the limbic system of the brain. This is the "emotional switchboard" of the brain, where these inhaled molecules create impressions associated with past experiences and emotions. The limbic system is directly connected to the parts of the brain that control such basic metabolic elements as heart rate, blood pressure, breathing, memory, stress levels, and hormone balance.

Thus, essential oils may provide one of the fastest ways to achieve medicinal or psychological effects.

Leading scientific researchers have found that calming oils, such as orange, jasmine, and rose, change the brain waves into a rhythm that produces a sense of well-being. Similarly, the stimulating oils of basil, black pepper, rosemary, and cardamom work by inducing a change in the rhythm of the brain waves to produce an increased energy response. Even scents too subtle to be consciously detected can significantly affect central nervous system activity and a person's responses.

A word of caution to keep in mind when purchasing essential oils: As many oils have been diluted to create fragrances and to process food, it is best to ensure that you are getting truly pure essential oils by purchasing from a supplier who specializes in essential aromatherapy oils. Cheaper formulations are often impure. Pure essential oils are expensive because it can take as much as 1,000 pounds of raw plant material to make a single pound of pure essence. However, just a few drops will go far, making aromatherapy very cost-effective in the long run.

HOW AROMATHERAPY IS USED

Aromatherapy is ideal for use at home, as long as you avoid excessive or direct topical use of potentially irritating or allergenic oils, such as clove, cinnamon, oregano, and savory. Essential oils can be inhaled, applied to the skin, or, in rare cases (and under the supervision of a specialist), ingested.

Diffusers

Diffusers are devices designed to disperse microparticles of essential oil into the air. They are ideal to charge the air with the mood-lifting or calming qualities of an oil. There are different types of diffusers. Many operate on electricity. Others utilize heat from a candle or lamp. To use a diffuser, simply follow the manufacturer's directions.

External or Topical Application

Oils are very easily absorbed through the skin, and therefore are an ideal addition to baths, and massage oils. Used in this manner, they can act to stimulate or calm the individual and his or her skin. Essential oils can also be used in compresses to soothe, reduce swelling, and help to prevent infection. Topical application of a diluted solution is an easy, effective alternative for many skin conditions. Remember, most essential oils should *not* be applied directly to the skin. They should be diluted in water or a carrier oil first. (See Part Three for more information about preparing aromatherapy treatments.)

Floral Waters

Floral waters, made by adding a drop or two of essential oil to distilled water, can be sprayed into the air or onto sensitive skin to create a therapeutic effect.

Ingestion

Essential oils are highly concentrated. They are very strong compounds, and many are potentially toxic if swallowed. Because of this, essential oils are *rarely* ingested. When they are, this must be done under proper medical guidance only. It is imperative that you *do not* attempt this on your own.

ESSENTIAL OILS IMPORTANT IN DERMATOLOGY

Chamomile (Roman)

Chamomile can be recognized by its apple-like scent. It heals the skin by reducing swelling and inflammation, and by fighting infection. Studies have shown that it reduces dryness, itching, redness, and sensitivity in irritated and inflamed skin. It is also calming and uplifting, and is a sleeping aid.

Everlasting

Everlasting has tissue-regenerating properties that are useful in the treatment of scars. It is also a strong anti-inflammatory agent and can prevent swelling and bleeding with bruises. It should be used topically only in concentrations of 2 percent or less.

Eucalyptus

Eucalyptus has a fresh, camphor-like scent. It is commonly used to regulate overproductive sebaceous (oil) glands, to cool and prevent sweat evaporation in acne, and to control body odor. It also decreases inflammation, disinfects, and fights bacterial, viral, and fungal infections. It is a common insect repellent. It can also be diffused in the air or rubbed on the wrists and temples to effect an immediate relaxation response, to energize, and to increase mental clarity.

In large amounts, eucalyptus can be toxic, so take care not to use too much. Eucalyptus oil can also irritate sensitive skin, so don't apply it to your skin unless it has been greatly diluted.

Geranium

Geranium has a green, sweet scent that is sometimes rosy, sometimes minty. It has antifungal and antiviral properties and fights infection. It stops the bleeding of cuts and wounds, and stimulates both the lymphatic and circulatory systems, promoting the elimination of wastes. Geranium also stimulates new skin-cell growth and it tones and tightens skin tissue, imparting a healthy glow. It simultaneously calms and energizes. You should avoid it if you have low blood sugar, however, as it can lower blood sugar levels.

Lavender

Lavender is one of the most popular essential oils used in aromatherapy, and has a fresh fragrance. It is a very helpful aid for rapid healing, and is soothing if applied directly on acne, burns, small wounds, and insect bites. It stimulates new cell growth, fights infection, and reduces inflammation. Lavender also balances oil production of the skin and scalp and helps repair damaged hair.

Added to the bath or sprayed on the bed sheets, lavender reduces tension and helps one to relax. If you have low blood pressure, take care using it in the bath, as lavender oil lowers blood pressure.

Myrrh

Sweet, spicy-smelling myrrh oil encourages new cell growth and reportedly prevents and treats wrinkles. It soothes and softens rough, cracked, or chapped skin. Myrrh reduces inflammation, fights bacterial and fungal infections, and helps wounds to heal. It also improves skin circulation, thereby improving the complexion. Myrrh oil should not be used during pregnancy, as it stimulates menstrual flow.

Neroli

Neroli oil, which is derived from bitter orange tree blossoms and has a somewhat sharp, citrusy fragrance, has rejuvenating properties for the skin, increasing local circulation and stimulating new cell growth. It is also used to prevent stretch marks and minimize other scars. Neroli is useful for treating skin conditions that are linked to stress, such as psoriasis and eczema, as it calms the emotions as well as soothing dry, irritated, and sensitive skin.

Tea Tree

Tea tree oil is derived from a tree, *Melaleuca alternifolia,* that is native to Australia. In addition to its distinctive pungent aroma, it has antibacterial, antiviral, and antifungal properties, so it is useful in healing wounds, acne, rashes, and warts. It also kills insects and is a good bug repellent. Caution must be taken in using tea tree oil, however, as it may be irritating if applied directly to sensitive skin.

POSSIBLE SIDE EFFECTS OF ESSENTIAL OILS

Some pure essential oils cannot be applied directly to the skin, as they are too irritating to the skin. These oils must first be diluted with a carrier oil, such as almond, coconut, olive, or sesame oil. These strong oils include basil, cinnamon, lemon, lemongrass, peppermint, and thyme essential oils. About 5 percent of the population will get an allergic dermatitis reaction if clove or cinnamon oil is applied to the skin. Recently, there was also a clinical case report of allergic airborne contact dermatitis from the essential oils of lavender, jasmine, rosewood, laurel, eucalyptus, and pomerance used in aromatherapy. With the increasing use of aromatherapy, we might expect an increasing number of such reports. If you will be using essential oils on your skin, always apply just a drop of *diluted* oil and allow it to dry, to be sure that you won't have an allergic or irritant reaction when applying it to larger areas.

In addition, applying essential oils of angelica, bergamot, cumin, lemon, lime, orange, tangerine, or verbena on areas of skin that will be exposed to sunlight is not recommended. These oils heighten the skin's sensitivity to the sun and a photodermatitis, or sunburn-like reaction, may result on exposed areas.

Some essential oils are potentially toxic to a developing fetus, so they should be *avoided* during pregnancy. These include essential oils of basil, clary sage, hyssop, juniper, marjoram, myrrh, and sage.

Homeopathy

Homeopathy is a system of healing that uses remedies consisting of highly diluted extracts of natural substances, including plants, minerals, and animals. The remedies are designed to stimulate the body's natural healing response, and are specifically matched to different symptom patterns, or profiles, of illness unique to each individual. Interest in homeopathy has been increasing in America, on the part of both medical doctors and the public. This is due in part to its low cost and virtually nonexistent risk of unwanted side effects, and because it is a system of medicine already used by more than 500 million people worldwide. Homeopathy is particularly effective for treating chronic illnesses and for self-care of minor conditions, including skin eruptions, but can also be helpful for acute problems and as a preventive measure. So let's take a look at the fundamentals of homeopathy, its history, and the homeopathic remedies that have been found to be most helpful for skin problems.

AN INTRODUCTION TO HOMEOPATHY

In the late 1700s, Dr. Samuel Hahnemann, a German physician, proposed the principles of homeopathy, which have held to this day:

1. The Law of Similars. Often abbreviated as "like cures like," this principle was based on Hahnemann's discovery that a substance that causes certain symptoms when taken in large doses by a healthy person can cure those same symptoms when taken in minute, dilute doses.
2. The Law of Infinitesimals (or Law of Potentiation). Simply, the more a remedy is diluted, the greater its potency.
3. The holistic medical model. Each person's experience of illness is unique, so the appropriate therapy needs to be determined by the person and his or her symptom pattern, not by the disease.

Actually, the Law of Similars was known among Ayurvedic physicians 2,000 years before Hahnemann did his work, and it was rediscovered by Hippocrates in the fourth century BC while he was studying the medicinal effects of herbs. In another form, the Law of Similars forms the theoretical basis for the development of vaccines by Edward Jenner, Louis Pasteur, Jonas Salk, and others, which are in use worldwide today. Our bodies are immunized by the administration of trace amounts of a disease component, usually a virus, to induce the body to develop an immune response to the actual disease. Conventional medicine treats allergies in a similar manner, by injecting minute quantities of a suspected allergen to increase a person's natural tolerance to that allergen.

In conventional pharmaceutical chemistry, the higher the dose of the chemical, the greater the effect. In homeopathy, the opposite is true: The more dilute a substance is, the higher its potency, the greater its effect on the body's vital force, and the greater the medicinal effect. It is also thought that the high dilution of the active ingredients minimizes the risk of dangerous or bothersome side effects.

Homeopathic remedies are prepared through a process of diluting the material with pure water or alcohol and *succussing,* or shaking it vigorously. Potency depends on how many times a remedy has been succussed. Any solution diluted to 1-in-10 strength and succussed more than twenty-four times (which would give it a potency designated as 24x or higher) will have no chemical trace of the original substance remaining. Yet these remedies are the most potent. This is explained by the laws of quantum physics and the growing field of energy medicine. Some researchers believe that the specific electromagnetic frequency of the active ingredient is imprinted in the homeopathic remedy during the process of successive dilution and succussion. The distinguished Italian physicist Emilio del Giudice proposed that water molecules form structures capable of storing minute electromagnetic signals. According to this theory, a homeopathic treatment conveys an electronic "message" to the patient's body. This matches the specific electromagnetic frequency of the illness unique to that person, and stimulates his or her body's natural healing response. What Dr. Hahnemann may have been doing in his research was unknowingly matching the frequencies of the extract with the frequency or pattern of the patient's illness.

Recent research confirms these theories. Dr. Wolfgang Ludwig, a German biophysicist, has shown that homeopathic remedies give off measurable electromagnetic signals, with specific frequencies dominant in each different homeopathic substance. A separate study using nuclear magnetic resonance (NMR) imaging showed distinctive readings of subatomic activity in twenty-three different homeopathic remedies, while no readings of any subatomic activity were demonstrated in any of the placebos. With the recent surge of interest in quantum physics and energy medicine, this is very exciting news indeed.

Dr. Hahnemann's third principle of homeopathy is that an illness is specific to the individual, based on the mental, emotional, and physical aspects of the patient's symptoms and personality. For example, there may be a hundred symptom patterns associated with one general complaint such as itching, and there is a corresponding unique remedy for each specific type of itching. Therefore, the homeopathic practitioner must first go through a process called profiling, or recording all of the physical, mental, and emotional characteristics of the patient's current state, which will determine the remedy to be used. Next, the homeopath consults vast books (or, today, computer programs) called repertories that contain compilations of the findings of thousands of tests done over the past 200 years that record how healthy individuals react to different substances. This helps him or her to determine the remedy that most closely matches the total picture of the patient's specific constellation of symptoms.

Homeopathy is thought not only to alleviate identifiable symptoms, but also to reestablish the body's internal order at the deepest levels. Like other illnesses, some skin diseases are felt to be manifestations of internal or constitutional disorders. Dr. Constantine Hering, the nineteenth-century father of American homeopathy, felt that the homeopathic healing process began with the emotional and mental aspects of the illness and then moved to the physical manifestations. He also postulated that the healing process began at the deepest levels of the body and moved to the extremities, and that healing progressed from the upper to the lower body. Hering's Laws of Cure also include the premise that healing progresses from the most recent disorders to the oldest, in reverse chronological order. Thus, in homeopathy, the process of getting better begins by eliminating the immediate symptoms, then moving on to the older, deeper layers of underlying symptoms and emotions. Many of these deeper layers of symptoms are thought to be residues of fevers, emotional or physical trauma, and chronic diseases that were suppressed or treated unsuccessfully by conventional therapy or the patient him- or herself. A "healing crisis"—a situation in which the patient gets worse before he or she gets better—often occurs as the deeper stages of homeopathic healing are reached, and many underlying emotions and pains are reexperienced. However, once these conditions are treated, it is felt the person will be more thoroughly cured.

Homeopathic remedies include single-ingredient and combination remedies. Single-ingredient remedies are generally named after the scientific Latin term for the original source ingredient. Combination homeopathic formulas contain a mixture of several remedies to cover a large number of different symptoms for an acute problem. Single and combination remedies look the same, as all are available in small tablets or pellets, or are combined to make tinctures, lotions, or ointments for external application. The body is thought to use what parts of the remedies it needs and eliminate the other parts, which reportedly have little negative effect.

HISTORY OF HOMEOPATHY

In the late 1700s, Dr. Hahnemann had become frustrated by the ineffective and harmful practices of bloodletting and blistering then used for the treatment of many diseases. He experimented by taking cinchona, a Peruvian bark known as a cure for malaria, and found that he quickly developed the periodic fevers symptomatic of malaria. Hahnemann then theorized that if taking a large dose of cinchona created symptoms of malaria in a healthy person such as himself, then maybe this same substance, taken in a smaller dose by a person with malaria, might stimulate the patient's body to fight the disease. In other words, he felt the symptoms were not the illness, but part of the body's defensive effort to eliminate the underlying disease. The homeopathic medicine would make it easier for the body to recognize the underlying illness and mobilize its defenses against the disease. Hahnemann's theory was also based on his belief in the presence of a vital force in the body, the underlying life force that animates the body. He proved his treatment theory correct over years of experimentation with hundreds of homeopathic substances. In the 200 years since Hahnemann, other researchers have added more than 3,000 additional homeopathic remedies to his arsenal.

Homeopathy actually has a long history in the United States. It was popular here in the mid-1800s and early 1900s. Dr. Constantine Hering, a student of Hahnemann, brought the practice of homeopathy to the United States. Hering started the first homeopathic medical school in America in 1835, in Allentown, Pennsylvania. Homeopathy became popular so quickly that the first national medical association, the American Institute of Homeopathy, was formed nine years later, in 1844.

Just three short years later, however, the American Medical Association (AMA) was formed, and denounced homeopathy as a delusion. AMA members were not to associate with homeopathic doctors either professionally or socially, and a deep schism arose between practitioners of the two approaches to healing.

Despite this rivalry, homeopathy still thrived in America during the second half of the nineteenth century, due in part to its success in treating cholera and yellow fever. It was widely followed, with John D. Rockefeller, Thomas Edison, and Samuel Clemens (Mark Twain) among homeopathy's best known adherents. Indeed, 15 percent of all American physicians were practicing homeopathy by 1900, and there were twenty-two homeopathic medical schools and almost one hundred homeopathic hospitals in the United States. At the same time, however, the AMA and the pharmaceutical companies formed a strong financial and ideological bond, and the practice of homeopathy had nearly disappeared as a force in American medicine by 1930. From the 1930s until recently, there were no homeopathic hospitals and only two homeopathic medical schools in the United States.

HOMEOPATHY TODAY

Homeopathy is experiencing a resurgence of popularity in America, and is being recognized by many as a beneficial alternative approach to medicine. This is demonstrated by current sales of homeopathic medicines of approximately $150 million a year in the United States.

In a recent article published in the *British Medical Journal,* more than 100 controlled clinical studies relating to homeopathy performed between 1966 and 1990 were reviewed. In over 75 percent of the cases, homeopathic therapies were found to be beneficial in treating a wide range of health conditions. Similarly, in a 1997 article published in the prestigious medical journal *The Lancet,* U.S. and German researchers reviewed data from 89 independent studies comparing homeopathic treatments with placebos. A review of all these studies showed that homeopathic remedies were almost two and a half times as likely to have a positive effect on the underlying illnesses as were the placebos. Homeopathy was also found to be more effective than placebos, although to a lesser degree, when the 26 best designed studies were analyzed.

Approximately 3,000 health-care providers in the United States currently practice homeopathy. The U.S. Food and Drug Administration (FDA) recognizes homeopathic remedies as drugs and regulates their manufacturing, labeling, and dispensing. Official acceptance and integration of low-cost homeopathic treatments into the American health care system could have a huge impact on lowering the national cost of health care.

Homeopathy continues to be popular in Europe. In Britain, homeopathic hospitals and outpatient clinics are already part of the national health system, and Parliament has declared homeopathy a postgraduate medical specialty. In Germany, there are about 6,000 practitioners; in France, about 5,000. All French pharmacies must carry homeopathic remedies along with conventional drugs, and more than 17 million French people see only homeopathic physicians for all of their medical needs.

Homeopathy is also widely practiced today in India, Mexico, Argentina, and Brazil. In all, an estimated 500 million people worldwide now routinely receive homeopathic treatment, and the World Health Organization has stated that homeopathy should be integrated with conventional medicine to provide better health care around the globe.

HOMEOPATHIC REMEDIES COMMONLY USED FOR SKIN PROBLEMS

Apis mellifica

Prepared from whole honeybees or bee venom, *Apis mellifica* (or, simply, *Apis*) is effective for the relief of sting-type symptoms characterized by rapidly forming red swellings that burn. It is used to treat insect bites and stings, hives, early stages of boils, frostbite, minor burns, and sunburns.

Arnica

Made from the whole fresh arnica plant, *Arnica* is important in the relief of bruising, swelling, and local tenderness after sprains or muscle injury. Externally, it should be applied only to unbroken skin. Homeopathically diluted arnica tablets are safe to take internally, unlike the more concentrated herbal preparations of arnica, which should only be applied topically to the skin. Do not confuse the homeopathic remedy with its herbal counterpart.

Calendula

Made from the whole calendula (pot marigold) plant, *Calendula* is important for the treatment of minor cuts, sunburns, and other minor skin irritations. Homeopathic calendula is usually used topically in the form of ointments, tinctures, oils, and soaps. However, it is also available in pellet and tablet form for internal use to help heal sunburns and scrapes.

Graphites

Graphite is a form of carbon, and the main ingredient in pencil "lead." Hahnemann discovered the graphite remedy after learning that workmen in a mirror factory were applying graphite to heal cold sores.

Graphites (the plural is used to designate the remedy) is used to treat skin complaints felt to be caused in part by an underlying metabolic imbalance. This includes weeping atopic eczema; psoriasis; thick, cracked, and misshapen nails; and hair loss. *Graphites* is also used in the treatment of keloids, hypertrophic (abnormally large or prominent) scars, and cold sores.

Graphites is one of the remedies associated with a personality type. *Graphites* types are thought to be anxious, timid, indecisive, and pessimistic. They are slow to react to external stimuli, and have low stamina. Plump, pale people with rough, dry, cracking skin are considered characteristic of the type.

Ledum

Prepared from the leaves and twigs of wild rosemary, *Ledum* is used in homeopathic dilutions to treat cold, numbing injuries or injuries that are relieved by cold. Puncture wounds, bites from mosquitoes or small animals, and persistent bruises are frequently treated with *Ledum*. This small evergreen shrub is very toxic, and thus is not used in herbal remedies, but only in very dilute homeopathic formulations.

Pulsatilla

Made from the poisonous pasqueflower, *Anemone patens, Pulsatilla's* medical applications were discovered by Hahnemann in 1805. It is often used for skin eruptions, especially for people who are sensitive and prone to crying.

Rhus toxicodendron

Derived from the leaves of the poison ivy plant, homeopathic dilutions of this remedy are used for red, swollen skin conditions, such as poison ivy, rashes, hives, and burns. It may sound strange to think of taking a remedy made from poison ivy, but remember the homeopathic Law of Similars—"like cures like." In homeopathic doses, this remedy is appropriate for conditions causing symptoms similar to those caused by exposure to the poison ivy plant.

Ruta graveolens

Ruta graveolens (or, simply, *Ruta*), made from flowering rue, is useful for bruised kneecaps and elbows. It is also good for any other injury that involves the periosteum, the tough connective tissue that covers the outside of the bones.

Urtica urens

Prepared from flowering stinging nettle, *Urtica urens* is a useful first-aid remedy for bites, stings, burns, hives, prickly heat, and other conditions that cause red, rashlike welts. It can be used topically or taken internally to help lessen the symptoms of these conditions.

Acupuncture and Acupressure

Acupuncture is part of traditional Oriental medicine, rooted in ancient China and mentioned as far back as 2697 BC in the *Huang-ti Nei-Ching,* or "The Yellow Emperor's Classic of Internal Medicine." Acupuncture is based on the Chinese belief that the flow of *chi*, or *qi,* the vital life energy thought to be present in all living things, needs to be balanced for good health. The opposing *yin* and *yang* forces within the body must be in balance, according to the Chinese view, before *chi* can get our spiritual, mental, emotional, and physical aspects to function normally. Acupuncture and acupressure are methods used to balance the *chi* within the body.

AN INTRODUCTION TO ACUPUNCTURE AND ACUPRESSURE

Chi is thought to circulate in the body along fourteen pathways, or meridians. Twelve of these pathways cross the trunk, limbs, and head in various directions, and go deep into the tissues. These twelve meridians are actually six pairs of meridians, because there are corresponding meridians on both sides of the body. The other two pathways go up the front and back. Each meridian is linked to specific organs and to each of the others. The energy flows continuously along one meridian and going into another in a clock-like cycle. An organ's normal functioning is dependent upon a normal energy level in its associated meridian. The meridians surface at various locations in the body. The spots where they do are acupuncture points (or acupoints) that can be stimulated to enhance the flow of *chi*. It is thought that there are more than 360, and perhaps as many as 1,000 acupuncture points.

Illness, according to this system, is a result of the failure of *chi* to flow properly. Blockages in the energy flow through a meridian can be due to injury, stress, poor nutrition and other poor health habits, exposure to toxins, infection, and various diseases. Energy blockage and imbalance between *yin* and *yang* affect not only the directly involved pathway, but also the interconnecting meridians and the organ systems they in turn serve. When special needles, finger pressure, applications of heat, or electrical or laser stimulation is applied to various combinations of the acupoints just under the skin, the flow of energy can be rebalanced and pain relieved or health improved.

According to traditional Chinese medicine (TCM), there are twelve skin regions. In each region, one of the twelve regular meridians and its branches are distributed. These meridians connect internally with organs and externally with the trunk, arms, and legs. TCM teaches that the location of skin lesions reflects problems within the associated meridians, which need to be balanced to treat the skin disorders and the body as a whole.

HISTORY OF ACUPUNCTURE

The practice of acupuncture has remained virtually unchanged since the time of the Yellow Emperor, almost 5,000 years ago. *The Huang-ti Nei-Ching* is still used today as one of the main references on acupuncture theory.

Acupuncture was introduced into the United States by Chinese immigrants in the mid-1800s, but it became widely known as a direct result of President Richard Nixon's trip to China in 1972. While in China, James Reston, President Nixon's press secretary, required an appendectomy, which to the amazement of the West was performed with acupuncture for anesthesia and postsurgical pain relief. By the end of the 1970s, acupuncture schools and practitioners had sprung up throughout the United States.

ACUPUNCTURE AND ACUPRESSURE TODAY

The World Health Organization recognizes acupuncture as a valid treatment modality and lists 104 different conditions that acupuncture can treat successfully. It is often used in conjunction with herbal remedies and recommendations for lifestyle changes.

There are about 3,000 physicians who practice acupuncture in the United States, up from only about 500 ten years ago. Twenty-one states limit acupuncture practice to medical doctors and chiropractors, while the others allow nonphysicians who finish a training course and pass a certifying exam to practice acupuncture. The skill of different practitioners varies considerably, so if at first the treatment doesn't work, you may consider trying another therapist before giving up on the treatment altogether.

Acupuncture is most commonly used for pain relief and surgical anesthesia, to treat stroke and addiction problems, and to improve immune function in people with HIV/AIDS, but it can also aid many dermatologic problems. It has been used successfully in dermatology to ease the pain of shingles, to tone down flare-ups of psoriasis or eczema, and to treat acne, boils, facial pigmentary changes, hair loss, herpes, hives, neurodermatitis, rosacea, skin ulcers, vitiligo, warts, and wrinkles. The future of acupuncture in the West looks very promising, as the practice provides benefits for quite a few disorders with very little risk and only very rare complications. At least eighty private insurance companies and state Medicaid programs now reimburse practitioners and patients for acupuncture treatments.

ACUPUNCTURE AND ACUPRESSURE FOR SKIN DISORDERS

In traditional Chinese medicine, states of ill health can broadly be classified as due to an excess or a deficiency of *chi* in one or more parts of the body. (Of course, an excess or deficiency anywhere eventually affects the entire body.) The pattern of onset of the disease and its signs and symptoms are important in determining the underlying causes. In addition, practitioners of TCM often use terms to describe illness that reflect a long cultural history of living in accordance with the laws and elements of nature. Thus, acute skin problems are often described as syndromes of excess caused by pathogenic wind, dampness, heat, and toxins associated with malfunction of the heart, lung, and spleen. It is believed that if the disease is to be resolved or improved, acupuncture to reduce these excesses is required. Chronic skin problems, on the other hand, are thought to be deficiency syndromes requiring reinforcing manipulation or mild stimulation with acupuncture, as well as ear needling. Insufficiency of blood flow in the skin is associated with pathogenic wind, and dryness is associated with liver and kidney deficiencies.

Skin diseases on the face are related to wind and heat—the accumulation of phlegm in the internal organs, and heat in the lungs and stomach. It is thought that selecting acupoints along the channels that pass through the face, as well as reaction points on the ears, will filter *chi* and the blood, and regulate the functioning of the internal organs.

The location and features of the skin lesions are thought to indicate either wind, fire, dampness, or stasis of *chi* or blood as the cause or causes of a disorder.

A practitioner of TCM takes into consideration the state of the whole body, as evidenced by changes in the tongue and pulse when making a diagnosis, and formulating his or her acupuncture treatment plan accordingly. Traditionally, the practitioner uses the patient's wrist to diagnose and test the eighteen radial pulses known to the Chinese. He or she feels for nine pulses on each side—three deep, three intermediate, and three superficial—and can use more than twenty-seven different characteristics to describe each pulse. More recently, a system of electrically evaluating the energy level of each meridian by measuring the conductance of each meridian's source point has been used as a reproducible method of making an acupuncture diagnosis. This method of diagnosis is known as Ryodoraku. Whichever way the diagnosis is made, the information obtained by the practitioner is supposed to show the status of the patient's *chi* and explain the patient's symptoms.

Western scientists believe that acupuncture works by stimulating the release of natural opiates called endorphins in the brain. There is thought to be neurochemical transmission of impulses at the acupuncture sites, separate from the vascular or lymphatic channels. Endorphins reduce a person's perception of pain much as a narcotic would. Westerners back up their explanation for acupuncture's effect with the experimental evidence that when animals are given a chemical that blocks endorphins, the animals don't respond to acupuncture.

After the diagnosis is made, specific needles are inserted in not more than twelve of the thousand acupoints on the body. Usually, the more skillful the acupuncturist, the smaller the number of needles he or she will have to use. Needles are usually hair-thin, made of stainless steel or copper, and only a slight pricking sensation should be felt when they are placed, usually about one-quarter inch deep into the skin. Needles are generally left in for twenty to thirty minutes, but treatments may last as little as seconds or as long as forty-five minutes. The effectiveness of acupuncture is related to the intensity of the needling sensation and its propagation along the channels. Most people are helped significantly with twelve to fifteen treatments. Side effects are possible, but very rare.

Ear acupuncture, or auriculotherapy, was developed in the 1950s by Dr. Paul Nogier, a French physician. He noted that several of his patients had tiny scars on their outer ears from electrical stimulation done by a local healer as a successful treatment for back pain. Dr. Nogier found that specific points on the outer ear, when stimulated, could affect other areas of the body. He discovered thirty basic auricular (ear) points that neurologically affected specific layers of the body and presented this research at the Munich Acupuncture Convention. His findings were confirmed by studies in China and Japan, and detailed Chinese ear acupuncture charts were devised. In 1989, auriculotherapy was recognized by the World Health Organization as a useful medical therapy. Like acupuncture involving other parts of the body, auriculotherapy is done through the use of acupuncture needles and staples, ear massage, or electrical or infrared stimulation. During ear acupuncture, the outer ear often becomes red and develops a burning feeling that may last for up to forty-five minutes after the needles are taken out. This is a sign of the effectiveness of the treatment. In the United States, auriculotherapy is currently used primarily for pain and addiction control, but its use can certainly be expected to expand in the future, perhaps for skin problems as well.

Additional forms of treatment can be applied to the acupoints with or without the needles. Some practitioners apply finger or hand pressure to the acupoints. This form, known as *shiatsu*, has been particularly popular in Japan for more than 5,000 years, and has been officially authorized there by the Japanese Ministry of Health and Welfare. Dr. Palle Rosted, a highly trained consultant in acupuncture at the Weston Park Hospital in England, described in a 1992 article in the *American Journal of Acupuncture* how he successfully uses laser treatment on acupuncture sites in very young children, in older adults, and in people of any age who are very afraid of needles.

Skin disorders that flare up in response to stress, anxiety, or fatigue respond best to acupressure, as it is thought to work by relaxing muscular tension and increasing circulation. Most dermatology treatments combine the use of local, trigger, and tonic acupoints. Pressure on local points increases circulation in the area of a skin eruption. Trigger points are used to stimulate the organs and glands controlling skin functions, which are thought to be the lungs, large intestine, liver, and stomach. Tonic points are used for whole-body rejuvenation, to fortify the immune system, to help with coping mechanisms for stress, and to increase emotional stability. Potent bilateral points for relieving skin disorders have such poetic names as *Sea of Vitality*, located at the back of the waist, three finger-widths away from the spine on each side; *Three-Mile Point*, found four finger-widths below each kneecap toward the outside of the shin, *Heavenly Pillar,* one-half inch below the base of the skull and one-half inch out from either side of the spine; and *Four Whites, Facial Beauty, Wind Screen, Heavenly Appearance,* and *Third Eye Point,* all of which are located on the face and head. Acne, eczema, hives, and poor complexion are said to be improved by applying acupressure to various combinations of these points.

Finally, an herb called *moxa* can be burned just above the point being treated to stimulate the acupoint and speed healing. This process is called *moxibustion.* Moxibustion is used mainly in the treatment of chronic eczema, neurodermatitis, and warts. Electrostimulation, other forms of heat, ultrasound waves, and laser beams can also be applied instead of needles to the acupuncture points.

POSSIBLE SIDE EFFECTS OF ACUPUNCTURE AND ACUPRESSURE

In general, undesirable side effects from acupuncture are rare, but some have been reported. Occasionally, a patient may feel lightheaded, nauseated, or even faint. Other adverse side effects, including abscesses, hepatitis-B infection, infection in the cartilage of the ear, blood or air in the lung cavity, and allergic reactions to the metal in the needles, have been reported, but so rarely that they have been written up as isolated case reports in the professional literature.

Other Skin Therapies

Today, stress is being blamed as a factor in the development of many emotional, mental, and physical problems. The skin is not immune to the effects of stress; in fact, signs of stress often show up first on our most visible organ, the skin. Thus, it is becoming increasingly important to integrate stress reduction measures, relaxation therapy, and meditation into our everyday life. Also, with the recent general acceptance of the fact that one's thoughts and feelings do affect one's physical health, the field of mind-body medicine has grown in influence. If you have skin problems, especially chronic ones, you may get tremendous physical benefit from doing your own emotional work, and from the use of cognitive-behavioral techniques, spirituality, prayer, hypnosis, and biofeedback. Let's take a look at these important ways in which we can increase our emotional health as well as our skin's physical health.

STRESS REDUCTION

Stress is the culprit in triggering or causing flare-ups of more and more diseases in our modern world. Skin diseases and problems are no exception. In fact, skin problems often are the most obvious indication that a person is suffering from too much stress.

Reducing stress in our lives not only can improve our quality of life, but also helps to speed recovery from many dermatologic problems. Many people are now learning relaxation techniques, meditation, and yoga, and have benefited from the myriad of good effects these techniques provide.

Take psoriasis as an example. In 1977, British researcher R.H. Seville reported that 44 percent of the 132 patients he studied had had a specific incidence of stress within one month before their first episode of psoriasis began. Drs. W. Susskind and R.J. McGuire found that stress was associated with the first onset of psoriasis in 40 percent of the group of twenty patients they studied. They also found that relapses were associated with stress in 70 percent of their study group of psoriasis patients. Dr. Capore and others recently reported in the *Postgraduate Medical Journal* that forty-four of their sixty-four British patients with chronic skin problems such as psoriasis and eczema had experienced a major life problem such as a severe illness or the death of a loved one just before, or at the same time that, their skin problems began. They found that talking about the stressful event helped the subjects' chronic skin conditions. Therefore, since anxiety and stress cause flare-ups of most skin conditions, learning stress reduction techniques is very important in helping to ease dermatologic problems.

RELAXATION THERAPY

Relaxation and meditation have been successful in aiding a number of medical conditions, especially those that have a great tendency to flare up with anxiety, are painful, or are directly related to an altered immune status. When the fight-or-flight adrenaline response is triggered too often in reaction to everyday real or perceived stresses or internalized emotions, the body's systems, including the immune system, are taxed, and health suffers. The goal of relaxation training in dermatology is to lessen the anxiety that can cause or worsen skin problems, to increase tolerance to pain and itching, and to divert attention away from the distressing skin symptoms.

Most relaxation techniques use progressive relaxation training (PRT), or the relaxation response. In PRT, you first learn to tense and relax your muscles, which are divided into seven groups for the purpose of these exercises. Next, you learn to tense and relax muscles in four groups at a time. Finally, you learn to tense and then let go of tension in all of the muscles of the body simultaneously, so that you fully relax.

Drs. A.D. Domar, J.M. Noe, and H. Benson, working in the Division of Behavioral Medicine at Beth Israel Hospital, Boston, reported in 1987 their experience with twenty-one control-matched skin-cancer patients in whom the relaxation response was practiced for twenty minutes a day from the time that they were told that they needed skin-cancer surgery to the day of the outpatient surgery. The control patients read for twenty minutes a day instead of performing the relaxation response. Neither group showed any increase in anxiety immediately before or after surgery on objective psychological or physiological measures. However, there were statistically significant subjective differences in that the relaxation-response group reported feeling their highest levels of anxiety prior to starting to practice the relaxation response, when they first found out about the proposed surgery. This differed from the control patients who read instead of practicing the relaxation response. They reported feeling most anxious during and after their surgery, not when they first found out about their need for skin cancer surgery. Therefore, Domar concluded that regular practice of the relaxation response can subjectively change the amount of distress a patient perceives when undergoing minor surgery for skin cancer. Relaxation methods have also been reported to significantly improve the symptoms of atopic dermatitis.

In 1994, S.C. Putt and colleagues at the Department of Psychology and Human Ecology at Cameron University reported excellent results of behavior modification (including monetary reward, relaxation procedures, and hair massage) in a young man with a five-year history of alopecia areata, a common autoimmune cause of hair loss thought to have both physiological and psychological causes. Putt's group compared seven months without treatment with seven months of treatment. Hair loss was greatly decreased after the first three months of massage, relaxation, and reward therapies, and there was actually new hair growth on the patient's scalp during the last four months of the study.

Although relaxation training has been criticized because the manner in which it affects skin disorders is not clearly understood and because controlled studies have not been done, it does offer promise for treating the symptoms of a large variety of dermatologic problems.

MEDITATION

Although meditation has been practiced for thousands of years, only recently have researchers proved that a person is able to achieve some voluntary control over his or her autonomic nervous system (the part of the nervous system responsible for such "involuntary" functions as breathing, circulation, and digestion) through meditation. It is through the autonomic nervous system that stress and perceived pain are reduced and health is improved with various forms of meditation. Meditation can also be a very useful aid to enhancing immunity, especially for people who have autoimmune diseases such as lupus.

More than 6,000 physicians in the United States recommend meditation to decrease anxiety and increase emotional stability, adaptability, an internal sense of control, and a sense of one's true self. All of these personal characteristics influence the health of your skin. Well-known proponents of meditation include Dr. Herbert Benson, Dr. Dean Ornish, and Dr. Joan Borysenko. Indeed, 80 percent of conventional medical doctors at a 1999 meeting of the American Association of Health Plans said they thought that meditation needs to be a standard part of medical training.

MIND-BODY MEDICINE

Mental health and physical health are intimately connected. One's thoughts, feelings, emotions, and expectations can have a huge effect on one's health. This is particularly true in the field of dermatology. The traditional medical establishment is now addressing this in increasing depth. Drs. M.R. Bilkis and K.A. Mark of the New York University Medical Center recently published suggestions for practical applications of mind-body medicine in dermatology in the American Medical Association's *Archives of Dermatology*. They presented for their audience of dermatologists practical methods for utilizing meditation, journal writing, affirmations, prayer, biofeedback, and hypnosis.

As an important interface between the internal and external, the skin responds to both internal and external stimuli, both sensing and integrating environmental cues and relaying internal conditions to the outside. We now understand the biochemical basis for this close relationship between the mind and the skin a little better. In the 1970s, the field of *psychoneuroimmunology* (PNI) emerged and scientifically verified the mind-body interrelationship. Researchers found that natural compounds in the body called neurochemicals normally secreted during different emotional states can cause changes in mood or feelings of pain or pleasure. Endorphins were among the first of these substances to be described. They are found in and affect the brain, the immune system, the endocrine system, the skin, and other areas of the body. Scientists have also discovered that the immune system too has the capacity to learn and remember, as the central nervous system does. Thus, intelligence is found in every cell of the body. In an article in the November 1998 issue of *Archives of Dermatology,* Dr. Sullivan and others did a review of what has been described as the neuro-immuno-cutaneous-endocrine (NICE) phenomena—in other words, the link between mental and skin health.

Mind-body medicine goes beyond PNI to encompass the view that energy is the underlying pattern of the universe. This is similar to Ayurvedic and traditional Chinese medicine philosophies, which view people as part of an interconnected universal energy field. Mind-body medicine recognizes that because each person is biochemically unique, the same disease can result from different causes in different people. Thus, individual paths to recovery may be different even if people have the same disease. A physical illness may start as an imbalance in one of the many interrelated parts of the self, such as a person's genetics, social support, diet, exercise, mental or emotional attitudes, lifestyle, or spirituality. Conversely, as a person makes a positive change and heals in one area, other areas of his or her life tend to improve as well.

In mind-body medicine, illness is seen as a message from the body that some aspects of a person's life are out of balance and need to be reexamined. It is seen as a warning signal alerting you to look beyond the immediate illness and reassess and heal your emotions, attitudes, and lifestyle. Illness is not seen as a failure and death is not seen as the enemy, as they are in conventional Western medicine. There is currently tremendous interest in the mind-body approach to medicine. Many people feel that the present Western medical model will soon become just a part of the holistic mind-body medicine of the future.

There are now comprehensive mind-body medicine programs at the medical schools affiliated with Harvard University, the University of Massachusetts, the University of Miami, Case Western Reserve University, the University of California at San Francisco, San Francisco State University, and Stanford University, as well as at Dallas's Parkland Hospital and the Menninger Clinic in Topeka, Kansas. Mind-body techniques include emotional work, cognitive-behavioral therapy, prayer, music therapy, hypnosis, guided imagery, biofeedback, and neurolinguistic programming. Many think that skin problems provide an excellent subject for studying psychophysiology and behavioral medicine because the skin is easily observed and changes in it can be measured noninvasively.

EMOTIONAL WORK

Healing involves emotional balance, with the release of negative emotions and the encouragement of feelings of well-being and self-control. Some naturopathic and homeopathic physicians and psychologists think that the skin serves as a direct guide to our emotions. As Debbie Shapiro points out in her book *Your Body Speaks Your Mind*, each emotion creates a response in the skin that can be electrically recorded and easily seen by others. Our skin blushes with love or embarrassment, sweats with fear, flushes with shame or anger, and breaks out in goosebumps with anticipation or fright. Some naturopaths link red, fiery rashes with an underlying fire in the form of suppressed anger or irritability. Oversensitive people are often thought to have sensitive skin, while insensitive personalities have been linked with being "thick-skinned." The feeling of being emotionally dried up, stuck, or numb is felt by Dr. M. Ullman, Ms. Shapiro, and others to be associated with dryness and cracking of the skin in some cases, just as oily skin can imply an excess of emotions. Conflicting emotions, repressed feelings, anguish, self-hatred, or inappropriate passions are thought to be expressed on the face in the form of rashes or blemishes.

Dr. Ted Grossbart, author of the very complete book *Skin Deep,* which is based on the research-based techniques he uses at the Mind/Body Program at Harvard University, where he works and teaches, thinks of emotions as a factor in all skin problems, and feels that all dermatologic problems have an emotional impact. For many skin problems he describes what he thinks are the most common underlying emotional conflicts and factors to explore and work on. He also describes comprehensive exercises to help people focus on the hidden role of their emotions in the formation and maintenance of their diseases. Dr. Grossbart further discusses techniques to reduce the emotional impact of bothersome symptoms of dermatologic illnesses.

COGNITIVE-BEHAVIORAL TECHNIQUES

Cognitive-behavioral techniques are based on the assumption that cognitions (thoughts), attitudes, beliefs, and expectations can determine a person's emotional reactions and, therefore, his or her physical reactions. In people with skin disorders, anxiety and attitudes toward the problem are thought to influence the experience of symptoms. Therefore, a change in thought patterns or cognition may be able to change the perceived experience of these disturbing skin symptoms. In cognitive therapy, you learn which of your negative beliefs are faulty and how to substitute more positive thoughts. You are also taught to use visual imagery and distractions to cope with stressful events, as well as ways to reinterpret your symptoms. Behavioral changes can also incorporate relaxation techniques and assertiveness training.

SPIRITUALITY AND PRAYER

Harvard Medical School researchers have been studying the benefits of mind-body interactions for more than twenty-five years. Their research has shown that repeating a prayer, word, sound, or phrase, and disregarding intrusive thoughts, slows a person's metabolic, heart, and respiratory rates, and also slows brain waves. These changes have been demonstrated to be effective for the treatment of chronic pain, anxiety, and mild depression. In fact, the effectiveness of these techniques was shown to have a direct correlation to the extent that the disease in question is caused or made worse by stress. It was also found that patients experienced increased feelings of spirituality as a result of going into this altered state, regardless of whether or not they used a repetitive prayer to do so. Subjects described their feelings of spirituality as experiencing the presence of a power, force, energy, or God close to them. This increased spirituality was in turn found to be associated with fewer medical symptoms and improved health.

There has been a recent renaissance in a spiritual approach to health. Research studies and practical approaches have recently been developed to integrate spirituality into conventional medical practice. Professional conferences in spirituality and healing in medicine are given around the country through the Mind/Body Medical Institute at Harvard Medical School and the Institute of Religion at the Texas Medical Center. Work by Drs. Herbert Benson, Larry Dossey, David Larson, and Dean Ornish, among others, is state of the art in this area. In the field of dermatology, there was a recent 1998 review article in *Archives of Dermatology* by Dr. R.J. Thomsen of the Los Alamos Medical Center in New Mexico discussing the role of spirituality in traditional and alternative medical practice. He also detailed the methods to use to grow spiritually, and how to apply spirituality to a dermatologist's medical practice. Thus, these topics are now reaching mainstream dermatologists and will continue to have an important impact.

HYPNOSIS

Hypnosis can be a very powerful tool for pain and anxiety relief. Hypnosis accesses the deepest levels of the mind and produces physiological changes in the autonomic nervous system. This in turn effects positive shifts in a person's behavior and his or her sense of well-being. Traditional hypnosis works with the increased suggestibility that takes place during a formally structured, deep trance. Posthypnotic suggestions to relieve pain work best when they are given to an individual in this state.

Hypnosis was devised by Austrian physician Franz Mesmer in the late 1700s. At that time, the practice was known as Mesmerism. The name was later changed to hypnosis based on *hypnos*, the Greek word for sleep. In 1955, the British Medical Association approved hypnotherapy as a valid medical therapy. The AMA did the same in 1958. More than 15,000 doctors now combine hypnotherapy with traditional therapies.

All hypnosis is considered a form of self-hypnosis, as a hypnotherapist is only the facilitator for a willing participant. Experts estimate that 10 percent of people are very susceptible to hypnosis, 65 to 70 percent are moderately susceptible (defined as being at least able to relax fully with the aid of hypnosis), and 25 to 30 percent are not susceptible. Hypnosis should not be done with anyone who has psychosis, an organic psychiatric condition, or an antisocial personality disorder, as it may worsen these conditions.

A frequently used approach to hypnosis is Milton Erickson's "altered state of mind," which is common in everyday life. Everyday trances, such as daydreaming or losing track of time while absorbed in reading or some other activity, are examples of this form of hypnosis. In a superficial hypnotic state, the patient willingly accepts suggestions but does not necessarily follow through on them. The main aim of hypnosis is to quiet the patient's conscious mind and to make the patient's noncritical unconscious mind more accessible, as it is there that suggestions have a better chance of being followed. A session of hypnosis generally lasts from sixty to ninety minutes, and a course of treatment is often six to twelve sessions given once a week.

Hypnotic suggestion has reportedly been used successfully in cases of atopic eczema, contact dermatitis, herpes, warts, neurodermatitis, psoriasis, hives, severe hair loss (such as alopecia areata), rosacea, itching, and chronic pain. As early as 1928, doctors at the University of Vienna used hypnosis to treat flare-ups of oral herpes in their patients. They also found that reminding patients under hypnosis of the emotional events that had been associated with the first outbreaks of herpes triggered new flare-ups.

In 1952, Dr. A. Mason reported in the *British Medical Journal* a now-famous case of hypnotic treatment of a sixteen-year-old boy with ichthyosis, or severely dry skin, from birth. Thick, blackened scales covered most of his body. The condition had been unresponsive to all prior treatments, including surgical skin transplantation. The boy was put under hypnosis and the hynotherapist made suggestions that different parts of his body would clear. Within two weeks, the thick black scales began to fall off and his skin cleared tremendously. Working independently of each other, researchers C.B. Kidd and J.N. Schneck in 1966 also reported cases of ichthyosis that responded to hypnosis with site-specific positive results.

Some people continue to doubt the effectiveness of hypnosis as an adjunct medical therapy because the mechanism by which it works is not well understood. However, researchers argue that studies have shown that hypnosis creates changes in stress-hormone levels, breathing, and blood pressure, as well as other shifts in autonomic nervous-system functions that bring about relief of symptoms. In fact, many hospitals have on their staffs a doctor or nurse who is also a trained hypnotherapist. Also, physicians and nurses are increasingly attuned to offering encouragement and positive expectations to unconscious patients who can still hear and remember suggestions.

BIOFEEDBACK

Biofeedback is a technique used to consciously affect many bodily processes that previously seemed beyond our control. Robert Adler, Ph.D., who is considered the father of psychoneuroimmunology, found that rats could be conditioned to suppress or improve their immune systems through conditioning to the taste of saccharin. Because the body cannot distinguish between actual events and those present in thought alone, conditioning is a very important link between the mind and the body. Canadian researcher Dr. John Basmajian has shown that people can learn to consciously control not only whole systems, but also individual muscle cells and neurons!

Biofeedback equipment measures skin temperature, blood pressure, or other bodily functions and produces an audio or visual signal to represent them. The patient learns to control the bodily process that is being monitored by first learning to control the pitch of a sound, the rate of a series of beeps, or a computer-generated image by using whatever thoughts, feelings, or sensations work for him or her. While the training involves specialized therapists and equipment, once you have learned the technique, you can use it anyplace, anytime. Biofeedback is different from generalized relaxation in that you focus on a specific response, rather than trying to relax the whole body at once.

Biofeedback-assisted relaxation can help to avoid the complications of poor circulation and delayed wound healing in people with diabetes. Drs. B.I. Rice and J.V. Schindler of the Department of Health Education at the University of Wisconsin–La Crosse studied a group of forty diabetics and found that they could increase the temperature of their toes by 9 percent with the use of a general relaxation tape. However, they could increase the temperature of their toes a significant 31 percent with biofeedback-assisted relaxation. This is important in preventing diabetic foot and leg ulcers, which are very difficult to heal once they develop.

In 1989, Sedlacek cited cases in which psoriasis cleared with thermal biofeedback. He thought that biofeedback helped skin to heal by having a positive psychoneuroimmunologic effect in restoring and maintaining a balanced and calm central nervous system and brain. Researchers H.H. Hughes and colleagues, and L.J. Benoit and E.H. Harrell also achieved great improvement in several patients with psoriasis using biofeedback training. In 1994, M. Goodman of the University of Maryland described a case of a fifty-six-year-old woman whose psoriasis of the arms had failed to respond to standard medical treatment for seven years. After thirteen weekly one-hour finger and hand thermal biofeedback treatments, all eleven original one- to three-inch psoriatic lesions had cleared, and any new lesions that had begun to form during the treatment had disappeared without visible scarring. The woman continued to be symptom-free, taking no psoriasis medications, one year after the biofeedback treatment had ended. Goodman hypothesized that the biofeedback therapy worked by stimulating the nervous system to increase blood circulation to the affected areas.

In 1992, Dr. Shinrigaku performed an interesting study on the effects of thermographic biofeedback on itching. A group of twenty-six people had yam glue applied to their forearms to cause itching. Each subject was given biofeedback information on his or her computer screen. The color of the screen changed with the temperature change in each of the subjects' forearms as they practiced biofeedback techniques. Those who were told to decrease their skin temperature subjectively reported less itching, although they actually did not objectively change their own temperature. Those who were instructed to increase their skin temperature ended up subjectively raising the intensity of their itching. This study suggests that the use of thermographic biofeedback might be useful for severe itching that does not respond to other measures.

NEUROLINGUISTIC PROGRAMMING

Practitioners of neurolinguistic programming (NLP) study the verbal and nonverbal expressions of an individual's thinking patterns. They then try to alter the patient's beliefs about healing so that he or she can make better choices in behavior, especially in regard to health.

First, the practitioner observes the language patterns, eye movements, postures, gestures, and tone of voice of the patient. These indicate the way the person processes and interprets information and beliefs. Next, the programmer tries to separate the individual's identity from that of his or her chronic disease. He then asks the client to envision being in a specific state of good health, using touch or visual or auditory methods to create a positive association, or nervous system anchor, to that healthy state. The brain, once limiting beliefs are redirected, then triggers the necessary immunologic responses to guide the patient's body to health.

NLP has been helpful in reducing anxiety and in re-imprinting, especially in chronic diseases. Therefore, it can be tried in cases of intractable eczema or psoriasis. It too is cost-efficient and simple, thus further bringing it to the attention of business and insurance people, who strongly influence the economy of our health-care system.

PART TWO

Common
Skin
Problems

Introduction

Part One of this book introduced you to the basic practices of conventional dermatology, as well as to various alternative medical therapies that can be applied to dermatology. These include nutritional therapy, herbal medicine, aromatherapy, homeopathy, acupuncture, stress-reduction techniques, mind-body medicine, and others. Finally, a section on general recommendations gives advice for commonsense helpful measures that apply regardless of what type of treatment you are using.

In Part Two you will find an alphabetical listing of common skin problems and diseases, with both conventional and alternative medical therapies that may be useful for treating them. A brief description of the skin disorder is followed by recommendations for prevention, conventional medical approaches, nutritional therapy, herbal remedies, aromatherapy, homeopathy, stress reduction, mind-body medicine, electrotherapy, or light or sound therapy, depending on which of these treatments are useful for a particular problem.

Depending on your symptoms and your affinity for various approaches to health care, together with your health care practitioner you can integrate your therapy to combine the best of what conventional and alternative medicine have to offer you.

Troubleshooting Guide
Symptoms and Possible Causes

The guide below lists some of the more common skin symptoms, together with possible causes, to help you decide which sections in this book may be most helpful to you. Although you may be experiencing one or some of the symptoms listed here, you may or may not have any of the illnesses mentioned. Disorders are listed here because they *can* cause the particular symptom, and they are listed in alphabetical order, not in order of the likelihood of occurrence. This chart is not meant to substitute for the advice of a qualified health-care provider. Always consult with your doctor or other practitioner for a professional diagnosis.

Symptom	Possible Cause(s)
Bulla (large blister)	Burn; contact dermatitis; drug reactions; friction; insect bite.
Mouth ulcers	Canker sores; cold sores; drug reaction; skin cancer (squamous cell carcinoma).
Nodule (large bump), red and inflamed	Abscess; skin cancer (basal cell carcinoma); boils; fungal infection.
Papules (small bumps), various colors	Acne (common); drug reaction; insect bite; keloid; mole; rosacea; skin cancer (basal cell carcinoma or squamous cell carcinoma); systemic lupus erythematosus; wart.
Pimples	Acne (common acne, acne caused by cosmetics, medication-induced acne, steroid acne); rosacea.
Pustule (bump filled with pus), localized	Boil; cold sore; drug reaction; fungal infection; genital herpes.
Pustules (bumps filled with pus), widespread	Acne (common or steroid acne); fungal infection; insect bites; shingles.
Rash that forms lines	Contact dermatitis; insect bites; shingles; warts.

Rash that itches	Atopic dermatitis; contact dermatitis; drug reaction; dry skin; fungal infection; hives; insect bites; mycosis fungoides; seborrhea; sun-sensitivity disorder.
Scaling skin	Chemical contact; drug reaction; dry skin; sunburn; sun-sensitivity disorder.
Spot, brown	Drug reaction; freckle; mole; darkening of the skin following a rash; sun sensitivity disorder.
Spot, white	Chemical exposure; systemic lupus erythematosus; lightening of the skin following a rash; vitiligo.
Ulceration	Bedsore; burn; fungal infection; leg ulcer; trauma.
Vesicles (small blisters)	Athlete's foot; cold sores; genital herpes; insect bite; shingles.
Wheal (flat, firm elevation of the skin with irregular borders)	Hives.

Abscesses

An abscess, or carbuncle, is a large, deep, tender, hot, red nodule that surrounds several hair follicles and drains pus through several points to the skin surface. Abscesses are extremely contagious and potentially serious, as they can lead to blood infection. They form only in areas where there are hair follicles, most often in the armpits and on the buttocks, face, scalp, neck, and trunk. An abscess can be painful, especially if it is in a location that presses on nerves or bone. When an abscess heals, there is usually scarring. If an abscess ruptures, masses of pus and a "core" of harder material comes out. People with abscesses quite commonly run fevers.

The most common bacteria found in carbuncles is *Staphylococcus aureus* (staph). Other bacteria also may cause abscesses, depending on the location of the abscess and the immunity of the patient. Less commonly, viral, parasitic, or fungal abscesses may form. In some cases, abscesses may be a sign of an underlying immune problem or other disease. People with alcoholism, cancer, HIV/AIDS, or malnutrition, and those on chemotherapy are especially susceptible to developing abscesses.

CONVENTIONAL TREATMENT

■ Keep the area clean with an antimicrobial soap such as chlorhexidine.
■ Apply hot, wet compresses to help relieve the pain and bring the abscess to a point. This will make it easier for your health professional to lance the abscess.
■ *Do not* squeeze the bump. If it does not rupture or go away by itself, consult your doctor.
■ Your doctor will probably cut open the abscess, empty out the contents, and allow it to drain. *Do not* try to cut it open yourself. If it is large, your doctor may pack the remaining cavity with gauze. Local antibiotic creams are usually applied to the site of the wound.
■ Always seek professional medical advice, especially if you also have a fever, chills, and/or malaise.
■ An oral antibiotic that is effective against Staphylococci, such as dicloxacillin (sold under the brand names Dynapen, Dycill, and Pathocil) or amoxicillin/clavulanate (Augmentin) may be prescribed. If you have had

recurrent abscesses, have not done well with prior antibiotics, have a fever and malaise, are immunocompromised, or have abscesses that involve the central face, muscle, or deep tissues, a Gram stain and bacterial culture will be done to determine what kind of bacteria are causing them and which antibiotics are likely to be most effective. If you are very ill or have a serious underlying disease, hospitalization and intravenous antibiotic therapy may be appropriate.

■ If abscesses keep returning, your doctor will look for an underlying disease. People with certain chronic diseases are thought to carry staph bacteria in their nasal passages or groins and continually reinfect themselves. Bacterial cultures of these sites are taken and if staph bacteria are found, treatment will usually include applying mupirocin ointment (Bactroban Nasal) in the nasal passages twice daily, plus a a course of the antibiotic rifampin (Rifadin, Rimactane).

■ If an abscess develops around the mouth or on the lips, surgical drainage is not used because of the risk of the infection spreading to the brain through the bloodstream. Instead, the abscess is cultured and an appropriate systemic antibiotic prescribed.

DIETARY MEASURES

■ Increase your intake of fluids. Drink water throughout the day.

■ Drink a glass of water with the juice of a fresh lemon and one teaspoon of chlorophyll on rising and before bed.

■ Limit your consumption of food products containing white sugar and white flour.

■ Foods rich in vitamin A, such as yellow-orange fruits and vegetables and dark green leafy vegetables aid in the rapid healing of abscesses. Try to have at least four different types of green vegetables a day.

■ Foods rich in zinc, including oysters, sunflower seeds, and pumpkin seeds, also speed healing of abscesses and should be included in the diet.

NUTRITIONAL SUPPLEMENTS

■ The following supplements help to heal the skin quickly, boost the immune system, and fight against inflammation.

- Vitamin A. Take 25,000 international units daily for two weeks.
- B-complex vitamins. Take a vitamin-B complex that supplies 100 milligrams of each of the major B vitamins daily.
- Beta-carotene. Take 50,000 international units daily for two weeks.
- Vitamin C with bioflavonoids. Take 5,000 milligrams daily.
- Zinc. Take 50 milligrams daily for two weeks.

HERBAL TREATMENT

Herbal mixtures can be applied topically to the abscess to rapidly draw out pus and limit infection locally. Herbs can also be made into teas and drunk to speed healing of the abscess.

■ Garlic boosts the immune system and fights inflammation. It can be taken in capsule form.

■ Calendula ointment can to applied to the skin overlying the unbroken abscess to decrease inflammation and act as an antiseptic.

■ Goldenseal and calendula are available as creams and can be used to draw out the boil. These topicals also help to stimulate regeneration of the damaged tissues. Leave a thin layer of either or both creams on the boil for twelve to twenty-four hours.

■ Slippery elm and eucalyptus oil help to draw out the pus. Mix together 25 grams of dried slippery elm, 3 drops of eucalyptus oil, and enough boiling water to form a thick paste. Apply the hot paste to the abscess and leave it on until it cools. Repeat until the pus is discharged. Marshmallow leaf or figwort can be used in the same way to draw out pus.

■ A tea made from two parts wild indigo to one part each of echinacea, pasque flower, and poke root can be taken internally three times a day to speed healing or applied externally to limit infection.

■ Astralagus tea helps to enhance immunity. Drink up to eight glasses a day.

AROMATHERAPY

■ Essential oil of echinacea, myrrh, or tea tree can be applied to the abscess to limit infection. These oils have a direct antimicrobial effect and increase the number of white blood cells fighting the infection in and around the abscess.

▨ Bergamot, chamomile, clary sage, or lavender oil can also be used to draw out the abscess.

▨ Tea tree oil can be applied topically to fight bacteria and fungi. A few drops diluted in a couple of tablespoons of any vegetable oil should not irritate the skin, but the pure oil may irritate the skin. Never take it internally.

HOMEOPATHY

Unless otherwise specified, use homeopathic remedies as recommended on the product label.

▨ Different homeopathic remedies are often used at different stages in these skin infections:
  • At the first stage, when the lesion is rapidly forming, red, and tender, take one dose of *Belladonna* 6c, 12c, or 30c every one to two hours, up to a total of ten doses, until the pus is released.
  • At the second stage, when the lesion becomes increasingly large and pus-filled, take one dose of *Hepar sulfuris* 6c, 12c, or 30c every one to two hours, up to a maximum of ten doses. This remedy is also good for darkish blue, extremely painful abscesses with a slower onset.
  • For persistent eruptions, take one dose of *Silicia* 12c or 30c four times a day until you notice an improvement.

▨ Add 10 drops of *Hypericum* tincture to 1 cup of warm water to make a compress to relieve the pain and encourage healing. Apply a compress to the affected area for fifteen minutes four times a day.

▨ *Arsenicum album* 30c is good for carbuncles with cutting, burning pain that improves when heat is applied.

▨ *Lachesis* 30c is good for very sore, purplish, slowly developing abscesses with thin, dark pus.

▨ *Mercurius solubilis* 30c is recommended for shiny, red, throbbing abscesses in glands.

▨ *Rhus toxicodendron* 30c is helpful for dark red, intensely painful, pus-filled swellings.

- *Sulfur* 12c is good for chronic, very itchy abscesses with profuse, thin discharges.
- *Tarentula cubensis* 30c is recommended for painful carbuncles with black cores in the presence of serious illness or toxicity.

ACUPRESSURE

See Acupressure Points in Part Three for the locations of these points on the body.

- To release muscular tension that prevents good local blood flow to the abscess, press the Golden Points closest to the sore. Repeat twice daily. The Golden Points are twenty points around the body often used for common illnesses and injuries.

GENERAL RECOMMENDATIONS

- Rest the affected area and avoid external friction and trauma.
- Wash your hands frequently.
- Use clean washcloths, and change towels and sheets daily.

Acne

Acne is an inflammatory condition of the skin characterized by the presence of blackheads, whiteheads, pimples, and cysts. Acne vulgaris (common acne) often begins during the teenage years, and is typically worse in boys. About 85 percent of teenagers are bothered by some degree of acne. Other types of acne may be caused by externally irritating cosmetics, chemicals, and oils; heat and humidity; ingestion of certain drugs, such as corticosteroids, phenytoin (Dilantin), lithium, and high-progestin birth control pills; food sensitivities; hormonal imbalance; or hormonal fluctuations such as those that occur in puberty, pregnancy, or menopause. Acne can even be found in normal newborn babies, but the pimples go away within a few weeks without treatment. Acne becomes rare after the age of fifty.

A number of factors cause or contribute to the development of acne. The sebaceous (oil) glands, located at the root of each hair follicle, start overproducing sebum when levels of androgens rise in adolescence. Androgens are commonly referred to as "male hormones," but are actually present in adults of both sexes. Skin bacteria, especially *Propionibacterium acnes,* are also factors in the formation of acne lesions, as enzymes secreted by the bacteria break down sebum, resulting in accumulations of irritating free fatty acids in the sebaceous gland. Natural-medicine proponents think that acne is in part the result of blood being too acidic, a condition brought about by eating refined foods, sugar, chocolate, and lots of dairy products, sweets, fat, and cholesterol. Naturopaths also believe that acne is the result of poor elimination of toxins via the large intestine and kidneys.

Acne is made worse by the use of oil-based cosmetics and moisturizers, poor diet, nutritional deficiencies, allergies, lack of exercise, stress, environmental pollution, hot weather, emotional problems, and the onset of menstruation. There seems to be a genetic component as well, as parents with a history of severe acne often have children with the same problem.

Whiteheads, blackheads, pimples, pustules, and cysts can form wherever sebum and debris on the skin clogs pores, most commonly on the face, neck, chest, back, and shoulders. A blackhead is an open comedone (a pore filled with dark, dried oil and shed skin cells). A whitehead is a clogged, closed comedone. A papule, or pimple, is a red bump that forms around a ruptured pore that has released its oil, debris, and bacteria into the surrounding skin. If a papule becomes inflamed enough, a pustule (pus-filled bump) forms. If inflammation is severe and extends below the surface of the skin, cysts can develop. In very severe cases, the pores may become permanently dilated or heal with scarring. Dermatologists classify acne according to four grades of severity—designated GI, GII, GIII, and GIV—depending on the number and type of lesions present. The type of treatment chosen is based on this grading system.

Although most teenagers have acne, it is often a good idea to treat it aggressively, as this is an age when attractiveness to the opposite sex and peer acceptance is of the utmost importance. Avoidance or ridicule by peers because of uncontrolled acne can be devastating to an adolescent's self-esteem and have far-reaching consequences. Physical scars as the result of untreated acne can also persist for many years.

CONVENTIONAL TREATMENT

■ Cleansers and topical agents are usually tried first, and may be sufficient to control mild cases of acne. You should thoroughly cleanse your skin in the morning and at night using a mild medicated soap. Avoid scrubbing, irritating, and drying out your skin.

■ Alpha- and beta-hydroxy acids are gentle exfoliants that can help people with very mild acne. They are available in many different over-the-counter lotions designed to help the skin shed surface cells, open blocked pores, and keep sebum moving evenly onto the skin's surface.

■ Benzoyl peroxide is an ingredient in many nonprescription and prescription gels, creams, lotions, and soaps. It helps to open and clean out clogged pores and limit the growth of bacteria on the skin and in the pores, and thus is useful for pimples and pustules. It can be very drying, however, especially in the gel form, and may cause redness, scaling, and irritation. It is therefore best to start with a low-strength water-based cream and apply it only once every other day at first to make sure that there is no irritation from the benzoyl peroxide product. If there is none, you can slowly increase the strength and frequency of application of the benzoyl peroxide cream to whatever level your skin can tolerate without getting itchy, red, flaky, or inflamed.

■ Drying agents, such as those containing sulfur or lime sulfur solution, salicylic acid, resorcinol, and benzoyl peroxide are used to cause a continuous mild drying and peeling of the skin. This may work quickly and effectively if you have mild pustular acne and are reluctant to try anything stronger.

■ Topical antibiotics available with a prescription, including topical erythromycin (Erygel, Erythra-Derm, and others), clindamycin (Cleocin T), meclocycline (Meclan), and tetracycline (Achromycin, Topicycline), are particularly useful for mild pimples and pustules. They help to get rid of *Propionibacterium acnes.*

■ Tretinoin (Retin-A) has until recently been the topical medication of choice for blackheads and whiteheads. Many dermatologists prescribe it for pimples as well. It works by increasing skin-cell turnover in normal hair follicles and blackheads and whiteheads, thus opening up and pushing out the debris from blackheads. The solution and gel forms can be drying and irritating. Either form makes the skin more susceptible to sunburn and sun damage, so you must take care with other drying agents and sun and heat exposure. The lowest strength (0.025 percent) cream is quite mild and is better for dry skin with acne. Start by using only a small amount every other night, after washing your skin and drying it thoroughly, for twenty minutes. You may increase the strength and frequency of application as tolerated. Tretinoin increases the penetration of other topicals by temporarily thinning the skin and dilating the capillaries, so there is a beneficial synergistic effect when it is used in combination with other topical medications. However, benzoyl peroxide may inactivate tretinoin, so those two medications should not be used together. Recently, the patent on tretinoin expired, so generic formulations have become available. In addition, several better formulations of tretinoin cream have entered the marketplace. For example, Retin-A Micro 0.1-percent gel contains microspheres that deliver full-strength tretinoin in a gentler way, without as much irritation. It can be put on the face directly after washing, instead of after waiting twenty minutes as with Retin-A. Avita is another newer formulation of tretinoin cream or gel that has the same efficacy but causes much less irritation than the most potent Retin-A gel (0.025-percent strength). It is intended to be used for acne only. Most people start to see improvement in their acne within two weeks, and the improvement continues for about six weeks.

■ Adapalene (Differin) gel is a newer high-strength retinoid therapy that is much gentler than tretinoin. It is best for blackheads and whiteheads.

■ Tazarotene (Tazorac) gel is another topical retinoid treatment. It is excellent for deep whiteheads and blackheads, oily skin, and inflammatory acne papules and pustules that have not responded to milder therapies. It is not as unstable as tretinoin in the presence of light, and therefore not as photosensitizing. However, it can still be irritating, and a noncomedogenic (non-pore-clogging) moisturizer and sunscreen should also be used daily. Tazarotene gel should not be used by women who may become pregnant, so if you are a woman of childbearing age, you must use a reliable method of birth control. With nightly use of tazarotene gel, you should see improvement in your acne starting at four weeks and continuing for twelve weeks.

▓ Azelaic acid (Azelex) cream may be prescribed for mild to moderate acne. Azelaic acid is a natural compound found in wheat. It works to normalize the keratinization process in the skin that blocks the pores, and also has antimicrobial activity. It is most effective when used together with topical benzoyl peroxide, erythromycin, or tretinoin, although acne does improve when azelaic acid is used alone. Azelaic-acid cream should be applied to blemishes twice a day for twelve weeks to determine its maximum effectiveness.

▓ If proper cleansing and topical treatment are not enough, an oral antibiotic may be prescribed. Oral antibiotics such as tetracycline (Achromycin V), erythromycin (ERYC, Ilotycin, and others), minocycline (Dynacin, Minocin), doxycycline (Doryx, Vibramycin, and others), ampicillin (Omnipen, Polycillin, and others), cephalosporins, and sulfa drugs are often prescribed by dermatologists for more severe acne with many papules and/or pustules. These are often very helpful, but one cannot stay on antibiotics forever.

▓ For women who have acne and also need birth control, hormonal therapy may be useful, especially if the acne is thought to be driven by a hormonal imbalance. Birth control pills with 50 micrograms of estrogen and low progesterone can help to control acne and are sometimes prescribed for just that purpose in women. Examples include Demulen 1/50, Demulen 1/35, Loestrin 1/20, Ortho-Novum 7-7-7, Triphasil, and Tri-Norinyl. In more severe cases in older women, antiandrogens such as spironolactone are sometimes used.

▓ Isotretinoin (Accutane) is frequently used for severe acne. It usually yields great results that can markedly improve a person's self-image and self-esteem. Isotretinoin is a strong derivative of vitamin A that significantly reduces the glands' production of sebum and shrinks the oil glands. However, it can cause side effects, including very dry skin and mucous membranes, sore muscles and joints, bone changes, rising levels of cholesterol and blood fats, elevation of liver enymzes, and headaches. Close monitoring by a physician is necessary. Often, more than one course of treatment is necessary for very severe, chronic cases. However, people are often pleased with the results, so they are willing to put up with the side effects and risks. The biggest risk concerning isotretinoin concerns pregnancy. This drug causes birth defects, so it cannot be used if you are planning to get pregnant just before, during, or just after the course of treatment. Some doctors are reluctant to prescribe it for women of childbearing age in any case. If you are female, of child-bearing age, and take this drug, a doctor may insist that you have a pregnancy test before starting, that you use not one but two methods of birth control simultaneously, and that you submit to monthly pregnancy tests.

■ For very severe acne, a dermatologist may prescribe isotretinoin (Accu-tane) and prednisone (also sold under the brand names Deltasone, Orasone, Sterapred, and others), which may be taken orally or injected directly into the lesions.

■ Physical therapies for acne include liquid nitrogen, acne surgery, and corticosteroid shots. Dabbing liquid nitrogen very lightly on acne lesions causes a mild shedding of skin and improvement, especially of discrete acne cysts. Acne surgery consists of using a comedone extractor to carefully re-move the contents of blackheads and whiteheads. It also includes draining pustules and cysts through a small incision. Inflamed, painful cysts also heal very quickly with local corticosteroid shots directly into the lesions. How-ever, this is not a method for long-term control of acne, only for emer-gency shrinkage of large, painful lesions.

■ Chemical peels, dermabrasion, scar excision, and collagen injections are helpful for deep scarring resulting from severe acne. With dermabrasion, af-ter local anesthesia is given, a high-speed mini-sander is used to remove the top layer of scarred skin. The new skin grows back without as much scar-ring. However, this procedure poses the risk of your skin healing with light or dark spots, and it is not painless. With chemical peels, a mild, moderate, or strong acid is used to peel off the top layer or layers of skin. The new skin heals without superficial acne scars and with an evening out of overall skin tone and coloring. Local swelling, redness, and sun sensitivity are to be expected. Many deep ("ice pick") scars are too deep for dermabrasion, and are better treated by being individually excised by a skilled dermatologic surgeon. After excision, the skin is closed. Collagen injections can also be used to temporarily fill deep acne scars.

- Drink at least six to eight glasses of pure filtered water a day.
- Eat a nutritious, well-balanced diet with lots of raw yellow-orange and leafy green vegetables, at least four to five servings a day. Carrots, beets, celery, cucumber, lettuce, and spinach are especially helpful, and should be eaten raw, cooked, or juiced.
- Lean protein sources, fiber-rich foods, whole grains, whole fruits, and complex carbohydrates are also important components of a good diet, and are very important for clear skin.
- Food sensitivities can cause flare-ups of acne and need to be evaluated. Blood tests for food allergies that cause delayed reactions are available. Immediate food sensitivities can be discovered through the careful use of a food diary in which you record everything you eat and your skin's apparent reactions. Suspect foods can then be avoided.
- Limit animal and hydrogenated fats as much as possible. This means cutting down on dairy products, margarine, fatty meats, and fried food.
- Avoid foods containing additives, preservatives, alcohol, aspartame (NutraSweet), caffeine, and refined sugar as much as possible. Especially avoid candy and carbonated soft drinks.
- Too much iodine can irritate pores and cause flare-ups. Limit your consumption of foods containing high levels of iodine, including iodized salt, fast foods, sea vegetables, kelp tablets, milk, and shellfish.

NUTRITIONAL SUPPLEMENTS

- Beta-carotene is used by the body to make vitamin A and helps to heal the skin. Take 25,000 international units daily.
- The antioxidant vitamins C and E, zinc, and selenium, are important in combating free radicals and, therefore, the inflammation in the skin. Vitamin C also helps to strengthen connective tissue and thus help skin stay blemish-free. Zinc is also important in maintaining normal blood levels of vitamin A, aids in the normal functioning of the oil-producing glands, and helps to heal skin and mucous membranes. Take 500 to 1,000 milligrams of vitamin C with bioflavonoids three times daily; 400 international units of vitamin E daily; 25 milligrams of zinc with 1 milligram of copper twice a day, with meals; and 200 micrograms of selenium daily.

■ Vitamin B may help for premenstrual or mid-menstrual-cycle acne. Because the B vitamins should be taken together, take a supplement that supplies 100 milligrams of each of the major B vitamins daily.

■ Chromium helps decrease sugar cravings and keep blood sugar balanced so you are not driven to consume loads of sugary junk food. Take 200 micrograms of chromium twice daily.

■ Flaxseed and primrose oil are good sources of omega-3 essential fatty acids (EFAs). Acne may be a manifestation of EFA deficiency. Take 2 teaspoons of flaxseed or primrose oil daily.

■ Calcium and magnesium relax a stressed nervous system and are helpful for those who experience flare-ups due to nervousness. These minerals also reduce sugar cravings, which may perpetuate acne. Take 750 milligrams of calcium and 375 milligrams of magnesium twice daily, between meals.

■ Acidophilus and bifidus restore the friendly bacteria in your intestines, cleansing and strengthening your digestive system to function more efficiently. This results in the presence of fewer toxic metabolites that can show up on the skin. Take one dose of acidophilus and bifidus twice a day, between meals.

HERBAL TREATMENT

■ Calendula soap, made from marigold flowers, is good for helping to clear blemishes. Wash with it twice a day, using warm water alternating with cold water.

■ A combination of calendula and witch hazel also makes an excellent cleanser. Mix equal parts of liquid calendula extract and distilled witch hazel and apply this to the lesions three times a day.

■ Make a goldenseal and tea tree oil paste by mixing ½ teaspoon of powdered goldenseal root with 12 drops of tea tree oil. Apply the resulting paste to the acne lesions and leave it on for twenty minutes minutes before rinsing it off. Repeated twice a day, this has been found to be extremely effective.

■ A combination astringent lotion made by mixing equal parts of liquid marigold and chickweed extracts and distilled witch hazel can be applied to blemishes three times a day.

■ Use a clay masque for deep cleansing. Mix 1 teaspoon of green clay in a little water, until a paste is formed. Apply this to areas of oily skin and leave it on for fifteen minutes before washing it off with warm water.

- Lemon juice diluted in water has an antiseptic effect when applied twice a day.
- The following herbs have been noted to help acne when taken orally:
  - Burdock root. Take 500 milligrams three times a day.
  - Echinacea and goldenseal. Take 500 milligrams of echinacea with 300 milligrams of goldenseal three times a day.
  - Grapeseed or pine bark extract. Take 250 micrograms three times a day.
  - Blue flag, cleavers, echinacea, figwort, and poke root. Make a tea containing equal parts of these herbs, and drink a cup three times a day to help support the metabolism of fats and carbohydrates, and to promote healthy elimination.
  - Red clover, echinacea, nettle, burdock root, dandelion root, licorice root, and ginger. Make a tea containing four parts red clover, two parts each echinacea, nettle, burdock root, and dandelion root, and one part each licorice root and ginger. Drink one cup three times a day to aid in eliminating toxins.

AROMATHERAPY

- Benzoin, chamomile, clary sage, frankincense, myrrh, patchouli, and peppermint oils are anti-inflammatory oils that decrease irritation and swelling.
- Bergamot and rosemary oils are balancing oils, which normalize oil production in the skin.
- Basil, cedarwood, cypress, frankincense, juniper, lemon, neroli, patchouli, peppermint, rosewood, tea tree, thyme, and ylang ylang are astringent oils that reduce the oiliness of the skin.
- Eucalyptus, everlasting, and sandalwood have both anti-inflammatory and balancing properties.
- Geranium and palmarosa oils are both balancing and astringent.
- Lavender and orange oils are anti-inflammatory, balancing, and astringent.
- One drop of pure tea tree oil can be applied directly to each acne lesion twice a day. Results may be as good as those achieved with benzoyl peroxide.

HOMEOPATHY

■ The most commonly used remedy for mild to moderate acne with whiteheads, blackheads, and small papules and pustules is *Kali bromatum* 12x or 6c. Take one dose three to four times a day until the lesions improve, for a total of up to fourteen days. This remedy is particularly helpful if you are the kind of person who is fidgety and restless, while awake and asleep.

■ *Hepar sulfuris calcareum* 6c, taken three times a day for up to fourteen days, is recommended for more severe acne with large pustules and scarring.

■ *Pulsatilla* is commonly used for overweight girls who may have a hormonal imbalance when they start their menstrual period. The usual recommendation is to take one dose of *Pulsatilla* 6c three times a day for up to fourteen days.

■ Other symptom-specific remedies to be taken twice a day until improvement include:

- *Antimonium crudum* 6c, for small red facial pimples accompanied by thirst and indigestion.
- *Antimonium tartaricum* 6c, for pus-filled pimples.
- *Berberis* 6x, for persistent acne associated with rough skin.
- *Calcarea sulfurica* 6c, for weeping pustules that form yellow crusts that are slow to heal.
- *Ledum* 6c, for red pimples, especially at the root of the nose.
- *Sanguinaria* 6c, for girls with acne and very light menstrual periods.
- *Silicea* 6c, for skin with acne-like lesions that scar easily.
- *Sulfur* 12x or 6c, for chronic red, sore infected acne associated with rough, hard skin, overwashing, diarrhea, and profuse sweating.

ACUPUNCTURE/ACUPRESSURE

See Acupressure Points in Part Three for the locations of these points on the body.

■ There are reports in the literature of success in treating acne with acupuncture. In a 1990 article, Dr. Xu Yihou reported treating eighty cases of acne with acupuncture, with an over-75-percent cure rate. Treatment was most effective for people with less severe papules and pustules, and was much less effective for severe acne with deep nodules and cysts. In 1993, Dr. Liu Jin reported treating ninety-eight cases of adolescent papular-pustular acne (none with deep nodules or cysts) with acupuncture with excellent results. He regarded over half of the cases as cured, and over 40 percent as improved, with only two failures. Thus, the total effectiveness was calculated to be 98 percent. Consult a qualified acupuncturist if you are interested in trying this type of treatment.

■ Different Chinese medical practitioners suggest strengthening meridians to increase the elimination of toxins that cause acne flare-ups, release facial tension that blocks circulation, relax the nervous system, and stimulate the pituitary gland. To effect these changes, press four or more of the following points on both sides of the body for three minutes three times every day:

- Large Intestine 1, 4, 11, or 20;
- Bladder 2, 10, 23, or 47;
- Stomach 2, 3, 6 or 36;
- Triple Warmer 23;
- Small Intestine 18;
- Gallbladder 20;
- Spleen 10;
- Liver 3; and
- the Forehead Point.

  Caution: Do not use the Large Intestine 4 in pregnancy.

OTHER THERAPIES

■ Doing breathing exercises outdoors in the fresh air and sunlight is very helpful.

■ Learn relaxation and/or meditation techniques to reduce stress. (See Part Three for suggested techniques.)

■ Yoga can be helpful, as there are specific poses which increase the blood flow to the face. (See Part Three.)

■ Lymphatic drainage massage helps to drain accumulated toxins and clear severe acne.

■ Reflexology—massage of the hands and feet focusing on parts that correspond to the liver, kidneys, intestines, adrenal glands, thyroid, and diaphragm—is useful in the treatment of acne.

■ Imagining clear skin without acne three times a day for five minutes at a time can also be helpful. (See Guided Imagery in Part Three.)

■ If emotional issues are triggering your acne and causing you other problems, seek the advice of a qualified counselor.

GENERAL RECOMMENDATIONS

■ Get regular exercise, preferably outdoors in the fresh air and sunlight. Exercise strenuously enough to break a sweat.

■ Get enough restful sleep each night.

■ Use drying astringents no more than once a week, being careful not to irritate your skin and thus worsen your acne.

■ Do not squeeze pimples, pustules, or whiteheads. This can cause infection and scarring.

■ Do not lean on or block acne lesions with your hands or other objects. This will make them worse.

■ If you wear makeup, use oil-free, water-based products. Remove any makeup completely every night before going to bed.

■ Use flesh-tinted anti-acne lotions such as Clearasil to cover acne instead of covering blemishes with makeup.

■ Avoid heavy, oily moisturizers. If a moisturizer is necessary, use only noncomedogenic, water-based formulations.

■ Wash your hair regularly, especially if it is oily. Do not use oily conditioners or hair gels. Try to keep your hair off your face.

Age Spots

Age spots, or liver spots, are flat brown spots composed of cellular debris known as lipofuscin, which accumulates due to years of sun exposure. The lipofuscin deposits clump together to produce brown spots known to doctors as *lentigines*. They are composed primarily of molecules partially destroyed by free-radical damage. These marks commonly develop on the face, neck, hands, back, and feet of middle-aged and older people. They are harmless, but many people find them distressing from a cosmetic point of view.

CONVENTIONAL TREATMENT

- Apply sunscreen with an SPF factor of 15 or higher to all sun-exposed areas every morning and reapply every several hours if you remain outdoors.
- Use cover-up makeup or concealer to hide any spots you find cosmetically displeasing.
- Apply a topical lightening agent such as hydroquinone (Eldoquin, Melanex) directly to the age spots with a cotton swab (Q-Tip).
- Glycolic acid and other alpha-hydroxy acids have also been used to exfoliate areas of dark age spots, revealing younger-looking skin underneath.
- Tretinoin (Retin-A) gel increases cellular turnover to peel away age spots and stop new spots before they get started. In a recent ten-month study of fifty-eight people with age spots at the University of Michigan Medical Center, most had lightening of their spots after one month, and 83 percent had significant lightening after ten months.

NUTRITIONAL SUPPLEMENTS

- Take a high-potency multivitamin and mineral supplement to ensure an adequate supply of all vital nutrients.
- Antioxidants, which reduce free-radical damage, are one of the newest treatments for age spots. The following antioxidant nutrients are recommended for age spots:

- Vitamin C. Take 500 to 1,000 milligrams three times a day. Also apply a 10-percent vitamin-C lotion to the spots every day.
- Vitamin E. Take 400 to 800 international units daily. Also apply a 5-percent vitamin-E cream to the spots every day.
- Beta-carotene complex. Take 50,000 to 100,000 international units daily.
- Selenium. Take 50 to 200 micrograms daily.

Using topical vitamin formulations allows much greater skin-cell levels of the nutrients than taking pills, capsules, or other oral formulas. These formulations are applied directly to the lesions only. For example, topical 10-percent vitamin C allows you to get approximately 30 times the level of vitamin C in the cells of the lesion than can be achieved by taking oral vitamin C.

HERBAL TREATMENT

- Aloe vera gel can be applied directly to the age spots several times a day.
- Kojic acid, a mushroom derivative that has been used in Japan for years, has been found to be as effective as hydroquinone for lessening the appearance of age spots, with less irritation and other side effects. Use it as directed on the label.
- Dab fresh lemon juice twice a day on the age spots with a cotton swab. It is thought that the mild citric acid is just strong enough to safely peel off the epidermis, revealing fresh new skin underneath.
- For a slightly stronger solution, mix together 1 teaspoon grated horseradish root, ½ teaspoon lemon juice, ½ teaspoon vinegar, and 3 drops rosemary oil. Dab this on your liver spots.
- Grapeseed extract is an antioxidant. Take 50 milligrams three times a day.

Athlete's Foot

Athlete's foot, or *tinea pedis*, is a common fungal infection of the feet. Over 30 percent of all Americans suffer from athlete's foot at some point in their lives, usually after puberty. Fungi thrive in warm, dark, and damp environments where there is little light or air, so people often get athlete's foot after walking barefoot on shower floors or in locker rooms, or after continually wearing sweaty socks. The fungi break down, and then live off, the skin cells of the feet. They are contagious and can spread quickly from person to person, especially in public swimming-pool areas or locker rooms. Fungi take a stronger hold on people whose beneficial intestinal flora are out of balance.

Athlete's foot frequently begins between the third and fourth toe webs, then spreads to the arches and soles of the feet. There can be small ulcers between the toes. The fungus causes redness, scaling, blistering, burning, and itching of the feet. It can also lead to a secondary bacterial infection. If the toenails are affected, there can be crumbling, thickening, and discoloration of the nails.

In mild cases, athlete's foot can usually be treated pretty well at home. However, if a secondary bacterial infection develops, if the nails are affected, if the case is chronic and severe, or if the affected individual has a compromised immune system, a doctor's expertise will be necessary. Your doctor can confirm the diagnosis of athlete's foot by looking at some loose scales of skin under a microscope and culturing skin scrapings for fungi.

CONVENTIONAL TREATMENT

■ Over-the-counter clotrimazole (Lotrimin), undecylenic acid (in Desenex and other products), and miconazole (Micatin, Zeasorb-AF) cream or powder is effective for early, mild cases of athlete's foot.

■ Prescription creams containing as ketoconazole (Nizoral), miconazole (Monistat-Derm), itraconazole (Sporanox), or fluconazole (Diflucan) are very effective, although expensive. A convenient terbinafine (Lamisil) spray has also been developed. More recently, oxiconazole (Oxistat) cream has been found to be safe for children as young as one month of age. This medication has convenient once-a-day dosing.

■ Recurrences can be prevented by washing the feet with selenium sulfide (Exsel, Selsun) or ketoconazole (Nizoral) shampoo several times a week.

■ Oral griseofulvin (Fulvicin, Grifulvin, Grisactin, Gris-PEG) is used for more severe, resistant cases that do not respond to topical treatments. This medication can cause gastrointestinal upset and, in rare cases, liver toxicity, so caution needs to be used. However, oral antifungals are necessary if the toenails are involved.

■ Oral ketaconazole (Nizoral), itraconazole (Sporanox), fluconazole (Diflucan), and terbinafine (Lamisil) are the newest oral drugs in the dermatologist's arsenal against fungal infections. They are quite expensive, but oral treatment is necessary if the toenails are involved.

■ If your feet sweat a lot, use medications such as aluminum chloride, or Drysol, on your soles to decrease sweating. This will make you less susceptible to getting athlete's foot.

DIETARY MEASURES

■ Eat a balanced diet with lots of vegetables.

■ Include in your diet plenty of yogurt and other acidophilus-containing foods.

■ Avoid coffee, cola, tea, and chocolate. These foods increase alkalinity of the skin, making it more desirable for fungi.

■ Avoid sugary foods, including honey and fruit juices. Fungi thrive on sugar.

■ Avoid yeasty foods such as beer and breads made with yeast.

NUTRITIONAL SUPPLEMENTS

■ Acidophilus supplements replenish the "friendly" bacteria that inhibit pathogens such as fungi. Take 1 teaspoon of acidophilus powder or two capsules on an empty stomach twice a day.

■ Take a multivitamin that includes the B vitamins and vitamins A and E daily.

■ Vitamin C increases immunity against fungi. Take 3,000 milligrams of vitamin C with bioflavonoids daily.

■ Zinc increases immunity, inhibits fungi, and helps to heal skin tissue. Take 50 milligrams daily, with food.

■ Methylsulfonylmethane (MSM) is a good source of sulfur, which is believed to fight fungi. It is now available in cream or spray form to apply topically to affected areas.

HERBAL TREATMENT

■ Apple-cider vinegar applied to a washcloth can be rubbed between your toes to relieve the itch and remove scales and dead skin.

■ Calendula cream, ointment, or tincture diluted in warm water has antifungal, astringent, and healing properties, and can be used two to three times a day.

■ Drinking a cup of chamomile tea three times a day, and also applying the tea directly to the affected area with a cotton ball three times a day, should help.

■ Garlic extract is one of the best herbal antifungals. Take 6 teaspoonfuls each day. In addition, you can put raw garlic in a blender and apply it to the rash three times a day with a cotton ball. Dust your feet and shoes with garlic powder daily. Garlic's antifungal properties have been documented by clinical studies, which show that people taking garlic have blood serum levels with significant antifungal activity.

■ Ginger tea, made from 2 ounces of fresh ginger root simmered in 8 ounces of water for twenty minutes, contains more than twenty different antifungal compounds. Drink a cup of ginger tea three times a day. You can also make compresses by soaking cotton in the tea and apply them to the affected area for five minutes three times a day.

■ Goldenseal is a good antifungal agent. Add 5 drops of the tincture to juice and drink it three times a day. Or simmer 6 teaspoons of the dried herb in a cup of water for twenty minutes to make tea. Strain out the herbal matter and apply the tea to the rash with a fresh cotton ball three times a day.

■ Drink a cup of lemongrass tea three times a day, and also apply the used tea bags to the affected area. This should help athlete's foot to clear faster.

■ Licorice contains at least twenty-five fungicidal substances. Add 6 teaspoons of powdered licorice root to a cup of boiling water and simmer for twenty minutes. Strain out the herbal matter, and apply the tea to the areas of athlete's foot with a cotton ball three times a day.

■ Olive leaf extract has antifungal properties and helps to fortify the immune system. Take 250 milligrams three times a day.

■ Pau d'arco tea may be sipped three times a day to increase the body's immunity and enhance lymphatic drainage.

■ A mixture of 2 tablespoons of pau d'arco tincture, ¼ teaspoon each of tea tree and lavender tincture, ⅛ teaspoon of peppermint tincture, and 4 ounces of vinegar can be added to enough warm water to make a healing foot bath. Use this treatment three times a day, drying the feet thoroughly afterward.

■ Turmeric oil, diluted with two parts water to one part turmeric oil, can be applied to the affected area with a cotton ball three times a day to speed healing of your fungal infection. Additionally, you can take 300 milligrams of turmeric extract orally three times a day.

■ Some commercial antifungal lotions combine herbals with pharmaceuticals to get the benefits of both. Also, mixtures of antifungal herbs work synergistically, or much better, than single herbs. One such product combines tolnaftate, myrrh, tea tree oil, aloe vera, calendula, rosemary, and thyme.

AROMATHERAPY

■ Add 10 drops of tea tree oil to a pan of warm water to make a therapeutic foot soak. Soak your feet for twenty minutes three times a day. Dry your feet completely afterward. You can then apply a few drops of oil directly to the rash. If you find it irritating, dilute it with an equal amount of vegetable oil. You can also paint tea tree oil on affected toenails twice a day to keep the fungus at bay. Remember never to drink this oil.

■ Myrrh, which has antifungal and astringent properties, can also be made into a footwash. Add 10 drops of myrrh oil or 1 milliliter of tincture of myrrh to a pan of warm water. Soak your feet for twenty minutes three times a day. Dry your feet completely afterward.

Caution: Do not use myrrh during pregnancy.

HOMEOPATHY

■ *Silica* is the mainstay of homeopathic treatment for athlete's foot. It is particularly good if you have cracks between your toes and are producing lots of smelly sweat. Take it as recommended by the manufacturer.

■ Rub a few drops of homeopathic *Thuja* directly on the affected area twice a day.

ACUPRESSURE

■ Apply slight pressure for ten seconds at the base of the little toe where it joins the fourth toe. Repeat this three times twice a day.

OTHER THERAPIES

■ Ultraviolet light, in the form of a heat lamp or sunbathing, helps to dry up the fungus.

GENERAL RECOMMENDATIONS

■ Wash your feet twice a day, then dry them completely, using a new towel each time.

■ Wear white, 100-percent cotton socks and change them at least daily so that they stay dry. Wash your socks in chlorine bleach to prevent reinfection.

■ Place cotton balls in the webs between your toes to keep them open and dry.

■ Wear open sandals whenever possible to allow air to circulate between your toes.

■ Air out your shoes and sprinkle a powder containing an antifungal such as tolnaftate (Aftate, NP-27, Tinactin, Ting, Zeasorb-AF) inside them during flare-ups and afterward, to prevent recurrences.

- Wear shoes when walking in gyms or pool locker rooms.
- Do not share your socks or shoes with anyone.
- Do not scratch your feet. This can only spread the fungal infection and increase the risk of a secondary infection.

Bedsores

Bedsores, or decubitus ulcers, are deep skin ulcers that form after long periods of bed rest or immobility. They are especially common in people who are disabled, comatose, elderly, or malnourished, and those with decreased sensation in the affected areas due to nerve damage. They usually develop after two weeks of immobilization of the affected parts of the body. Heels, buttocks, hips, and shoulder blades are most commonly affected. Bedsores are very painful, especially if they extend deeply and spread.

In areas where there is pressure over bony prominences, local circulation is markedly reduced and cells in the overlying tissue die from a lack of nutrients and buildup of cellular toxins. Bedsores start superficially, affecting only the top layer of skin, but can grow and spread very rapidly to involve the deep tissues—as far down as the bone, if untreated. Secondary infection can develop and spread into the surrounding skin and, in severe cases, the bloodstream, with accompanying fever and chills.

If caught early and treated aggressively, bedsores usually start to heal within one week. There are many alternative treatment modalities that can replace or supplement conventional methods of preventing and healing bedsores.

CONVENTIONAL TREATMENT

■ The wound should be cultured for bacteria, fungus, yeast, and viruses, especially if there is pus on the surface.

■ A paste of dextranomer beads and polyethylene glycol (Debrisan), the enzyme elastase, or a 20-percent benzoyl peroxide solution can be used to chemically clean ulcers.

■ Dead tissue and debris must be removed manually from the base of ulcers with a forceps and scissors.

■ Synthetic dressings such as Vigilon or DuoDERM can be placed over the ulcers and changed every two to three days.

DIETARY MEASURES

■ Proper nutrition is crucial for the healing of bedsores. Eat a healthy diet, with plenty of fruits, vegetables, and protein. Also include plenty of fiber to keep the bowels moving.

■ Drink at least six to eight glasses of pure water daily.

NUTRITIONAL SUPPLEMENTS

■ Take a high-potency multivitamin daily to ensure an adequate supply of all vital nutrients.

■ The following nutrients help to speed healing and build up overall nutritional status:

- Beta-carotene. Take 25,000 international units daily.
- The B-complex vitamins. Take a supplement providing 100 milligrams of each of the major B vitamins daily.
- Vitamin C with bioflavonoids. Take 3,000 milligrams daily. If diarrhea occurs, cut back on the amount until you reach a level you can tolerate.
- Vitamin D. Take 400 international units daily.
- Vitamin E. Take 400 international units daily.
- Zinc. Take 50 milligrams daily, with 2 milligrams of copper.

■ To supply protein needed for healing, take a free-form amino-acid supplement as directed on the product label.

HERBAL TREATMENT

■ Daily sponge-bathing with warm water and mild calendula, vitamin E, or aloe vera soap is recommended.

■ Aloe vera gel, ointment, or cream is effective for healing bedsores in their earliest stages.

■ Calendula cream, if applied at an early stage, is very soothing and healing.

■ The following herbs may be applied directly to a bedsore in a powder or paste form to speed healing: comfrey root, echinacea, goldenseal, raw honey, myrrh, pau d'arco, slippery elm, and suma.

■ A good salve can also be made from 1 teaspoon of goldenseal powder, vitamin E oil squeezed from two 400-international-unit capsules, zinc oxide, and olive oil to make a paste. This should be applied to the sores three times a day.

■ Another popular combination to mix and apply directly to the bedsore calls for vitamin E cream, aloe vera gel, comfrey ointment, and calendula cream combined to make a paste.

HOMEOPATHY

■ *Arnica* applied externally to the bedsore is helpful in the first stage of skin breakdown.

■ *Hepar sulfuris* is best for the stage when the bedsore is red and inflamed but does not have much of a discharge.

■ Bedsores that are slow to heal, inflamed, and discharging a thick yellow pus benefit from *Calcarea sulfurica* or *Silica*.

■ *Calendula, Chamomilla, Hamamelis, Hypericum perforatum, Lachesis, Mercurius solubilis,* and *Phosphorus* are helpful for painful, slow-to-heal decubiti.

ACUPRESSURE

See Acupressure Points in Part Three for the locations of these points on the body.

■ Pressing the back Bladder points, Gallbladder 34, Large Intestine 4, Liver 3, and Stomach 36 improves circulation. This helps to bring necessary nutrients and take away toxins from the decubiti. Gently apply pressure for three minutes to any of these points that can be easily reached three times a day.

OTHER THERAPIES

■ Low-intensity pulsed direct electrotherapy has been shown to significantly improve healing. In 1993, Dr. J.M. Wood and colleagues found that the electrical current caused a rapid change in calcium in the top layer of the skin, enhancing the growth of new skin cells and fibroblasts to produce collagen for wound healing. A. Stefanovska and others found that medium to severe pressure sores in spinal-cord injury patients healed twice as fast with low-frequency pulsed current therapy as without it.

■ Experiments with using high-voltage pulsed electrical stimulation instead of low-intensity direct current to speed healing of bedsores have found that this treatment also speeds healing. Pulsed high peak power electromagnetic field therapy may also be effective.

■ Ultraviolet light in the form of a heat lamp is often useful in drying up wet, soupy bedsores.

■ Massaging around affected areas frequently using the hands or rubbing alcohol on cotton increases local blood flow, supplying the area with necessary nutrients and removing harmful cellular toxins.

GENERAL RECOMMENDATIONS

■ Lots of fresh air and good natural light in the room aid in healing.

■ Loose-fitting cotton clothing is recommended. Tight clothing causes further friction and breakdown of the skin.

■ Anyone who is immobilized or bedridden should be moved from side to side or, if possible, sat up every hour so that pressure is not always on the same areas. The bed should be kept clean and dry. The head of the bed should be elevated less than 30 degrees.

■ A specialized foam "egg-crate" mattress can help prevent bedsores. These mattresses have pockets of air that lessen pressure on each part of the skin surface.

■ A person with bedsores should be mobilized as soon as possible.

Bites and Stings, Insect and Spider

We have all experienced the pain, itchiness, and reddened swelling associated with bee, hornet, or wasp stings or gnat, flea, fly, ant or mosquito bites. Mosquitoes are probably the most common insect to bite humans. When they bite, they inject some of their saliva into the skin, causing an allergic reaction and itching. If you have a severe reaction, you will develop large red welts and a low-grade fever.

Bees loose their stingers at the time of their attacks, but wasps and hornets keep their stingers for the next assault. Fleas bite humans only incidentally, preferring to infect and live off household pets. Their bites are usually only slightly irritating, causing a small red bump or a welt. Fire ants are vicious, since they attach to the skin with their mouthparts and move around while repeatedly stinging their victims. The place where their mouth attaches become a red bump, and small blisters and, later, pustules form at the points of the stings. Fire ants are problematic because they attack their victims in large numbers.

Ticks prefer wooded areas, and are most likely to bite in the spring and summer. The local reaction to a tick bite is usually a small red bump, an allergic response to the tick's saliva or mouth parts. Bites from deer ticks pose and additional risk, as they can pass on Lyme disease. The initial symptoms of Lyme disease are a growing round rash at the site of the bite and, possibly, flulike symptoms. Later, more severe nervous system and joint symptoms may develop. Also, the rare person gets Rocky Mountain spotted fever from a tick bite infected with a microorganism known as *Rickettsia rickettsii*.

Scorpion stings usually produce painful swellings accompanied by nausea, fever, and vomiting. If seizures or increased blood pressure develops, emergency care is necessary. Most North American spiders have no interest in biting anyone, as they prefer to be left alone, and relatively few people are unfortunate enough to have been bitten by a brown recluse or black widow spider. Black widows like to live in woodpiles and brushy ground debris. Brown recluse spiders are common in the midwest and southwest, outdoors, and in attics and unused closets. If you suffer a bite from a venomous spider, you need emergency medical attention.

For most people, bites and stings cause minor discomfort. For some individuals, however, a severe allergy to bites and stings can make them quite dangerous. If you have ever had an allergic reaction to an insect bite or sting, seek immediate emergency medical treatment if you are bitten or stung again, especially if you develop wheezing or difficulty breathing.

CONVENTIONAL TREATMENT

■ Remove any bee, hornet, or wasp stinger with the back of a knife blade or by scraping it out with your fingernail. Do not pull the stinger out directly. Stingers are barbed, and doing this can squeeze more venom into the wound.

■ To remove a tick, do not try to pull it off with your fingers. Instead, use a pair of tweezers to grasp the head, and pull back slowly and firmly.

■ Cleanse your wound site with rubbing alcohol, apply a topical antibiotic such as bacitracin, and cover with a sterile dressing.

■ An oral antihistamine such as diphenhydramine (Benadryl, Diphenhist, and others) or chlorpheniramine (Chlor-Trimeton, Teldrin, and others) can help relieve the itching and swelling of a bite.

■ A low-dose over-the-counter cortisone cream such as Cortaid can be applied to the area for several days as needed to relieve itching.

■ If your reaction to the bite or sting is severe, or if the bite is from a brown recluse or black widow spider or scorpion, seek the help of a qualified physician immediately.

■ Depending on the severity of the reaction, a physician may prescribe topical or oral steroids. Antivenin is available for black widow spider bites.

■ If you have a history of severe reactions to bites or stings with swelling of the airway and difficulty breathing, you should keep an epinephrine kit on hand to use in a crisis, wear a Medic Alert bracelet to let emergency personnel know of your allergy, if necessary, and go to the emergency department of the nearest hospital immediately if you are bitten or stung. Your physician may recommend a desensitization program as well.

DIETARY MEASURES

■ Drink plenty of fluids to flush out toxins.

■ Take 1 gram (1,000 milligrams) of pantothenic acid as soon as possible after a bite. Then take an additional 500 milligrams every hour until the pain and swelling subside.

■ Vitamin C with bioflavonoids helps to reduce toxicity and inflammation. Take 5,000 milligrams a day, in divided doses, for two days. If you develop loose stools, cut this dosage in half. Vitamin C can also be applied topically to reduce inflammation. Mix vitamin-C powder with just enough water to make a paste, and apply it as often as needed.

■ Calcium and magnesium help to calm a nervous system on edge from the pain of a bad bite or sting. Take 250 milligrams of calcium with 125 milligrams of magnesium two or three times a day for four days.

■ To help prevent insect bites, take a B-vitamin complex twice a day starting three days before an outdoor trip and continue to take it throughout the trip. B vitamins are excreted through the skin and are believed to act as a repellent.

HERBAL TREATMENT

■ Aloe vera gel topically soothes stinging areas where bugs have bitten. Aloe vera extract can also be taken internally. Make sure you take only a food-grade aloe vera extract, not one designed to be used on your skin.

■ Calendula gel or cream is also useful. It helps to soothe the stinging and burning of the bite.

■ Cold packs of clay, cabbage, comfrey, plantain, tobacco, or baking soda locally are helpful in soothing the pain of bee and wasp stings.

■ Echinacea extract can help relieve pain and itching. Immediately after a bite or sting, take 250 to 500 milligrams, and take an additional dose every two to three hours for the rest of the day. Then take a dose three to four times a day for up to five days, as needed. German medical studies done as far back as 1952 and 1955 showed that echinacea inhibits the enzyme hyaluronidase, which is injected by the insects and breaks down body tissues at the site of the bite or sting. Liquid echinacea extract can also be applied directly to the bite.

■ To help prevent bites and stings, try the following natural bug repellents:
  • Citronella oil can be applied directly to the skin when out in bug-infested areas.

- Garlic capsules, 500 milligrams twice a day started 3 days before a wilderness trip and continued throughout the duration of the trip, help to keep bugs away.
- Pennyroyal oil is also a good natural bug repellent. However, do not use it during pregnancy.

AROMATHERAPY

▪ Apply a single drop of bergamot, blue chamomile, lavender, echinacea, goldenseal, pine, or tea tree essential oil directly on the affected area to help soothe the burning and pain of the bug bite or sting. Tea tree oil is usually the favored oil. Or, if you prefer, add 10 drops of the essential oil you like best to a quart of cold water and soak a clean cotton cloth in the mixture. Apply the resulting compress to the bite for ten to fifteen minutes four times a day.

▪ Witch hazel, which has gentle astringent and anti-inflammatory properties, can be applied to the affected areas several times a day for one to two days to help relieve itching. Adding 8 drops of peppermint oil to a 4-ounce bottle of witch hazel makes it even more soothing. Peppermint contains menthol, an antiseptic that irritates the skin just enough to calm the itching sensation. Shake the bottle well before using and apply the mixture with a cotton ball as needed. Store it in a cool, dark place.

▪ Commercial products combining the essential oils of citronella, echinacea, nettle, and rosemary are available to help with the sting of bug bites.

▪ Peppermint essential oil works well to discourage ants. Make an anti-ant spray by mixing eight ounces of water with 1 teaspoon of peppermint oil in a spritzer bottle. Shake well before spraying on counter tops, along baseboards, on windowsills, in cabinets, and anywhere else you see ants.

HOMEOPATHY

A 1995 randomized study of sixty-eight healthy volunteers done at the London School of Hygiene and Tropical Medicine found that mosquito bites treated with homeopathic gel were less inflamed when compared with untreated bites. However, bites treated with placebo gel also responded somewhat. More controlled studies need to be done on different types of bites and stings, testing different homeopathic remedies at varying strengths. Anecdotally, several homeopathic remedies have been found to be very effective at preventing bites and reducing the pain, swelling, and poisonous effects of bites and stings.

■ *Apis mellifica* 6c, 9c, 12x, or 30x is for rapidly swelling, burning, stinging bites that feel better with the application of ice. It is especially good for bee and wasp stings, as *Apis* is derived from the honeybee. Take one dose every fifteen minutes, up to a total of four doses.

■ *Cantharis* 30c is good for bee or wasp stings if they look especially red and angry.

■ *Carbolicum acidum* 30c is recommended for severe allergic reactions to bee stings and black widow spider bites. Take one dose every thirty to sixty minutes.

■ *Hypericum* 30c is especially good for bee or wasp stings accompanied by pain shooting up the involved limb.

■ *Lachesis* 30c is best for bites that turn bluish and feel better when cold is applied.

■ *Ledum* 6c, 9c, 12x, or 30x is especially helpful for brown recluse spider bites or bee or wasp stings that are cold and numb and relieved by cold applications. Take one dose every fifteen minutes, up to a total of four doses.

■ *Natrum muriaticum* 6x, applied topically, lessens the itching and burning of a bite.

■ *Urtica urens* 30c is good for the itching, burning, and stinging pain that accompanies a bite.

■ As insect repellents or as treatment for a bite or sting, the following tinctures can be applied externally:
  • For bee stings, *Apis mellifica, Ledum,* or *Urtica urens.*
  • For gnat bites, *Calendula* or *Hypericum.*
  • For wasp stings, *Arnica* or *Ledum.*
  • For all types of bites and stings, Rescue Remedy. This is available in cream form as well.

■ *Pyrethrum* tincture or spray can be used as a general insect repellent.
■ *Staphysagria* 12c can be taken orally as a mosquito repellent.

ACUPRESSURE

See Acupressure Points in Part Three for the locations of these points on the body.

▪ Pressing the Liver 3 point for three minutes helps the liver remove toxins from a bite or sting, calms the nervous system, and strengthens your immune system. Liver 3 is located on the top of the foot, in the web between your first and second toes, just after the small bones of the foot join the rest of your foot. Place your fingers under your foot and apply pressure to the Liver 3 point perpendicularly with your thumb. Take care not to press on the tendons and blood vessels, but in the hollow between the bones and tendons. Repeat on the other foot, and then as needed.

▪ Stimulating the Liver 1 acupoint improves the circulation in the lower abdomen to help eliminate toxins from the sting or bite. This point is located on the inside of the big toe, at the corner of the toenail. Press this acupoint using the edge of the fingernail from your thumb or index finger. Repeat on the other big toe, and then as needed.

▪ Pressing Bladder 65 acupoint for three to five minutes can help your bladder remove toxins from a bite or sting, and can reduce the pain. Bladder 65 is on the outside edge of the foot, in the depression under the bone just beyond where your fifth toe joins the rest of your foot. Supporting your foot with your fingers under your sole and your thumb on top of your foot, apply pressure to the Bladder 65 point using your index finger. Your fingernail should be edge-up underneath the bone and angled toward your fifth toe. Repeat on your other foot, and then as needed.

GENERAL RECOMMENDATIONS

▪ Apply ice to the site of a bite or sting to immediately reduce pain, swelling, and itching.

▪ Mix 2 teaspoons of baking soda and 2 teaspoons of Epsom salts with just enough water to make a paste. Apply the paste to a bite or sting and leave it on for twenty minutes to reduce pain, swelling, and redness. Or mix meat tenderizer with water to form a thick paste and apply to the bite or sting. There is an enzyme in the meat tenderizer that breaks down the venomous material and provides relief within a few minutes.

■ For wasp stings, apply vinegar immediately.

■ To help prevent insect bites, take the following commonsense precautions:

- Wear light-colored long pants, long-sleeves, gloves, and shoes in infested areas and when gardening.
- Avoid wearing fragrances, perfumed suntan lotion, and shiny jewelry when spending time outdoors.
- Apply a commercial insect repellent such as Cutter's or Off with DEET.
- Spray your clothing with permethrin, or Nix, as an insect repellent.

Body Odor

We have all had the experience of being around someone with strong and displeasing body odor. It's impossible to forget. No one wants to be remembered for such an undesirable characteristic.

Unpleasant body odor, or bromhidrosis, is most frequently due to excessive perspiration from the eccrine or apocrine sweat glands. This in turn causes an overgrowth of bacteria on the skin. The bacteria break down the top layer of skin cells and the sweat, forming chemicals that produce the unpleasant smell.

Apocrine bromhidrosis rarely occurs before puberty, since the apocrine sweat glands virtually do not function before then. As most apocrine sweat glands are located in the armpits, this is the smelliest area. People in groups that tend to have larger numbers of apocrine sweat glands, such as people of African ancestry, are affected to a greater extent than those who tend to have fewer apocrine sweat glands, such as older adults and people of Asian descent. Poor hygiene, of course, is another reason unpleasant smells come off the body. Diet can also be a factor. Sweat containing high levels of garlic, curry, or other spices also has a repellent odor. Taking certain medications can cause bad body odor, too.

Excessive eccrine sweating of the feet, most common in young men, is another common cause of bad body odor. Bromhidrosis from the feet occurs when the thick, warm, sodden skin becomes a breeding ground for numerous bacteria. Eccrine bromhidrosis can also occur in areas where skin contacts skin, especially between the thighs. This can be made worse by obesity and diabetes.

Other, more serious causes of offensive body odor include nutrient deficiencies, such as zinc deficiency; underlying medical problems such as genetic metabolic disorders, liver disease, or diabetes; and gastrointestinal problems such as parasites or chronic constipation. You should seek your physician's expertise to screen for these problems if excessive sweating, poor hygiene, or a spicy diet are not factors in causing the unpleasant body odor.

■ Wash thoroughly once or twice a day with an antibacterial or deodorant soap. Pay special attention to your feet, which are most affected by their warm, airless environment. Effective cleansers that kill off bacteria usually contain chlorhexidine (Hibiclens) or povidone-iodine (Betadine).

■ Shaving the armpits frequently can be very helpful.

■ Mild over-the-counter deodorants containing aluminum, zirconium, or zinc salts are generally the first line of defense against excessive eccrine sweating and bacterial growth.

■ Prescription drying agents containing aluminum chloride such as Xerac AC can be applied every night to underarms in more severe cases.

■ Applying a strong drying agent such as 20-percent aluminum chloride lotion (Drysol) to the underarms every night is prescribed in more severe cases.

■ Topical antibiotics such as gentamicin cream (Garamycin, Gentamar, G-Myticin) can be used in the armpits.

■ A scopolamine patch (Transderm-Scop), applied behind the ear and changed every three hours, may be prescribed as a drying agent.

■ For excessive foot sweating and odor, treatment with aluminum chloride solution is a starting place. Also, soaking the feet every day in Burow's solution at a 1-to-40 concentration decreases the number of bacteria on the feet. Formaldehyde-containing sprays and creams can be applied locally once or twice a day to reduce the amount of sweat produced by the feet. Using foot dusting powders and changing your socks often also helps control the smell.

■ Iontophoresis is one of the most effective methods of treating smelly feet resulting from excessive eccrine sweating. This involves the use of a device called a Drionic unit, which uses tap water and can be bought without a prescription. To use it, you simply place your feet on a water-soaked pad for several minutes every day. A very low electric current runs through the pad and stops the sweat glands from perspiring. The procedure is painless—most people feel nothing at all.

■ In severe cases, local surgery to remove the apocrine or eccrine sweat glands is possible.

DIETARY MEASURES

▪ Eat a wholesome, balanced diet rich in raw foods.

▪ Be sure to drink eight glasses of filtered water a day.

▪ In the morning and before bed at night, drink one glass of filtered water with the juice of a fresh lemon and one teaspoon of chlorophyll.

NUTRITIONAL SUPPLEMENTS

▪ The following supplements have been found to be helpful for body odor:

- Vitamin A. Take 25,000 international units daily for two weeks.
- Vitamin-B complex. Take a supplement containing 100 milligrams of each of the major B vitamins daily. Also take an additional 50 milligrams of vitamin B_6 (pyridoxine) daily and 50 milligrams of vitamin B_1 (thiamine) twice a day while the problem exists, then cut back to 20 milligrams every other day for three weeks.
- Vitamin C. Take 3,000 milligrams daily.
- Zinc. Take 50 milligrams daily.

HERBAL TREATMENT

▪ Alfalfa tablets contain a lot of chlorophyll, which has a deodorizing effect.

▪ Chlorophyll, available in soft gel capsules and chewable tablets, helps reduce embarrassing body odors.

▪ Parsley also is a good source of chlorophyll. Munching on several sprigs of parsley a day can help with body odor.

AROMATHERAPY

▪ Make an herbal spray deodorant by combining 5 drops each of sage, coriander, and lavender essential oils with 2 ounces of distilled witch hazel. Shake before each use.

■ Skin brushing daily with a natural bristle brush, followed by a bath to which a few drops of sage oil has been added, can be helpful.

HOMEOPATHY

■ *Hepar sulfuris calcareum* can be used for bad body odor.
■ *Sulfur* also can be taken for bromhidrosis.

ACUPRESSURE

See Acupressure Points in Part Three for the locations of these points on the body.

■ Chinese practitioners treat excessive perspiration causing body odor by strengthening the cooling meridians and dampening the heat. Press acupoints Bladder 64 and 66 and Kidney 3 and 8 on both legs for three minutes three times a day until improvement is seen. Bladder 64 is on the middle outside of the foot, just under the large bone before the heel. Bladder 66 is on the outside of the foot, just in the middle of the 5th toe. Kidney 3 is on the inside of the ankle, just behind the large bony prominence. Kidney 8 is just above and in front of the bony prominence of the ankle.

OTHER THERAPIES

■ Crystal deodorant stones are said to be equivalent to six cans of spray deodorant. These can be used on the underarms and feet. They are available either unscented or with herbal scents added.
■ Instead of using aluminum-based commercial antiperspirants, you can apply baking soda under the arms and between the toes.

Boils

A boil, or furuncle, is a bacterial infection with pus that develops around a hair follicle. Boils are very contagious and potentially serious if the infection spreads. A boil starts out as a tender, red, hot, tense bump and develops a yellowish point within 2 to 4 days. Boils are very painful, especially if they occur in skin that cannot move freely. The boil can burst open, discharging pus but relieving some of the pain. Unfortunately, boils heal with scarring.

Boils usually occur in areas that are hairy or that are exposed to lots of movement and friction. These include areas under the belt and on the neck, face, scalp, underarms, and buttocks. Boils can become chronic and come back time and again in the same areas.

The most common bacteria found in boils is *Staphylococcus aureus* (staph bacteria). They may be caused by other types of bacteria, however, depending on the location of the boil and the individual's immune function. In rare cases, boils may be a sign of an underlying immune problem or other disease. People with diabetes, alcoholism, cancer, or HIV/AIDS, and those on chemotherapy are especially susceptible to developing boils.

CONVENTIONAL TREATMENT

- Keep the area clean with a soap containing an antimicrobial agent such as chlorhexidine.
- Apply hot, wet compresses. These help to relieve the pain and bring the abscess to a point, which makes it easier to lance open.
- *Do not* squeeze the bump, as it may spread the infection. If it does not rupture or go away by itself, let your doctor cut it open, remove the contents, and allow it to drain. *Do not* try to cut it open yourself. If it is a large boil, the doctor may pack the remaining cavity with gauze. Local antibiotic creams are usually applied to the site of the wound.
- Always seek professional medical advice, especially if you also have a fever, chills, and/or malaise.
- An antibiotic that is effective against *Staphylococci,* such as dicloxacillin (Dynapen, Dycill, Pathocil) or amoxicillin/clavulanate (Augmentin), may

be prescribed. If you have had recurrent boils, have not done well with prior antibiotics, have a fever and malaise, are immunocompromised, or have boils that involve the central face, muscle, or deep tissues, a Gram stain and bacterial culture will be done by the doctor to determine which bacteria are causing the problem and which antibiotics are likely to be most effective.

■ If you are very ill or have an underlying disease, hospitalization and intravenous antibiotic therapy may be recommended.

■ If the boils keep returning, a doctor will look for an underlying disease. People with chronic illnesses may carry staph bacteria in their nasal passages or groins and continually reinfect themselves. Bacteria cultures of these sites are taken and, if *Staphylococcus aureus* is found, mupirocin (Bactroban Nasal) ointment is used twice daily in the nasal passages. Also, a course of the antibiotic rifampin (Rifadin, Rimactane) is usually given for two weeks to eradicate the bacteria.

■ If a boil develops around the mouth or on the lips, surgical drainage is not used because of the risk of the infection spreading to the brain through the bloodstream.

DIETARY MEASURES

■ Increase your intake of fluids. Drink water throughout the day.

■ Drink a glass of water with the juice of a fresh lemon and a teaspoon of chlorophyll on rising and before bed.

■ Limit your consumption of food products containing white sugar and white flour.

■ Foods rich in vitamin A, such as yellow-orange fruits and vegetables and dark green leafy vegetables, aid in the rapid healing of boils. Try to have at least four different types of green vegetables a day.

■ Foods full of zinc, including oysters, sunflower seeds, and pumpkin seeds, also speed healing of boils and should be included in the diet.

NUTRITIONAL SUPPLEMENTS

■ The following supplements are helpful to help heal the skin quickly, boost the immune system, and fight inflammation:

- Vitamin A. Take 25,000 international units daily for two weeks.
- Beta-carotene. Take 25,000 international units daily for two weeks.
- B-complex vitamins. Take a balanced B-complex supplement daily.
- Vitamin C with bioflavonoids. Take 3,000 milligrams daily.
- Zinc. Take 50 milligrams daily for two weeks.

HERBAL TREATMENT

- Astralagus tea helps to enhance immunity. Drink eight glasses a day.
- Calendula ointment can to applied to the skin overlying an unbroken boil to decrease inflammation and act as an antiseptic.
- Garlic is a natural antibiotic and immune-system booster. It can be taken in capsule form.
- Goldenseal-root powder can be mixed with enough boiling water to make a paste and used as a topical poultice to draw out the boil.
- A mixture of 25 grams (2,500 milligrams) of powdered slippery elm, 3 drops of eucalyptus oil, and just enough boiling water to form a thick paste can be applied to the boil. Leave it on until the paste cools, then make a fresh batch and reapply it. Repeat this until the pus is discharged from the boil. Marshmallow leaf or figwort can also be made into a poultice to draw out pus.
- Tea tree oil can be applied externally to a boil as an antiseptic against bacteria and fungi. The pure oil will probably irritate inflamed skin, but a mixture of a few drops in a couple of tablespoons of any vegetable oil should not cause a problem. Do not take tea tree oil internally.
- A tea made from two parts wild indigo to one part each of echinacea, pasque flower, and poke root can be drunk three times a day to speed healing. The tea can also be applied externally to a boil to limit infection.

AROMATHERAPY

- Echinacea, myrrh, or tea tree essential oils can be applied to a boil to limit infection. These oils have a direct antimicrobial effect and increase the numbers of white blood cells fighting infection.
- Bergamot, chamomile, clary sage, and lavender oil can also be used to draw out the boil.

HOMEOPATHY

■ When the lesion is rapidly forming, red, and tender, *Belladonna,* usually in 6c, 12c, or 30c potency, is taken every one to two hours, up to a total of ten doses or until the pus is released.

■ When the lesion becomes increasingly large and pus-filled, it is often treated with *Hepar sulfuris* 6c, 12c, or 30c every one to two hours, up to a total of ten doses. This remedy is also good for darkish blue, extremely painful boils that develop more slowly.

■ For persistent eruptions, *Silicia* 12c or 30c four times a day until improvement is noted is often recommended.

■ *Arnica* 30c is good for crops of sore boils all over the body.

■ *Calcarea sulfurica* is for boils discharging pus.

■ *Echinacea* 12c is recommended for recurrent boils.

■ *Rhus toxicodendron* 30c is helpful for dark red, intensely painful, pus-filled swellings.

■ Ten drops of *Hypericum* tincture can be added to 1 cup of warm water to make compresses to relieve the pain and encourage healing. Apply a compress to the affected area for fifteen minutes four times a day.

ACUPRESSURE

See Acupressure Points in Part Three for the locations of these points on the body.

■ To release muscular tension that prevents good local blood flow to the boil, press the Golden Points closest to the sore. Repeat twice a day. The Golden Points are twenty acupoints around the body frequently used for common injuries and illnesses.

GENERAL RECOMMENDATIONS

■ Rest the affected skin and avoid external friction and trauma.

■ Wash your hands frequently.

■ Use clean washcloths and change towels and sheets daily.

Bruises

The pain, swelling, and varied skin discoloration of a bruise comes from damage to the soft tissues beneath the skin, usually due to an injury. Blood leaks from the small capillaries below the skin's surface into the surrounding tissues. The bruise usually turns from red to black-and-blue to yellowish-brown as the tissues reabsorb the leaked blood. Often there is some associated swelling and redness of the surrounding tissues.

Bruises are generally more common in children and women. Certain medications, including anticoagulants (blood-thinners), steroids, anti-inflammatory drugs, painkillers, and some antibiotics, can cause easy bruising. If you have bruises that do not fade after a week or that recur frequently without known injury, you need to see your physician. This can be a sign of internal organ, anemia, or bleeding problems; vitamin-C or bioflavonoid deficiency; malnutrition or obesity; or underlying stress that is depleting your body's stores of vitamin C.

You've probably seen cartoons of fighters using raw beefsteak to treat black eyes and other bad bruises. Well, there are plenty of other good natural treatments as well!

CONVENTIONAL TREATMENT

- Apply a cold pack to the bruise in the first fifteen minutes to help reduce the pain and swelling. Repeat about four times a day.
- Avoid taking aspirin or other anti-inflammatories that increase bruising.
- While a bruise is fading, you can use makeup to help cover it. A color corrector, concealer, foundation, then makeup can be applied over the bruise to help disguise its presence.
- If there is not an immediately obvious injury to explain bruising, a physician needs to do blood tests to rule out thyroid disease, connective tissue disease, blood disorders, or abnormalities in the adrenal gland or other internal medical problems as possible causes for the bruising.

DIETARY MEASURES

■ If you bruise easily, be sure to consume fish, green leafy vegetables, and buckwheat to supply vitamins D and K, which are used by the body for blood clotting. Vitamin D is readily found in fatty fish, including salmon and mackerel. Vitamin K is found in dark green leafy vegetables and alfalfa sprouts. The same vegetables are also a good source of iron, which is key for new red blood cell formation. Rutin, an important bioflavonoid for maintaining strong capillaries and increasing blood-vessel elasticity, is abundant in citrus fruits and buckwheat.

■ Include in your diet plenty of citrus fruits, and drink citrus juices and rose hip tea. These contain vitamin C, which is important for the maintenance of strong capillaries.

NUTRITIONAL SUPPLEMENTS

■ Nutritional supplements recommended for preventing and clearing bruises include the following:

- Vitamin C with bioflavonoids. Take 3,000 milligrams twice a day. You can also apply topical 10-percent vitamin-C lotion directly on the bruise. Vitamin C strengthens the collagen around blood vessels. Topical vitamin C has been shown to markedly decrease bruising as compared to placebo.
- Vitamin D. Take 400 international units daily.
- Vitamin E. Take 400 international units of a supplement containing mixed tocopherols daily.
- Vitamin K. Take 80 micrograms daily. You can also apply topical 1-percent vitamin-K cream directly on the bruise. Topical vitamin-K cream is probably the most effective vitamin treatment for bruises. Vitamin K promotes blood clotting and strengthens blood vessel walls, thereby helping to prevent bleeding.
- Iron. Take 15 milligrams daily.
- Zinc. Take 50 milligrams daily.

■ Arnica is highly recommended for the treatment of bruises by the Commission E, the body of experts that advises the German government about herbs. Arnica has pain-relieving, antiseptic, and anti-inflammatory properties. It is particularly good for bruises if the skin isn't broken. Make a soaking solution from 1 tablespoon of arnica tincture diluted in 1 pint of cool water. Apply a compress soaked in this mixture to your bruises for a few minutes several times a day.

Caution: Do not use arnica if your skin is scratched or cut, as it can cause arnica poisoning.

■ Bromelain, an active ingredient found in pineapples, inhibits inflammation and stimulates the anti-inflammatory response to a bruise. Take 150 to 450 milligrams three times a day on an empty stomach to speed the healing of bruises.

■ Cabbage leaves made into cold wraps soothe the pain and swelling of an early bruise.

■ Calendula lotion or ointment is very soothing for mild bruises.

■ Comfrey, also known as bruisewort, contains allantoin, a compound that speeds skin repair and promotes new cell growth. It also helps constrict blood vessels and has anti-inflammatory properties. Boil a handful of comfrey leaves, cool and strain the leaves, and then soak the bruised or swollen body part with a poultice made by wrapping the leaves in a light cloth, such as gauze or cheesecloth. Or apply commercially prepared comfrey ointment directly to the bruise. Quick action can prevent some of the discoloration.

Caution: Do not take comfrey internally, as it may be toxic to the liver.

■ Repeatedly applying crushed parsley leaves to the bruise is said to clear up black-and-blue marks within a couple of days.

■ Applying a slice of raw potato is also supposed to speed healing of the bruise.

■ St. John's wort oil has been endorsed by Commission E for treatment of bruises. Apply the commercial oil to the bruised areas two or three times a day to speed healing and reduce pain. Or steep 1 to 2 teaspoons of the dried herb in vegetable oil for a few days, then apply the oil directly to the bruise.

■ Witch hazel is an early American remedy that is good for bruises. Its leaves and bark are very astringent and drying.

AROMATHERAPY

■ Put a few drops of lavender oil on a gauze compress and place it on the bruise. Other essential oils that can be used directly on bruises include everlasting, geranium, ginger, juniper, marjoram, and thyme.

■ Rescue Remedy cream can be applied to bruises on unbroken skin to soothe and speed healing.

■ Rub the bruise with thyme oil and tea tree oil diluted in olive oil, alternately, one in the morning and the other in the evening, to aid in healing.

HOMEOPATHY

■ *Arnica* 30c is the most important homeopathic remedy for bruising. Take a dose two or three times a day for a few days immediately after an injury to relieve pain and help the body reabsorb blood.

■ *Bellis perennis* 30c is good for bruises with bumps and lumps remaining.

■ *Ferrum phosphoricum* 30c can help bad bruises. Take 4 tablets every fifteen minutes until the pain is relieved. Then take 1 tablet three times a day to decrease swelling and inflammation of a bad bruise. *Kali muriaticum* 30c can be used the same way.

■ *Hamamelis* tincture, ointment, cream, or lotion is astringent and very helpful when applied directly on bruises, as long as the skin is not broken.

■ *Ledum* 6c or 12c is the best remedy for a black eye and for any bruise that feels cold, lingers on, and feels better when cold is applied.

■ *Ruta graveolens* 6c is especially good for severe bruises involving the bone, such as the shin. Take 2 tablets every hour for three hours after an injury. Then take 1 tablet three times a day for up to 1 week.

■ *Salicylicum acidum* is good for bruises that are slow to heal.

ACUPRESSURE

See Acupressure Points in Part Three for the locations of these points on the body.

■ Press the Golden Point nearest the site of injury as soon as possible. Repeat twice a day. The Golden Points are twenty points located around the body that are commonly used for injuries and illnesses.

■ Using the backs of your hands, briskly rub your lower back for one minute as you breathe deeply. Repeat this twice a day. This stimulates both the inner and outer Sea of Vitality points, Bladder 23 and Bladder 47, at the same time. These are located on the lower back, two to four finger-widths away from the spine at waist level.

■ For a bruise on the upper body, rubbing Large Intestine 15 is good for relieving the swelling and pain. This point is located on the tip of the shoulder, in the depression between the the bones found when your arms are by your sides. Place your thumb over the collarbone for support and press the point with your index or middle finger, angled slightly upward toward the shoulder. Repeat on the other shoulder. Do this twice a day.

■ Pressure on Liver 3 helps to repair small blood vessels and to clear bruises. This point is on the top of the foot in the web between the first and second toes, just before the joints of the small bones of the foot. Place your fingers under the foot for support, and press perpendicularly with your thumb in the hollow between the bone, tendons, and the blood vessels. Repeat on the other foot. Do this twice a day.

Burns

When you get a burn, you know it! You can get burned by dry heat from a fire, stove, or the sun; moist heat from hot liquids or steam; chemicals; or electricity. Burns are classified as first-degree, second-degree, third-degree, and fourth-degree, depending on how many layers of skin and underlying tissue they involve. First-degree burns involve only the epidermis and are characterized by pain, heat, and redness of the top layer of the skin. Sunburn is usually a first-degree burn. Second-degree burns go through part of the skin layers under the epidermis, in the dermis. They are extremely painful with swelling, blistering, and seeping of fluids. A third-degree burn destroys the nerves and blood vessels, so there is little pain at first, but excruciating pain later. The skin may be charred black, white, yellow, or bright red. Fourth-degree burns penetrate the body to destroy underlying muscle, bone, and internal tissue. Loss of body fluids, electrolyte disturbances, and danger of infection are typical.

Depending on the location, extent, and cause of your burn, you may need emergency medical care. Burns of the face, palms of the hands, soles of the feet, and joints can cause serious problems, no matter how small their size or what their degree of severity is. A burn in any of these areas should always be checked out by a physician and watched. If a second-degree burn is larger than the size of a quarter, you should seek professional medical advice. Third- and fourth-degree burns are always medical emergencies, and professional help should be sought immediately. All burns should be watched until thoroughly healed for signs of infection.

CONVENTIONAL TREATMENT

■ First, stop the burning. Put out flames, wash off chemicals, or break contact with whatever is causing the burn.

■ Expose a mildly burned area to warm running water until the pain becomes bearable, for about ten minutes. Applying cold compresses or ice water is not recommended. These measures may be more soothing in the short run, but they lead to greater pain later.

- Never apply butter, petroleum jelly, or any other greasy substance to a burn. This only traps the heat and can cause a burn to deepen.
- While cooling the burn, remove any watches, rings, belts, or bracelets from the affected area before the burned skin swells around these items.
- Cover exposed mildly burned areas with a light sterile dressing over a thin film of a topical antibiotic such as silver sulfadiazine (Silvadene, SSD, Thermazene) or bacitracin. Do not cover the affected areas tightly, as this will trap heat and deepen the burn.
- Do not burst any blisters over the burns. Blisters are natural bandages that help the burn to heal.
- If you have a chemical burn, immediately flood the affected area with cool running water to dilute and wash away the chemical.
- If the burn affects your mouth, you should immediately consult your dentist to be sure the wound heals properly.
- Always go to the emergency room to be evaluated after an electrical burn, even if it seems to be minor. There may be deep burns and internal damage that you cannot see.
- Acetaminophen (in Tylenol and other products), ibuprofen (Advil, Nuprin, and others), codeine, or hydrocodone may be precribed for the pain.
- If a burn is deep, oral or intravenous antibiotics will be prescribed to prevent a secondary infection from setting in.
- Deep burns need to be cleaned and the dead skin removed in the emergency room. Do not remove any clothing that is stuck to the burn before getting to the doctor's. Keep warm to prevent shock. For severe burns, you will be admitted to a hospital burn unit and your fluid and electrolyte status will be carefully monitored and controlled. Artificial skin or tissue cultured from your own skin cells may be used in severe cases.

DIETARY MEASURES

- Burns greatly increase the body's need for protein and energy, as the injured tissues' requirements skyrocket and your metabolism speeds up. Eat lots of lean, high-quality protein foods.
- A diet high in green and yellow vegetables helps to provide enough beta-carotene and vitamin C, which are important in the healing process.

- Eat pumpkin seeds and oysters to supply much-needed zinc.
- Drink lots of filtered water to replace fluids lost through the burn.

NUTRITIONAL SUPPLEMENTS

- The following vitamins and other supplements are recommended for burns:
  - Beta-carotene, a precursor to vitamin A, helps burned skin to heal. It is also an antioxidant that fights free radicals, which are increased by burns. Take 10,000 to 25,000 international units daily.
  - Calcium is a vital mineral that needs to be replaced following a burn. Take at least 1,200 milligrams a day if burns cover 30 percent or more of the body, particularly if you are immobilized.
  - Vitamin C may decrease fluid loss after a burn, and is an important antioxidant. Take 1,000 milligrams daily. Vitamin C can also be applied topically. Mix 2 tablespoons of powdered vitamin C in ½ cup aloe vera gel and apply it to the affected area.
  - A study conducted at the University of Texas Burn Unit found that levels of vitamin E were at only 25 percent of normal after severe burns. To replenish this vital antioxidant, take 400 international units daily. To reduce scarring, vitamin-E oil or cream can also be applied twice a day once the burn has healed.
  - Zinc helps in wound healing. Take 50 milligrams daily.
  - Free-form amino acids supply dietary proteins. Take a free-form amino-acid supplement as directed by the manufacturer.

HERBAL TREATMENT

- Aloe is the most important herb for mild burns. Applying aloe vera gel directly from the fresh plant eases the pain and keeps the burn from turning white and blistering. Some people prefer commercial preparations because they smell better and go on more easily and neatly. Aloe gel works on several enzyme systems to decrease pain, reduce inflammation, speed wound healing, and stimulate new skin-cell growth. It also has antibacterial and antifungal properties, and increases the amount of blood bringing healing resources to the areas of burned tissue. Aloe is strong enough to relieve burns caused by radiation therapy for cancer. Many people keep an aloe plant on the kitchen windowsill in case of burns from cooking.

■ Calendula cream can be applied directly to a burn for soothing relief of pain, as well as for its antiseptic properties and prevention of scarring.

■ Comfrey cream can also used to help increase tissue regrowth and for its healing properties.

■ Echinacea stimulates the immune system to prevent and fight infection, which is common after a burn. Take 1 to 2 teaspoons of tincture of echinacea immediately after a burn. You can also apply a few drops directly to the burn to benefit from echinacea's mildly antiseptic properties.

■ Gotu kola, taken orally with vitamin C supplements, helps to speed healing of skin tissue by stimulating collagen synthesis.

■ Plantain is one of the most popular American folk medicines for burns. Juice from the fresh leaves of the plantain is very soothing when applied directly to mild burns.

■ St. John's wort oil is frequently helpful for reducing pain, inflammation, healing time, and scarring of first-degree burns. To make the oil, steep 1 to 2 teaspoons of the dried herb in a few ounces of vegetable oil for several days. Or you can apply a few drops of St. John's wort tincture to a burn.

AROMATHERAPY

■ Combine 4 ounces of aloe vera juice with ⅛ teaspoon of lavender essential oil in a glass spray bottle. Shake it and spray on the affected area as often as needed to soothe burned skin. For additional cooling relief, the bottle can be kept in the refrigerator.

■ Lavender oil alone can be dripped directly on the wound. It is said to have remarkable pain-relieving and burn-healing powers. Remember never to ingest essential oils, though, as even a small amount can be toxic.

■ Tea tree oil also soothes and sterilizes burns.

HOMEOPATHY

The homeopathic remedies listed here are useful for different types of burns. The usual recommendation is to take one dose every thirty minutes, up to a total of three doses.

- *Apis mellifica* 12x or 6c helps to heal a burn that bubbles and resembles a bee sting.
- *Arnica* 200c is used to prevent shock associated with burns.
- *Arsenicum album* 30c is used to aid blistering burns that feel better when heat is applied.
- *Belladona* 30x or 9c helps to reduce severe redness and throbbing pain.
- *Calendula* lotion is antiseptic and prevents scarring, especially in second-degree burns with blistering. Add 10 drops of homeopathic tincture to 1 cup of cold water and apply it directly to the burn or to the dressing over the burn to keep it moist and cool.
- *Cantharis* 30c can be taken every ten minutes after the first *Arnica* dose for pain relief in second- and third-degree burns. It is good for burns that blister and feel better with cool compresses.
- *Causticum* 30c is best for second- and third-degree burns with blistering.
- *Hypericum* lotion is antiseptic, and is recommended for second-degree burns. Add 10 drops of homeopathic tincture to 1 cup of cold water and apply it directly to the burn or to the dressing over the burn to keep it moist and cool.
- *Kali bichromicum* 30c is recommended for deep burns that are slow to heal.
- *Urtica urens* 30c is good for minor, stinging burns.
- *Urtica urens* lotion can be used for first-degree burns. Add 10 drops of homeopathic tincture to 1 cup of cold water and apply it directly to the burn or to the dressing over the burn to keep it moist and cool.

ACUPRESSURE

See Acupressure Points in Part Three for the locations of these points on the body.

- Press the Golden Points near the burned area at least three times a day to increase local blood flow, which will remove toxins and bring needed nutrients to the area.
- To relieve the pain of the burn and speed healing, press Bladder 65 on each foot for three minutes three times a day. This point is on the outside edge of the foot, in the depression under the bone just beyond the joint joining the fifth toe to the foot. With your thumb on top of the foot and

your fingers under the sole of the foot, use your index finger to apply pressure to the acupoint. Your finger should be pointed toward the fifth toe, with your nail edge pointing up underneath the bone.

OTHER THERAPIES

■ Electrotherapy may be helpful for promoting the healing of burns and the regeneration of normal-appearing skin.

Canker Sores

Canker sores, or aphthous ulcers, are painful small, craterlike ulcers. They are gray-based with red rims. They usually develop on the insides of the cheeks, the inner lips, and the loose parts of the gums, mouth, and lips. Less commonly, they can affect the esophagus and rest of the gastrointestinal tract. There is usually a burning and tingling sensation starting twenty-four hours before the ulcers actually form, and it is most helpful to start treatment as soon as this is felt. Canker sores can be so painful that they interfere with speaking, eating, and nutrition.

If they are less than one centimeter (about one-half inch) in diameter, they are called minor aphthous ulcers. These usually heal by themselves within a week or two. If they are greater than 3 centimeters in diameter, they are classified as major aphthous ulcers, and it often takes six weeks for them to finally heal. When they do, they leave scars. Both small and large ulcers often return, either singly or in crops.

Canker sores are the most common disorder to affect the oral mucous membranes, with between 20 and 50 percent of Americans affected. Women are more likely to be affected than men, usually starting in their twenties or thirties. Some people seem to have an inherited tendency to form canker sores.

Canker sores may be infectious, resulting from a local bacterial or viral infection. They commonly have one or more triggers, including food allergies, acidic mouth conditions, minor injury to the tissues of the mouth, smoking, vitamin deficiencies, stress, extreme heat, fever, and premenstrual and postmenopausal hormonal changes. People with poorly functioning immune systems are also very susceptible to canker sores.

CONVENTIONAL TREATMENT

■ Over-the-counter medicines such as Zilactin and Anbesol can be used to numb the pain.

■ Topical 2-percent lidocaine (viscous Xylocaine) may be prescribed. Swishing 1 teaspoonful around your mouth, then spitting it out, numbs the pain of the ulcers. This can be used frequently during the day, as needed for pain, and is recommended before meals to reduce the discomfort of eating.

▨ Various oral antibiotic suspensions and solutions can be swished in the mouth for two minutes, then swallowed. Choices include penicillin VK suspension, clindamycin (Cleocin T), and tetracycline.

▨ Topical steroids formulated for use in the mouth, such as 50-percent fluocinonide (Lidex) in orabase, may be applied to mouth ulcers three times a day. Less commonly, injections of triamcinolone are given directly into the mouth ulcers.

▨ Your physician may look for gastrointestinal disease or other "hidden" disease that causes vitamin deficiency. Some people also have gluten sensitivity, an intolerance to wheat that results in breakdown of the intestinal lining if wheat products are eaten, causing the gut to be "leaky" and lose nutrients.

▨ Hormonal therapy such as progestin injections are used to control mouth ulcers that occur premenstrually on a regular basis.

▨ If attacks of major ulcers are severe, oral steroids given when the tingling and burning recur can sometimes abort a flare-up. Oral corticosteroids may also be used during the course of severe ulcerations to speed healing.

▨ Drugs that alter the immune response, such as azathioprine (Imuran), dapsone, or colchicine, may be used in extremely severe cases.

▨ Thalidomide (Thalomid) may be extremely effective for very serious major aphthous ulcers that have failed to respond to other treatments. This drug causes birth defects; it must not be used by pregnant women.

DIETARY MEASURES

▨ Food allergens, especially wheat and milk, are responsible for almost 40 percent of cases of canker sores. Try eliminating these foods from your diet for several weeks to see if the problem resolves. Keep a food diary and look for correlations between what you eat and flare-ups of canker sores.

▨ Avoid acidic foods, such as citrus fruits, sugar, vinegar, chewing gum, alcohol, dairy products, meat, spicy foods, chocolate, caffeine, and toothpaste containing sodium lauryl sulfate, all of which irritate canker sores.

■ Canker sores may be due to a deficiency of vitamin B_{12}, folic acid, zinc, the amino acid lysine, or iron, so these nutrients may need to be supplemented aggressively. The following supplements are recommended for people with canker sores:

- Vitamin B_{12}. Take 1,000 micrograms daily. Also take a vitamin-B complex with 100 milligrams of most of the major B vitamins three times a day, with meals.
- Vitamin C with bioflavonoids. Take 1,000 milligrams three times a day, with meals.
- Zinc. Take 50 to 100 milligrams a day.
- Iron. Take 15 milligrams a day.
- Folic acid. Take 400 milligrams twice a day.
- L-Lysine. Take 4 grams (4,000 milligrams) daily for the first four days, then cut back to 500 milligrams three times a day. Take this supplement on an empty stomach.

■ Supplementation with acidophilus powder or capsules to restore the healthy balance of bacteria in the mucous membranes of the mouth is often helpful.

■ Applying the oil from one vitamin-E capsule directly to the sores helps to clear the lesions more quickly.

HERBAL TREATMENT

■ Aloe vera juice, available by the gallon, swished around in your mouth three times a day like a mouthwash, often yields good results. Aloe contains salicylates, which are anti-inflammatory and relieve pain, and it also has mild antibacterial properties.

■ Chlorophyll is a blood detoxifier. Chlorophyll tablets are sometimes chewed for the treatment of canker sores.

■ A soothing antiseptic mouth rinse can be made of ½ teaspoon of goldenseal powder and ¼ teaspoon salt dissolved in 1 cup of warm water. Use this as a mouth rinse four times a day. Goldenseal helps reduce inflammation of mucous membranes, and has also been shown to have antibacterial properties.

■ Licorice is soothing and has antiviral and antibacterial properties. It provides relief for the pain and contains both tannin and glycyrrhizin, which help to speed the healing of mouth sores. Swish iicorice root tea around in your mouth twice a day.

■ Myrrh was used by early American settlers as a treatment for mouth sores. Today, Germany's Commission E, which does research on herbal treatments, has endorsed powdered myrrh for the treatment of canker sores. Myrrh contains tannin, an antiseptic with antibacterial and antiviral action. Just open a capsule of myrrh and dab a little powder directly on the sores.

■ After brewing a cup of regular black, raspberry, sage, peppermint, or licorice tea, take the bag and tuck it in your mouth, covering the sore. Tea contains tannic acid, which is the active healing ingredient in the over-the-counter drug Zilactin.

HOMEOPATHY

■ *Hypercal*, a mixture of *Calendula* and *Hypericum*, can be made into a mouthwash with one part tincture and three parts water that has been boiled and cooled. Use it frequently, swishing it around in your mouth and massaging it into the gums. Use this in combination with the appropriate internal remedy.

■ *Mercurius solubilis* is the major mouth-ulcer remedy, especially for ulcers on the gums, on the tongue, and in the mouth. It is best for ulcers associated with an increase in saliva and a flabby, indented tongue.

■ *Natrum muriaticum* 12c is recommended for the onset of mouth ulcers. It is particularly helpful for those who have recurrences of cold sores after a disappointment or a grief that is not expressed. Take a dose three times a day for two days.

■ *Nitricum acidum* is best for painful ulcers on the edge of the tongue associated with bad breath, an increase in saliva, and gums that bleed easily.

ACUPRESSURE

See Acupressure Points in Part Three for the locations of these points on the body.

■ The Small Intestine and Liver meridians should be strengthened to help keep necessary nutrients and get rid of toxins in food. Press the Liver 3 and Small Intestine 10 points on both sides of the body for three minutes three times a day until the ulcers have healed. Liver 3 is located on the top of the foot, in the web between the first and second toes, just before the small bones of the foot join the rest of the foot. Small Intestine 10 is on the upper outer back, just where the armpit meets the upper back.

■ Stomach 4 and Large Intestine 4 promote good oral hygiene. Stomach 4 is located at each corner of the mouth. Rest your thumbs against the jawbone and locate the acupoints with your middle or index fingers. Apply pressure to the corners of the mouth, pressing against the teeth and gums underneath. Repeat this twice a day. Large Intestine 4 is located in the center of the triangle made between the small bones of the thumb and index finger. Press deeply and perpendicularly into the point using the thumb of the opposite hand. Repeat using the other hand. Do this twice a day.

■ Bladder 10 helps to relieve the discomfort of the mouth ulcers. These points are located on the nape of the neck, just below the hairline, two fingerwidths on either side of the spine, in the depressions inside of each trapezius, or large neck muscle. Press this point on both sides of the body for three minutes three times a day.

GENERAL RECOMMENDATIONS

■ Rinse your mouth with warm salt water, holding the salt water on the sores for several minutes, three times a day.

■ Placing ice directly on the sores can help dull the pain.

Cold Sores

Cold sores, or fever blisters, are blisters caused by the herpes simplex virus 1 (HSV-1) and can occur anywhere around the mouth. They are transmitted by direct contact with the skin or mucous membranes of someone who already has cold sores. This generally takes place in childhood or early adulthood. When the sores heal, the virus remains dormant in local nerve cells. In about two-thirds of cases, they return in the same area at a later time. Cold sores are often thought of as a stress-related illness, as the transmission of the virus is a function of immune status, and flare-ups usually occur at times of some kind of stress. The virus can be reactivated by colds, hot weather, nutrient deficiencies, hormonal fluctuations, fatigue, fever, and other illnesses. By the age of fifty, more than 90 percent of the U.S. population has had cold sores at least once.

Before the lesions appear, there is usually tingling, itching, throbbing, and burning pain at the site where the rash will later develop. Then painful small, tense blisters on red bases develop, either singly or in clusters. During the initial episode, there may be almost no symptoms at all, but often people experience accompanying fever, fatigue, neckache, and swelling of local lymphatic glands. Within a few days to several weeks the blisters burst, dry out, encrust, and go away. The rash is contagious from the time of the first tingling until the blisters have healed over with a yellowish crust. Because the virus sheds during the tingling stage, before any sore is visible, cold sores are often spread unknowingly.

CONVENTIONAL TREATMENT

■ Viscous Xylocaine may be prescribed to relieve pain of cold sores. This is a 2-percent lidocaine solution that is swished around in the mouth several times a day.

■ Acyclovir (Zovirax), valacyclovir (Valtrex), and famcyclovir (Famvir) are prescription antiviral medications that may be used to prevent and heal flare-ups of cold sores.

■ Topical penciclovir cream (Denavir) also may be prescribed for the treatment of cold sores.

■ The amino acid lysine inhibits the growth of herpes viruses, while another amino acid, arginine, makes the virus grow very rapidly. While cold sores are active, you should eat a diet containing a relatively higher amount of lysine compared with that of arginine. Dairy foods, fish, seafood, chicken, turkey, eggs, black beans, lentils, soybeans, brewer's yeast, potatoes, and other foods rich in lysine should be the mainstay of the diet. Foods high in arginine, like most cereal grains, seeds, nuts, peanut butter, chocolate, coconut, beer, raisins, and gelatin should be avoided.

■ Avoid immune-weakening foods such as sweets, alcohol, coffee, tea, and junk food.

■ Avoid acidic citrus fruits and juices, which burn the mouth and slow healing.

NUTRITIONAL SUPPLEMENTS

■ When a flare-up starts, take 1,500 milligrams of supplemental L-lysine daily for two weeks. Lysine is also available in a cream form that can be applied directly on the blisters every few hours. Lysine Lipclear Coldstick SPF 21 is a product containing lysine; vitamins A, D, and E; and fourteen different immune-system boosters and natural antiseptic herbs to protect and heal the lips from cold sores and sun damage, which can cause flare-ups.

■ Dissolve ½ teaspoon of acidophilus powder in 2 ounces of warm water to balance the acidity of the body and thereby speed healing. Take this mixture twice a day, between meals.

■ The following nutrients have also been found helpful to reduce the number and frequency of cold sores:

- A high-potency multivitamin. Take this daily as directed by the manufacturer.
- Beta-carotene. Take 10,000 international units daily.
- Vitamin B complex. Take a formula containing 100 milligrams of the major B vitamins daily.
- Vitamin C with bioflavonoids. Take 3,000 to 8,000 milligrams daily, divided into three doses.
- Vitamin E. Take 200 to 400 international units daily. Vitamin-E oil can also be applied directly to the sores three times a day.

- Zinc. Take 50 milligrams daily. Zinc can also be applied topically in the form of zinc oxide.
- Flaxseed oil. Take 1 tablespoon daily.
- Selenium. Take 100 micrograms daily.
- Quercetin. Take 1,000 milligrams daily.

HERBAL TREATMENT

■ Echinacea and goldenseal make an antiviral, immune-stimulating, detoxifying herbal combination that is helpful in the treatment of cold sores. Take ¼ teaspoon each of echinacea and goldenseal tinctures in tea or juice three times a day. Or combine equal parts of echineacea, Siberian ginseng, nettle, and goldenseal tinctures and take ½ teaspoon of this mixture three times a day to strengthen your immune system and make it less vulnerable to infection.

■ Garlic has antiviral properties. Take two capsules twice a day for a week. Or simply add a few minced garlic cloves to pasta or salad every day that your cold sores are active.

■ Lemon balm, also known as melissa, has anti-herpes properties and is felt by some to be a first-choice herbal treatment. Make lemon balm tea by steeping 2 to 4 teaspoons of the herb in a cup of boiling water. Apply the tea to the cold sores with a cotton ball four times a day. In Europe, a lemon balm ointment containing 700 milligrams of dry leaf material per gram of ointment is widely used.

■ Lemon balm is only one of the herbs in the mint family that are effective anti-herpes agents and contain at least four antiviral compounds. Other members of this family include hyssop, oregano, rosemary, sage, and thyme.

■ Diluted calendula, myrrh, tea tree oil, slippery elm, St. John's wort, and licorice can also be used topically to aid in healing. You can brew a strong tea from any of these herbs and dab it on your cold sores with a cotton ball after it cools.

AROMATHERAPY

Aromatherapy helps with herpes by improving immunity, relieving stress, and easing the pain and discomfort.

■ At the first signs of an outbreak, chamomile, clary sage, eucalyptus, geranium, lavender, lemon, myrrh, rose, or tea tree oil can be applied directly to your cold sores using cotton balls. This will speed healing and reduce the severity of the outbreak. Be careful not to swallow the essential oils.

■ Erpace is a commercial lip balm that combines essential oils of chamomile, oregano, and marjoram, and has a convenient roll-on applicator for the treatment of cold sores.

HOMEOPATHY

■ *Natrum muriaticum* 12c or 30c is the best choice if sores are on the lips, the corners of the mouth, or around the mouth. It is also useful if cold sores are due to sun exposure or a grief reaction.

■ *Rhus toxicodendrum* 30c or *Sepia* 30c can be used twice a day for cold sores on the lips.

■ *Hypercal*, a mixture of *Calendula* and *Hypericum* tinctures, is very soothing and healing. Dilute 1 part tincture to 3 parts cooled boiled water and apply it to cold sores frequently.

■ Rescue Remedy is an all-purpose soothing and healing remedy made from flowers. It can be applied externally as needed for pain relief.

ACUPRESSURE

See Acupressure Points in Part Three for the locations of these points on the body.

■ Press Spleen 7 for three minutes as often as needed to help relieve the itching. The Spleen 7 acupoints are located halfway up the inner calves, just slightly to the front of the body.

OTHER THERAPIES

■ As cold sores are considered a stress-related illness, relaxation techniques including meditation, yoga, and massage help reduce the incidence of recurrence.

■ Psychotherapy, hypnosis, and visualization can all have positive effects in chronically recurring, severe cases.

GENERAL RECOMMENDATIONS

■ Wash your hands frequently.

■ Don't share utensils, glasses, or towels.

■ If you have cold sores, take steps to prevent contact that may spread them to others, especially pregnant women.

■ Use a sunscreen with a sun protection factor (SPF) of 15 or higher. Sun exposure may trigger recurrences.

■ As much as possible, limit exposure stressors that may set off recurrences.

■ Put ice on the lesions for ten minutes, then take it off for five minutes. Repeat this sequence to help relieve the pain.

■ Use a blow-dryer on the blisters to help dry them up.

Cuts and Scrapes

Cuts and scrapes are breaks in the skin that are inevitable in the course of life. They can be painful, interfering with movement and activities. Cuts can bleed profusely, especially if they are on the head, face, hands, mouth, or feet, where there are many blood vessels close to the surface of the skin. They can become infected, especially if they are on the face, fingers, and hands, which are not normally covered with clothing.

Cuts can leave scars. Special attention should be given to those on the face and lips so that there will be no noticeable lasting skin defect. Cuts on the lips often require stitches to heal properly. Stitches may be required to close larger wounds elsewhere to effect minimal scarring. The more severe the cut, the more underlying tissues may be involved and the longer it may take to heal.

You can treat minor cuts and scrapes at home with basic first aid. However, if the pain from a cut is severe, if bleeding cannot be stopped, if redness and tenderness develop around the wounds, if a cut is deep or long, or if it involves your lips, consult your physician or go to the emergency room of the nearest hospital immediately.

CONVENTIONAL TREATMENT

- Stop bleeding by elevating the wound and applying direct pressure.
- Cleanse and disinfect the wound with soap and water.
- A tetanus shot may if necessary if the wound was caused by a rusty or dirty object and it has been more than ten years since your last booster shot.
- A butterfly bandage or stitches may be needed to close the wound edges.
- Topical or oral antibiotics may be prescribed to prevent or treat infection.

DIETARY MEASURES

- Eat a balanced, whole-food-based diet, with adequate protein for good wound healing.

NUTRITIONAL SUPPLEMENTS

■ The following vitamin and mineral supplements are recommended to aid in rapid healing:

- Beta-carotene. Take 25,000 international units a day.
- Vitamin B$_6$ (pyridoxine). Take 50 milligrams a day.
- Vitamin C. Take 3,000 to 5,000 milligrams a day.
- Vitamin E. Take 400 international units a day.
- Zinc. Take 50 to 100 milligrams a day.

■ If the cut is superficial, after cleaning you can cover the cut with a mixture of zinc oxide cream and vitamin-E oil.

HERBAL TREATMENT

■ Calendula gel or ointment stimulates fast healing at the skin's surface, and is a good choice for a nice clean wound. It is been endorsed by Commission E, the body of experts that advises the German government about herbs, for reducing inflammation and promoting wound healing.

■ Clove oil is high in eugenol, a compound that is both an antiseptic and a painkiller. You can sprinkle powdered cloves on a cut to prevent infection.

■ Comfrey roots and leaves contain allantoin, which stimulates cell division and speeds wound healing and scar formation. You can take some fresh leaves and rub them directly on your cuts and scrapes. You can also find commercial cream formulations of comfrey in many health food stores. Do not to take comfrey internally, however.

■ Echinacea is also Commission E-approved as a topical treatment for superficial cuts. This herb has powerful immune-stimulating properties. You can also drink a cup of echinacea tea three to four times a day to strengthen your immune system to speed healing.

■ Goldenseal contains several antiseptic compounds. You can apply a poultice of crushed goldenseal root to any minor cuts.

■ Yarrow is excellent for stopping bleeding. Just sprinkle powdered yarrow extract onto the cut. Yarrow leaves and flowers have been used since ancient Roman times for their blood-clotting, anti-inflammatory, and pain-relieving qualities.

■ There are a number of herbal first-aid creams available, including calendula in echinacea-and-comfrey combinations; calendula blended with white sage, elder flower, and chickweed; and calendula mixed with goldenseal, propolis, and myrrh to make topical botanical antiseptics.

AROMATHERAPY

■ Widely used by Australian aborigines, by early American settlers, and as a disinfectant during World War II, tea tree oil is now one of the most popular germicidals for cuts that are likely to become infected. It contains a compound known as terpinen-4-ol, a powerful antiseptic that works against bacteria and fungi. Dilute a few drops of the pure oil in a couple of tablespoons of any vegetable oil before applying to your cut. If it is irritating, dilute the mixture further with the vegetable oil. Remember never to take tea tree oil internally.

HOMEOPATHY

■ A dose of *Arnica montana* 200c can be taken immediately after a severe cut, and repeated twelve hours later. It can be followed either by a dose of 30c potency three times a day or by one of the other remedies discussed below. *Arnica* is good for sore, bruised wounds to the head or muscles, especially after dental treatment or surgery.

■ *Calcarea sulfurica* 30c, one dose three times a day, is good for cuts that are oozing pus.

■ A dose of *Calendula* 30c twice a day promotes healing of any cut, especially very painful ones with pus.

■ *Hepar sulfuris* 30c is best for inflamed wounds with redness, pain, and tenderness to the touch.

■ *Hypericum* 30c is good for severe shooting pain going through the affected limb. It is best for ragged severe wounds with extensive damage to the underlying tissues, including puncture wounds, surgical incisions, and episiotomies.

■ *Ledum palustre* 30c is best for wounds to the palms or soles caused by splinters, nails, or surgery.

■ *Silica* 30c is good for inflamed wounds with the dirt or foreign body still inside and a forming lumpy scar that breaks open and is painful.

■ *Staphysagria* 30c is best for cuts made by sharp instruments to nerve-rich parts of the body.

■ Lotions made from 10 drops of the following homeopathic remedies diluted in 1 cup of cold water are helpful for moistening the dressing over a cut:

- *Calendula* lotion. This helps to fight infection.
- *Hypericum* lotion. This is best for severely lacerated wounds.
- *Hypercal* ointment, cream, tincture, or lotion, a combination of *Calendula* and *Hypericum*. This is excellent for soaking and covering wounds.
- Rescue Remedy. This flower cream can be used directly on cuts as well to heal and soothe them.
- *Symphytum* is a good all-purpose ointment or cream most helpful for minor, clean cuts.

ACUPRESSURE

See Acupressure Points in Part Three for the locations of these points on the body.

■ After the wound is cleaned, press the Golden Points nearest the cut to promote healing by relaxing the muscles around the wound and increasing local circulation. There are 20 Golden Points used for common injuries and illnesses around the body.

GENERAL RECOMMENDATIONS

■ In many folk medicine remedies from around the world, raw honey is dabbed on a cut because it dries to form a natural bandage. Scientific studies have shown that honey also speeds healing of cuts.

Dandruff

Mild dandruff is actually a normal, very common condition in which dead skin cells fall from the scalp. The most frequent cause of dandruff is seborrheic dermatitis. When the sebaceous glands make too much sebum, it dries into flakes and obstructs the sebaceous ducts. In turn, the sebaceous glands produce even more sebum, trying to force out the obstructions and clear a passageway to the skin's surface. Itchy, greasy flakes of dried sebum and dead skin cells are sloughed off from the scalp. They fall into the hair and onto the shoulders, causing more embarrassment than discomfort.

As many of us know only too well, dandruff worsens in the cold, dry winter months. Dandruff may also be complicated by an overgrowth of the persistent yeast *Pityrosporum ovale*. This yeast is usually found living in hair follicles, but it can overgrow, adding to the problem.

CONVENTIONAL TREATMENT

- A zinc pyrithione shampoo such as Zencon or Sebulon can be massaged into the scalp and affected parts of the face for at least five minutes a day before rinsing out.
- An anti-dandruff shampoo containing selenium sulfide, menthol, or salicylic acid may be more effective than zinc pyrithione. You can switch back and forth between shampoos if one loses its effectiveness.
- Coal-tar shampoos such as Ionil T and Polytar are stronger, but also have a strong smell. They also should be massaged into the scalp for at least five minutes before rinsing out. Be aware that coal tar can darken light-colored hair.
- Using ketoconazole (Nizoral) shampoo and applying ketaconazole cream to the affected areas are newer therapies that are directed against the yeast *Pityrosporum ovale*.
- Hydrocortisone creams and lotions are often prescribed to control itching and redness.

DIETARY MEASURES

■ Eat a high-fiber, whole-foods-based diet.

■ Avoid saturated and hydrogenated fats, refined sugars, and processed foods.

■ Include soy foods in your diet. Soybeans are a rich source of biotin, which is important for healthy skin and hair.

NUTRITIONAL SUPPLEMENTS

■ Biotin is most important for preventing and treating dandruff. Take 6 milligrams a day.

■ Vitamin A and beta-carotene can help to clear dandruff. Take 10,000 international units of vitamin A and 20,000 international units of beta-carotene daily for two weeks.

Caution: Do not take these doses of vitamin A and beta-carotene if you are pregnant. Consult with your doctor.

■ Vitamin B_{12} has been found to be helpful in clearing dandruff. Take 1,000 micrograms a day.

■ Vitamin-E oil, massaged into the scalp for at least ten minutes and then shampooed out, is helpful for softening the scalp.

■ Essential fatty acids (EFAs) reduce the skin's dryness. Take 1,000 milligrams of flaxseed oil twice a day.

■ Probiotics such as *Lactobacillus acidophilus* and *Bifidobacterium bifidum* help to create an internal environment conducive to healthy bacteria and help to fight yeast infection.

■ Selenium has antioxidant properties and has been found to be helpful for dandruff. Take 100 micrograms twice a day.

■ Kelp tablets provide trace nutrients needed for a healthy scalp. Take two tablets in the morning and one at lunch.

■ Zinc helps to prevent and heal dandruff. Take 50 milligrams a day.

HERBAL TREATMENT

■ A thyme dandruff rinse can be made by boiling 2 tablespoons of dried thyme in 1 cup of water for ten minutes. Strain and cool before pouring the mixture over clean, damp hair. Massage in gently, and do not rinse out.

■ A rosemary dandruff rinse can be made by boiling 2 tablespoons of dried rosemary in 1 cup of water for ten minutes before straining and cooling. Rosemary has astringent and antiseptic properties and increases circulation locally.

■ Burdock-root oil massaged into the scalp lessens dandruff.

■ Pine tar shampoos are available commercially to help with dandruff.

■ For a warm oil conditioner that also lessens itching, heat almond, calendula, vitamin E, or sesame oil and gently comb the oil into your hair. Wrap a towel around your head and leave the oil on for at least fifteen minutes before shampooing and rinsing out. Using a fine-toothed comb, gently comb away the loosened scales.

AROMATHERAPY

■ Mix 6 drops each of bay oil, lavender oil, and sandalwood oil with 6 ounces of warm sesame oil. Part your hair in one-inch sections and apply the warm oil mixture to the scalp with a wad of cotton. Wrap your head in a towel for at least thirty minutes to allow the oils to soak into scalp. Shampoo the hair thoroughly twice afterward with dandruff shampoo.

HOMEOPATHY

■ *Sulfur* 30x or 9c, taken twice a day for two days, helps to alleviate dandruff. This is especially useful if you are a person who is usually hot and relatively restless.

■ *Thuja* 30x or 9c, taken twice a day for two days, is especially helpful if you are a cooler and calmer sort of person.

ACUPRESSURE

See Acupressure Points in Part Three for the locations of these points on the body.

■ Applying pressure to the Gallbladder 20 points improves circulation to the head. These points are located at the back of the head, in the depression between the bottom of the skull and the neck muscles, three finger-widths on either side of the spine. Using your thumbs, apply acupressure to these points, angling upward under the edge of the skull.

■ Pressing Large Intestine 4 works on the head, skin, and face. These points are located in the center of the triangle between the small bones of the index finger and thumb. Press the point gently with the thumb of the opposite hand for one minute. Repeat on the opposite hand. Do this twice a day.

■ Pressing Large Intestine 11 helps to relieve itching and to tone the skin. The points are found in the depressions at the end of the skin creases, toward the outside of the elbows when the elbows are bent. Press with the thumbs for three minutes three times a day.

GENERAL RECOMMENDATIONS

■ Don't pick at or scratch your scalp.

■ Using a good moisturizer after shampooing is very helpful for a dry scalp.

■ A popular folk treatment entails applying a warm mixture of two parts apple-cider vinegar with one part water to your scalp. Cover with a towel for thirty minutes, then wash out.

Dermatitis (Rashes)

The term *dermatitis* means "inflammation of the skin," and is used to describe many different types of rashes. The skin may itch, flake, scale, thicken, ooze, crust, and/or redden, depending on the type of dermatitis. Dermatitis can develop anywhere on the body. Certain locations are typical for different forms of dermatitis.

Atopic dermatitis, or eczema, the "itch that rashes" is a chronic, common problem that affects many people and for which there are many possible therapies. It is discussed in its own section (*see* Eczema). Contact dermatitis is probably the most common type of dermatitis. It is caused by irritation or allergy to something the skin comes in contact with. Types of contact dermatitis include irritant contact dermatitis, allergic contact dermatitis, and photoallergic contact dermatitis. A common type of allergic contact dermatitis is the rash of poison ivy, oak, and sumac. These also are described in their own section (*see* Poison Ivy, Oak, and Sumac). Seborrhea (seborrheic dermatitis) is another distinct type of dermatitis, and is discussed in its own section as well.

Less common and well known types of dermatitis include *asteototic eczema, dyshidrotic eczema, exfoliative dermatitis, lichen simplex chronicus, neurodermatitis, nummular dermatitis,* and *stasis dermatitis.* Asteototic eczema occurs when the skin becomes so dry that it gets red, itchy and inflamed. Dyshidrotic eczema is a recurring, very itchy rash of vesicles (small blisters) on the palms and soles. Flare-ups may be triggered by excessive sweating and anxiety. In exfoliative dermatitis, large areas of the skin can scale and peel off. This can be due to a drug reaction, infection, or cancer, and can be life-threatening.

Lichen simplex chronicus is characterized by a single or a few thickened, scaly, dry, itching patches which the person is constantly rubbing or scratching. It is a form of neurodermatitis that starts with scratching, and has a large psychological component, usually anxiety or depression. The scratching in turn produces lesions, more itch, and more scratching. Especially common during dry winter months, nummular dermatitis causes coin-shaped itchy, scaling patches, usually on the lower legs. Stasis dermatitis is another problem of the lower legs. In this disorder, the blood from the veins is slow in returning to the heart, there is swelling around the ankles, and the skin becomes reddened, thick, scaly, and itchy.

Other forms of dermatitis are due to drug allergies. Still others are due to food allergies. Some types of rashes are signs of nutrient deficiencies. Infections, underlying diseases, pregnancy, physical factors, and cancer can also cause dermatitis. Also, some rashes are less commonly known types of diseases that affect only the skin. An experienced dermatologist can help you discover the cause of your rash if it is not immediately obvious and it persists.

CONVENTIONAL TREATMENT

■ Search for the cause of your dermatitis. Eliminate any factors you think may be causing or aggravating the rash.

■ Topical combinations of ¼ to ½ percent menthol and phenol, such as Sarna lotion, are soothing.

■ Calamine lotion is available over the counter to calm itching.

■ Topical formulas containing pramoxine, such as Pramagel, also help to control the itch.

■ If the rash is not severe, and there are not accompanying symptoms of fever or malaise, over-the-counter ½-percent hydrocortisone cream can help to soothe the rash.

■ An over-the-counter antihistamine such as diphenhydramine (Benadryl, Diphenhist, and others) or chlorpheniramine (Chlor-Trimeton, Teldrin, and others) can help relieve the itch of the rash.

■ Seek professional help if the rash does not improve and resolve quickly. Your doctor may prescribe hydroxyzine (Atarax, Hyzine-50, Vistaril) or a nonsedating antihistamine such as cetirizine (Zyrtec).

■ Your physician may prescribe a topical steroid cream or, if your rash is severe, a short course of oral prednisone or a steroid shot to speed recovery and help relieve itching and pain.

DIETARY MEASURES

■ A diet of whole, unprocessed foods is highly recommended. Eat lean proteins, whole grains, beta-carotene-rich vegetables, beans, sea vegetables, alfalfa sprouts, whole fruits, sesame seeds, and sesame oil.

■ Drink fresh juices such as apple, beet, cantaloupe, carrot, celery, and cucumber.

■ Avoid animal fats, fried foods, junk food, sweets, spicy foods, citrus fruits, and anything containing artificial colorings and preservatives.

■ Drink eight glasses of pure filtered water a day.

■ Many different food allergies and vitamin deficiencies can produce dermatitis. Try an elimination diet to see if your condition improves when certain foods are removed from the diet. Good foods to eliminate first include milk, eggs, gluten-containing grains (barley, oats, rye, and wheat), shellfish, soy products, and nuts.

NUTRITIONAL SUPPLEMENTS

■ Vitamin deficiencies should be investigated and treated aggressively with supplements. Vitamin A deficiency causes the skin to become lumpy, scaly, and rough, looking like gooseflesh or "alligator skin." It usually affects the forearms and thighs first. Vitamin B_2 (riboflavin) deficiency causes the skin of the body to form dry, greasy scales and soreness and burning of the mouth and lips. Vitamin B_3 (niacin) deficiency, or pellagra, shows itself as scaly, dark pigment on areas of the body that are exposed to the sun, heat, and irritation. Biotin deficiency may appear as a dry, scaly dermatitis, together with hair loss and loss of hair color. Vitamin B_6 (pyridoxine), B_{12} (cobalamin), and pantothenic acid deficiencies also manifest themselves in the skin, but with less specifically identifiable symptoms. Vitamin C deficiency leads to dry, scaly skin in addition to small pinpoint bleeding under the skin, poor wound healing, breakdown of old scars, and swollen and bleeding gums. Essential fatty acid deficiency causes red, dry, scaly skin. The face is greatly affected, especially the areas around the nose, mouth, and eyes; the forehead; and the cheeks. The forearms and thighs also develop a red, scaly rash.

■ The following supplements are recommended for dermatitis in general:

• A multivitamin and mineral supplement. Take this daily.

• Beta-carotene. Take 5 milligrams three times a day.

• Vitamin B complex. Take a supplement containing 100 milligrams of most of the major B vitamins.

• Vitamin C. Take 1,000 milligrams three times a day.

• Vitamin E. Take 400 international units daily.

• Zinc. Take 25 milligrams twice a day, with food and 1 milligram of copper. Zinc can also be applied topically in the form of zinc oxide ointment to help relieve itchiness.

- Cod liver oil. Take 1 teaspoon twice a day.
- Flaxseed oil, evening primrose oil, or fish oil. Take 1 teaspoon or 500 milligrams three times a day. Evening primrose oil can also be applied directly on the cracked and sore areas twice a day to soothe and speed healing.
- Quercetin. Take 500 milligrams three times a day, with meals.

HERBAL TREATMENT

■ Naturopaths believe that when waste products build up and exceed the capacity of the liver and kidneys to get rid of them, the skin has to eliminate the wastes. This can result in dermatitis. The following herbs cause sweating, which naturopaths feel is a good way to excrete the toxins that are trying to get out of your body:
- Burdock root. Take 500 milligrams three times a day, with meals.
- Sarsaprilla root. Take it as directed by the manufacturer.
- Yarrow. Take it as directed by the manufacturer.

■ Naturopaths recommend one or more of the follow blood cleansers for dermatitis:
- Chaparral root. Take it as directed by the manufacturer.
- Dandelion root. Take it as directed by the manufacturer.
- Echinacea. Take it as directed by the manufacturer.
- Goldenseal. Take 500 milligrams three times a day, with meals.
- Pau d'arco. Take 500 milligrams three times a day, with meals.
- Poke root. Make a tea by steeping 1 tablespoon of the herb in a cup of water. Drink this twice a day.
- Red clover. Take 500 milligrams three times a day.
- Yellow dock root. Take it as directed by the manufacturer.

■ The appropriate specific herbal therapy depends on the cause, location, and type of rash. However, the following therapies will all help relieve itching, no matter what sort of dermatitis you have:
- Aloe vera gel and green clay soothe the skin.
- Chamomile cream, calendula lotion, or comfrey ointment should be applied directly to the itchy areas as often as needed, as their anti-inflammatory properties will help relieve your discomfort.
- Chickweed infusion can be used to bathe the area to stop itching.

- Cucumber purée, made from peeled, blended fresh cucumbers, can be applied directly to the affected area for three minutes to relieve your itching and pain.
- Jewelweed, also known as impatiens, can be boiled in a gallon of water, strained, and cooled. The liquid stops itching extremely well. In fact, in clinical trials, it has worked just as well as prescription cortisone creams. Note that while it is sometimes called impatiens, jewelweed is not the same plant that is sold as a flowering annual in home and garden centers.
- An herbal tea made from two parts each of agrimony and chamomile and one part each of stinging nettle and heart's-ease can be taken three times a day as an aid to soothing the itching. In addition to drinking the tea, dip a clean cloth into it and apply it as a compress to the affected areas for five minutes every half hour, as needed. Other plants containing natural antihistaminic compounds from which you can make a combination tea include basil, fennel, ginkgo, oregano, tarragon, tea, thyme, and yarrow. These teas should be used in compresses applied to the itchy areas, as well as drunk three times a day.

AROMATHERAPY

■ Many essential oils can help soothe inflamed skin, reduce itching, and relieve anxiety. They include benzoin, cedarwood, chamomile, elemi, everlasting, geranium, jasmine, juniper, lavender, myrrh, neroli, orange, patchouli, peppermint, rose, rosemary, rosewood, sandalwood, tea tree, thyme, and ylang ylang. To get some relief from your rash, try using these oils in baths, compresses, and oil mixtures. Always use only a few drops of these strong oils diluted in water or a carrier oil, and never apply them directly to your skin.

HOMEOPATHY

■ *Psorinum* 200x or 200c is good for rashes behind the ears, on the scalp, or in the bends of the joints. You may have a tendency toward respiratory problems, and the rash is often made worse by drinking coffee. Take one dose weekly for three weeks.

■ *Sulfur* 30x or 15c is good for dry, scaly skin that worsens with dampness, warmth, and spring weather. Take one dose three times a day for three days.

■ *Vinca minor* 6x or 3c is good for a sore, sensitive, itching skin rash. Take one dose three times a day for three days.

■ The appropriate homeopathic remedy depends on the cause, signs, and symptoms of the rash. However, the following two remedies will help relieve itching from any form of dermatitis:

- *Rhus toxicodendron* 30x or 15c is good for itching, especially if the discomfort is worse with cold or scratching. Take one dose four times a day, up to a total of eight doses.
- *Urtica urens* is a good choice for itching, especially if the itching improves with rubbing, or becomes worse at night, with heat, or with exercise. Take it as directed by the manufacturer.

ACUPUNCTURE

■ There are reports in the literature of success in treating dermatitis with acupuncture. Dr. Yang Qinglin published his satisfactory results of acupuncture treatments with cupping for ninety-six cases of localized neurodermatitis and forty-three cases of generalized neurodermatitis, or itching and red rash due to "nerves" and scratching. Of the total, he considered almost 80 percent to be cured, slightly less than 20 percent to be improved, and less than 10 percent to be unchanged with acupuncture therapies over the course of approximately six weeks. Consult a qualified acupuncturist if you are interested in trying this type of treatment.

ACUPRESSURE

See Acupressure Points in Part Three for the locations of these points on the body.

■ Press the Spleen 7 points at least three times a day to relieve the itching and heat from the rash. These points are located halfway up the inner calves, just slightly to the front of the body.

■ If the dermatitis is recurrent, press the Liver 3 points three times a day to strengthen the liver, which helps to filter toxins from the body. These points are on the back of the feet, about one finger-width up from the toe joints, between the first and second toes.

■ Applying pressure to the Bladder 18 points three times a day also strengthens the liver and helps to purify the blood, thus improving the skin's appearance. These points are located two finger-widths on either side of the spine, three-quarters of the way down the back.

■ Bladder 23 and Bladder 47 help to relieve eczema also. They are located in the lower back, two to four finger-widths away from the spine at waist level.

■ Pressure to the Spleen 10 points for three minutes three times a day helps to regulate blood flow and thus helps to relieve skin irritation. Spleen 10 is located on the inside edge of the top of the knee.

■ Applying pressure to the Large Intestine 4 and 11 points for three minutes three times a day helps to relieve itching. Large Intestine 4 is located in the webbing between your thumb and index finger at the highest spot of the muscle. Large Intestine 11 is located on the top, outer end of the elbow crease.

Caution: Do not use Large Intestine 4 if you are pregnant, as it may cause premature contractions.

OTHER THERAPIES

■ Reflexology can be helpful. Massaging the feet and hands in the areas representing the diaphragm, liver, kidneys, intestines, adrenals, and other glands is thought to help promote the excretion of the toxins that are causing the dermatitis.

■ Biofeedback, guided imagery, and relaxation techniques are very useful for forms of dermatitis that flare up in response to anxiety or stress.

GENERAL RECOMMENDATIONS

■ Keep your nails trimmed to limit scratching and spread of the rash.

■ Applying cool water and ice locally can provide immediate relief from itching.

■ Taking oatmeal or baking soda baths can temporarily calm itching.

■ Use only hypoallergenic skin-care products, mild soap, and warm water on your skin.

■ Wear loose cotton clothing to help avoid becoming overheated.

Dry Skin

If the skin lacks sufficient oil and moisture, the top layer becomes dry and flaky and may itch. Dry skin feels "tight" after washing, and it is usually thin and inelastic. There may be roughened or reddish patches. Dry skin shows signs of aging sooner than normal or oily skin does, with tiny surface wrinkles that usually go away if you apply a moisturizer.

Water from the body's cells is slowly and constantly moving to the surface of the skin, where it evaporates. About a pint of water leaves the body this way every day. The skin itself is made up of more than 70 percent water. If too much water evaporates, however, the top layer of the skin becomes dehydrated, its natural oils are depleted, and less water is then held in the skin. The effect snowballs and the skin rapidly becomes increasingly dry.

Dry skin becomes a bigger problem as we get older because the top layer of skin loses some of its ability to hold water in as we age. Thus, dry skin, or *xerosis,* affects more than half of the population over age sixty-five. Environmental factors that make the skin drier include cold weather, a dry climate, exposure to wind, and, especially, too much sun exposure. Excessive swimming, the use of drying soaps, and exposure to certain chemicals can also make the skin scaly and flaky. Also, not ingesting enough essential fatty acids and not drinking enough liquids can cause the skin to be dry.

Because there are many factors that contribute to dry skin, there are many things you can do to prevent or remedy it. Let's look at the many traditional and alternative techniques that are available.

CONVENTIONAL TREATMENT

■ Use creamy facial and body cleansers instead of soaps, which are drying. Choose products without dyes or fragrances.
■ Try to avoid using skin- or nail-care products that contain acetone, alcohol, benzoyl peroxide, camphor, citrus juices, eucalyptus, menthol, and mint, all of which are drying and/or irritating.
■ Shower or sponge-bathe with bath oil every other day, if possible. Avoid long hot showers. Frequent hot baths and showers strip away your skin's natural oils and dry out your skin.

■ Blot your skin dry with a fluffy towel after showering, then immediately apply a moisturizer.

■ Topical moisturizers with urea, glycolic acid, lactic acid, or the newer alpha-hydroxy acids should be applied to all areas of dry skin after washing or showering and reapplied as frequently as needed throughout the day to keep the skin from feeling dry. Recommended products include Aqua Care, Lac-Hydrin, Neutrogena, Purpose, and alpha-hydroxy acid ointments.

■ Apply a sunscreen with a sun protection factor (SPF) of 15 or higher to exposed skin to avoid further drying from the sun.

■ If your hands and feet are very dry, apply petroleum jelly (Vaseline) or mineral oil to them and cover them with gloves and socks before going to bed. The skin will feel much smoother and more supple in the morning.

■ A humidifier can be very helpful in the winter or in very dry climates. Remember to clean it frequently to remove any mold, bacteria, and minerals from hard water.

DIETARY MEASURES

■ Eat fish, rolled oats, and ground flaxseeds frequently. These foods are high in omega-3 essential fatty acids, which help the skin retain moisture.

■ Include in your diet plenty of carrots, tomatoes, green leafy vegetables, cantaloupe, and apricots. These foods supply carotenoids, from which the body manufactures vitamin A, which is essential for skin growth and repair.

■ Eat plenty of whole grains, legumes, wheat germ, and nutritional yeast. These are good sources of pantothenic acid, which is important in the synthesis of much-needed fats and oils.

NUTRITIONAL SUPPLEMENTS

■ Take supplemental essential fatty acids in the form of 2 tablespoons of flaxseed oil daily or 1,000 milligrams of evening primrose oil three times a day to remedy any deficiency of omega-3 and omega-6 EFAs.

■ Beta-carotene is an antioxidant and is important for overall skin health. Take 25,000 international units daily, unless you are pregnant.

■ The B vitamins also are needed for healthy skin. Take a vitamin-B complex supplying 100 milligrams of most of the major B vitamins daily.

■ Vitamin C is required for the synthesis of collagen, an important skin protein, and is a potent antioxidant. Take 2,000 milligrams of vitamin C with bioflavonoids daily.

HERBAL TREATMENT

■ Almond oil is moisturizing. Massage 1 tablespoon of the oil into dry facial skin immediately after applying a steaming hot washcloth. Sesame oil can also be used this way.

■ Make an avocado masque by puréeing half of a peeled, pitted ripe avocado and spreading the paste over your face and neck. Leave it on for thirty minutes. Remove it with lukewarm water followed by cold water, then blot your face dry.

■ Comfrey cream, calendula ointment, and aloe vera cream are good moisturizers for dry skin.

■ Products containing combinations of apricot, avocado, canola, evening primrose, hazelnut, kukui nut, olive, safflower, soybean, sunflower, wheat germ, and other herbal oils are available, and are soothing skin moisturizers.

■ Process ½ cup sesame seeds and ¼ cup water in a blender for three minutes. Strain, then apply the lotion to your skin. Leave it on for as long as possible before removing it with warm water followed by cool water, then blotting dry.

■ There are many herbal combinations available in pill and capsule form that are formulated to support smooth skin.

AROMATHERAPY

■ Add 10 drops each of essential oil of carrot seed, chamomile, lavender, neroli, and rosemary to 2 ounces of a carrier oil such as almond oil, olive oil, or sesame oil. Apply this mixture to your whole body daily after showering or bathing.

HOMEOPATHY

■ *Natrum muriaticum* 30c, taken twice a day for one week, is often helpful for dry skin.

ACUPRESSURE

See Acupressure Points in Part Three for the locations of these points on the body.

■ Pressing the Golden Points near the areas of dry skin may be helpful. This increases local circulation, improving the supply of oxygen and necessary nutrients to the area.

OTHER THERAPIES

■ Dry-brush your skin every morning to increase local circulation and lymphatic flow and to stimulate your sebaceous glands to produce more sebum. Dry-brushing also removes dead skin. Before bathing, use a bristle brush to gently rub your whole body. Brush in small circles. Start with the soles of your feet and move up your legs, arms, and trunk toward your heart. Finally, use a gentle face brush for your face, again brushing in small circles.

■ Reflexology, with special attention to the thyroid and adrenal gland reflexes in the hands and feet, has been found to be helpful for dry skin.

GENERAL RECOMMENDATIONS

■ Avoid excessive sun exposure. However, *moderate* sun exposure in the early morning or late afternoon spurs the body's synthesis of vitamin D, which in turn promotes healthy skin.

■ Do not smoke. Smoking decreases circulation to the skin.

Eczema

Atopic eczema, or atopic dermatitis, is a very common inflammatory skin problem characterized by extremely itchy patches of red, dry flaking skin and other itchy patches that are inflamed and oozing. A vicious cycle of first itching, then scratching, followed by rash formation that again triggers itching is a hallmark of the problem. It is part of an atopic, or allergic, state in which an individual is vulnerable to flare-ups of eczema, asthma, and hay fever. There is a huge genetic component to atopic dermatitis; 70 percent of those who have it have a positive family history of atopy. The incidence of atopy has been on the rise in the past twenty years, perhaps due to the increasing load of sensitizing agents in the environment. Recently, as many as one-third of British children were reported to have some form of atopy, and 20 percent of all British children were found to have atopic eczema.

In addition to a very itchy rash and dry skin, eczema is characterized by abnormal changes in the blood vessels of the skin, immunologic abnormalities, and an inherited tendency to be hypersensitive to allergens. These allergens do not even have to directly touch the skin to aggravate eczema. Foods, dust mites, pollens, and animal furs are common culprits.

There are three distinct variants of atopic eczema: an infantile form , a childhood form, and an adolescent or adult form. However, an intensely itching rash is a feature of all of these stages.

The infantile form of eczema develops more commonly in bottle-fed than breast-fed babies, starting as early as two months, and almost always developing by the age of two years. Sixty percent of all eczema dermatitis sufferers develop the rash by the age of one year. Red, extremely itchy, oozing, crusted lesions can involve the face, scalp, neck, and outer aspects of the arms and legs of the infant. This often improves by age five, but asthma or hay fever then develops in more than half of the children.

The childhood form of eczema may follow from the infantile form or arise on its own between the ages of four and ten years. The type and site of the skin rash changes to dry, scaling, thickened, red bumps and patches on the inner folds of wrists, elbows, knees, and neck. The rash often improves with age and disappears by puberty.

The adult form of atopic dermatitis often extends to involve the upper chest, the hands and feet, and the skin overlying joints. It is also associated with marked dryness of the skin, and there may be scarring if the itching and scratching has been long-standing.

Many cases of atopic eczema may be due to food sensitivities or allergies. Dairy products such as eggs, milk, butter, cheese, and ice cream head the list of possible allergens. Indeed, many experts consider a child with atopic eczema allergic to dairy products until proved otherwise. Often babies develop eczema as they are weaned from mother's to cow's milk. Breastfeeding for as long as possible, with the mother also avoiding dairy products, can delay or improve a baby's eczema, and is recommended for those with a family history of asthma, hay fever, food allergies, and eczema. A ten-year New Zealand study involving a group of 1,265 children that was published in the October 1990 issue of *Pediatrics* reported that children who were introduced to four or more types of solid foods before the age of four months were almost three times more likely to develop recurrent eczema than children who did not have any solid feeding until after four months of age. Other very common food allergens in atopic eczema include wheat, sugar, food additives, citrus fruits, tomatoes, yeast-containing foods, and even fish.

Other factors that can trigger flare-ups of atopic eczema include cold weather, humid conditions, sudden temperature changes, anger, and stress. Therefore, treatment must try to address these factors as aggressively as it does irritants and allergens. Treatment, whether conventional or alternative, is aimed at preventing and controlling flare-ups. In the past, many people with severe eczema turned to natural medicine only after years of conventional treatment with no results. Now more and more people are using alternative techniques initially to augment conventional treatments. If you follow an integrative approach to your skin problem, you need to make sure that each type of health-care provider knows of the other treatments being used, so that you can get optimal care without experiencing unwanted side effects or decreasing the effectiveness of individual treatments.

Natural therapists see eczema as a reflection of the internal state of a person's health, energy balance, lifestyle, and psychological stability, as well as a function of irritant and allergy-provoking substances. In addition to aiding skin symptoms directly, natural therapies aim to combat psychological trauma and stress, support a harmonious attitude toward all aspects of human relationships, encourage a healthy lifestyle, realign the body's energy balance and it's own natural healing mechanisms, and stimulate the elimination of toxins from the body.

A British survey in the mid-1980s found that allergic symptoms such as eczema were the second most common reason people went to alternative medical centers. In the same survey, nearly two-thirds of patients said they noted improvement with the natural therapies, and those that believed in the treatments were more likely to get a good result.

CONVENTIONAL TREATMENT

■ Identify and avoid any triggering irritants and allergens. These can include not only foods, but also skin creams, cosmetics, perfumes, soaps, household cleaners such as detergents and bleaches, glues and other chemicals, hair and clothing dyes, wool, synthetic fabrics, cigarettes, jewelry, dust mites, pollen, animal hair and feathers, and plants such as ragweed and chrysanthemums. Allergy testing and referral to an allergist can be helpful in determining and avoiding precipitating allergens.

■ Many hypoallergenic and natural products can be obtained through various mail-order catalogues specializing in skin and allergy-safe products. Such products are becoming increasingly available in health-food stores, drugstores, and regular retail outlets. Choose 100-percent cotton mattresses and box springs, organic cotton and linen sheets, blankets, mattress pads, pillows, clothing, and towels. Avoid wool clothing. Use natural, fragrance-free soaps, cleansers, laundry detergents, cosmetics, toothpastes, and deodorants. Avoid using fabric softeners.

■ Dealing with house dust is very important. Special bedding designed to block dust mites is available. Vacuum frequently, especially draperies and around the bed, which should be elevated off the floor. There are special vacuums that filter house dust mites, and carpets should be wet-washed. Wet mop uncarpeted floors. Wash curtains and bedding often in hot water with perfume- and dye-free detergent. Use hypoallergenic bedding, blankets and pillows. Cover the bedding with special barrier materials and wash the bedding regularly to get rid of dust mites. Pillows or favorite stuffed animals can be put in the freezer overnight to kill mites. Toys and clothes should be kept in chests and drawers and washed weekly, and furry toys removed entirely, if possible. Wooden or leather furniture is preferable to upholstered pieces, and wooden or tile floors are much preferred over carpets in an effort to eliminate dust, mites, and chemical irritants.

■ Measures to decrease exposure to tree and grass allergens and dampness are also important. Windows should be kept closed during the pollen season, but left open whenever weather permits. HEPA air filters, which filter over 99.9 percent of particles out of the air, air-conditioners, and extractor fans in kitchens and bathrooms to decrease condensation all help to minimize mold spores and pollen in the air.

■ Maintain a cool, stable temperature. Avoid extremes of temperature, high humidity, and dryness. A temperature of 68°F to 70°F, with a humidity of 70 percent, is optimum.

■ Use well-vented electrical appliances rather than coal or wood-burning heaters which produce polluting irritants.

■ Ionizers, small machines that produce a flow of negative ions, often help the air to feel much fresher. It is the negative ions naturally found in the air by the sea that accounts for the refreshing and invigorating feeling of taking a walk by the ocean. Ionizers can be especially useful if you have a lot of electrical appliances, air pollution, synthetic fabric furnishings, or stuffy central heating and air conditioning in the home.

■ Exposure to soap and bathing should also always be minimized, and abrasive washcloths avoided. Repeated washing and drying removes important water-binding lipids from the top layer of skin. When you do wash, use only tepid water. If you have a tepid tub bath, add moisturizing bath oil or an oatmeal product such as Aveeno, which is soothing. A nonirritating moisturizer should be applied immediately after showering to prevent water loss. Only nonirritating soaps, such as Cetaphil or Purpose, and creams, ointments, and bath oils that soothe and moisturize the skin should be used. If you must do work involving wet or irritating substances, apply a good barrier cream to your hands and wear cotton-lined rubber gloves.

■ Corticosteroid creams are the most common conventional treatment for atopic dermatitis. These creams are very effective at reducing the symptoms of eczema by decreasing inflammation, swelling, redness, and itching, thereby allowing affected skin to heal. However, topical steroid creams must not be overused or stopped abruptly. Overuse for a long period of time can lead to thinning of the skin, and abrupt discontinuation of potent steroid creams can lead to sudden severe worsening of the eczema. Natural medical practitioners may complain that steroids suppress the symptoms without dealing with the cause of the disease, but it can also be argued that eczema sufferers are oversensitive to substances normally present in the environment and, therefore, the disease is a symptom produced by this sensitivity.

■ Other conventional topical preparations include coal-tar products, which soothe itchy and inflamed skin and help to thin rough, thickened patches. In the past these were messy and smelly and they stained clothing, so they were not well loved by users. There is now a clear, greaseless, nonstaining, odorless formulation, Exorex cream, which has proved to be very helpful in the topical treatment of eczema.

■ If your lesions are oozing and weeping, Burow's solution may be recommended. This is a powder that is mixed with water to make wet-to-dry compresses to soothe and dry the moist, itchy patches. Burow's solution is available over the counter.

■ Other standard topicals include ichthammol, or shale ointment, for mild eczema; salicylic acid to reduce thick scales; soothing zinc oxide paste; and aluminum chloride soaks to help dry up infected, weepy skin.

■ If the scalp is affected, topical forms of steroids such as fluocinolone (Derma-Smoothe/FS for overnight, Synalar lotion after regular shampooing) help to relieve and quiet lesions.

■ Oral antihistamines such as diphenhydramine (Benadryl, Diphenhist, and others) and hydroxyzine (Atarax, Hyzine-50, Vistaril) are helpful to control itching. They can cause drowsiness, but this may help you to get a good night's sleep if you take the medication before bed. You should avoid alcohol when taking these medications, and use caution if driving. There are also nonsedating antihistamines, such as astemizole (Hismanal) and loratadine (Claritin), for use during the day.

■ If the skin is broken, secondary infections can develop. These are typically treated with topical or oral antibiotics or antifungals, depending on the infecting organisms. *Staphylococcus aureus* is the usual offending bacteria, and is readily treated with erythromycin (E-Mycin, ERYC, Ilotycin, and others), cephalosporins (cefaclor, cefixime, ceftriaxone, cephalexin, and others), or dicloxacillin (Dynapen, Dycill, Pathocil). Infections with herpes simplex must be watched for closely, as the herpes virus can spread to all the areas involving eczema and become a very dangerous problem.

■ Oral prednisone or shots of the steroid triamcinolone are reserved for treatment of very severe flare-ups of atopic eczema.

■ If a very difficult case of eczema does not respond to steroid shots, a physician may recommend using cyclosporine A (Neoral, Sandimmune, SangCya). This drug is a potent immune suppressor.

■ Ultraviolet-light treatment with specialized light boxes has been found to help some people with severe atopic eczema. UVB or UVA light, or a combination of both, can be used, with the dose carefully monitored and increased slowly. Sometimes a medication, psoralen, is given first to increase the effect of the UVA light. This form of treatment is termed PUVA therapy. Ultraviolet light treatment can be done at home or in the doctor's office.

■ Many conventionally trained dermatologists also recommend special diets, oral evening primrose oil, and desensitization treatment to help people with atopic eczema.

DIETARY MEASURES

■ Eczema can clear within a few days to several weeks after the offending food allergens are removed from the diet. Use an elimination or exclusion diet to pinpoint foods that cause flare-ups. There is also blood testing for delayed-sensitivity food allergens (foods that cause symptoms one to three days after the food is eaten). You can confirm a specific food allergy or intolerance by avoiding the suspect food for about a month after the eczema has cleared, then reintroducing it to see if skin symptoms reappear. If you start by eliminating multiple foods, you must reintroduce them separately to diagnose individual sensitivities. Sometimes, if an allergenic food can be avoided for several months after symptoms clear, sensitivity to it may lessen and it may be possible to include some of that food in the diet up to twice a week.

■ Many allergists suggest a rotation diet after the initial evaluation of the food allergens. In this approach, different foods are rotated into the diet over a period of four to seven days, so that the same food is not eaten twice during this period. This can increase your ability to tolerate foods to which you previously reacted, and decreases the risk of developing new food sensitivities that will result in a flare-up of eczema.

■ A less commonly used food allergy and eczema treatment is Miller desensitization, in which you put a few drops of a specific dilution of the food allergen under your tongue before actually being able to eat small quantities of the offending food without exacerbating the eczema.

■ Eat organic food whenever possible, and avoid processed foods, fast foods, junk food, alcohol, and foods containing artificial colorings, preservatives, and other additives. Clinical ecologists think that between 10 and 30 percent of people in industrialized countries have food and chemical sensitivities that sometimes manifest themselves as eczema. Abnormal intestinal bacteria or enzyme deficiencies may magnify the food sensitivities and subsequently the eczema. Vitamin deficiencies can also lead to flare-ups.

■ Most practitioners recommend a healthier whole-foods diet with less animal fat, caffeine, sugar, alcohol, and processed and junk food. The consumption of fresh fruits, vegetables, fiber, and polyunsaturated vegetable oils is encouraged.

■ Drink lots of juice made from black currants, red grapes, carrots, beets, spinach, celery, cucumber, parsley, green juices, and wheatgrass.

NUTRITIONAL SUPPLEMENTS

■ Take a multivitamin and mineral supplement daily to ensure an adequate supply of all basic nutrients.

■ Beta-carotene aids in tissue healing. Take 50,000 international units daily.

■ The B vitamins are necessary for skin health, nutrient absorption, and the body's ability to cope with stress. Take a high-stress formula containing 100 milligrams of most of the major B vitamins daily. Also take an an additional 50 milligrams of vitamin B_6 (pyridoxine) three times a day.

■ Vitamin C is an anti-inflammatory and helps in the formation of collagen. Take 1,000 milligrams of vitamin C with bioflavonoids twice a day, with meals.

■ Vitamin E helps with tissue healing. Take 400 international units daily. Vitamin-E oil can also be used topically. It is very soothing and helps to reduce inflammation of the skin.

■ Calcium and magnesium calm a stressed nervous system. Take 1,500 milligrams of calcium and 750 milligrams of magnesium daily. The magnesium is especially important if you are a woman whose eczema worsens before your menstrual period.

■ Selenium is an antioxidant and helps the body to use vitamin E more effectively. Take 50 micrograms daily.

■ Zinc is needed for a healthy immune response and helps wounds to heal more quickly. Take 25 milligrams twice a day, with food and with 1 milligram of copper.

■ Evening primrose oil and flaxseed oil are good sources of essential fatty acids (EFAs), and are helpful for many skin disorders. Take three capsules of evening primrose oil three times a day or 1 teaspoon of flaxseed oil twice a day. Many people with eczema have supplemented their diets with the omega-3 and omega-6 essential fatty acids with great success. Other sources of EFAs include black currant seed, safflower, and borage oils. Evening primrose oil appears to be most helpful for childhood eczema. Be patient when taking EFAs. Results may be slow in coming, taking up to three months and requiring as many as six capsules of evening primrose oil a day. Evening primrose oil can also be very soothing and reduce inflammation of the skin when applied topically.

■ A 1997 study reported that the hormone dehydroepiandrosterone (DHEA) is a potential treatment for eczema. Eczema is a type of immune problem, and DHEA regulates the cell enzymes that cause autoimmune reactions. Take 5 to 50 milligrams of DHEA daily.

■ Acidophilus encourages the growth of "friendly" bacteria in your intestines. This helps the barrier function of the stomach wall and therefore helps to minimize food allergies. Take ½ teaspoon of acidophilus powder in 2 ounces of water twice a day, between meals.

■ Many people with atopic dermatitis have low levels of digestive enzymes. Supplementation can improve both your digestion and the condition of your skin within a few weeks. Take digestive enzymes, including betaine hydrochloride and pancreatic enzymes, with meals.

■ Vitamin-E oil and evening primrose oil can be very soothing and reduce inflammation of the skin.

HERBAL TREATMENT

Herbal therapy is one of the mainstays of alternative treatment of atopic eczema, and teas, topicals, and infusions or tinctures are used. Some remedies are used to treat the skin directly, while others help relieve stress, are calming, or help to cleanse the bowel or kidneys.

■ Burdock aids in cleansing the system by promoting the excretion of toxins through the urine and bowel. This in turn helps to heal the skin. Take 4 milliliters of burdock tincture or 500 milligrams in capsule form three times a day.

■ A poultice made of warmed, crushed, fresh green cabbage leaves applied to the affected area and covered with a bandage is soothing.

- Calendula tea, ointment, or compresses relieve itching, blistering, and flaking, especially if the eczema is dry.
- Chamomile tea is soothing and calming and is great before bed to promote rest from the irritation and stress of eczema. Chamomile cream applied topically is very soothing and has an anti-inflammatory effect.
- Chickweed can be used to help soothe the itching of eczema. Place 1 tablespoon of chickweed oil in your bath water or use chickweed cream, ointment, or infusion.
- Goldenseal powder can be mixed with honey and eaten, or mixed with warm water and spread on involved skin to relieve eczema symptoms.
- Echinacea and goldenseal help to detoxify the blood. Take 250 milligrams of echinacea and 100 milligrams of goldenseal three times a day.
- Heart's-ease tincture or infusion contains cleansing saponins that perform a diuretic and laxative function. Heart's-ease ointment or cream has an anti-infectious effect locally on the affected eczematous skin.
- Licorice, in the form of 250 milligrams of deglycyrrhizinated licorice (DGL) twice a day, is an excellent natural anti-inflammatory.
- Red clover is good for cleansing the system, fighting infection, and combating stress. Take 500 milligrams or a cup of red clover tea three times a day.
- Skullcap has a calming effect. Take it as recommend by the supplement manufacturer.
- St. John's wort oil relieves inflammation and blistering when rubbed into affected skin.
- Stinging nettle cream or ointment is an astringent that increases local circulation when applied to the skin. The tea or tincture helps eczema associated with poor elimination through the bowel and kidneys.
- Witch hazel ointment or compresses can be used locally three times a day for its local astringent properties. At least two studies have shown that the leaf extract applied to the skin can heal atopic dermatitis.
- Several herbs can be combined into salves or teas for better results:
  - Mix ½ teaspoon each of pau d'arco tincture and goldenseal root and 8 drops each of tea tree oil and chamomile essential oil into 2 ounces of comfrey skin salve. Apply the mixture to affected areas twice a day.
  - Combine ¾ ounce each of dried heart's-ease, red clover flowers, stinging nettle, and burdock, and ⅜ ounce each of dried skullcap and fumitory. Steep a little less than an ounce of the resulting mixture in a pint of water to make a tea three times a day. This mixture cleanses the system of toxins, calms jangled nerves, and soothes inflammation.

- A cup of tea made by mixing equal parts of figwort, nettle, and red clover can be drunk three times a day for its cleansing, calming, and astringent affects.
- Mix ½ teaspoon each of burdock root, pau d'arco bark, sarsaparilla root, and licorice root. Place the mixture in 3 cups of water, simmer for ten minutes, steep for ten minutes, then strain and drink. Do this three times a day.
- Make a tea from equal parts of chamomile, cleavers, and stinging nettle, and drink as an infusion three times a day.
- Mix equal parts of the tinctures of burdock, cleavers, and figwort. Take 1 teaspoon of this mixture three times a day.

▪ Emu oil (also known as kalaya oil) and pine tar soap are other remedies that have been said to help to clear eczema. Neem lotion or cream, a major ingredient in skin-care products in India for over 4,000 years, has also been described as very helpful for the itching and redness of eczema, with antiseptic, anti-inflammatory, and immune-enhancing properties.

AROMATHERAPY

▪ Essential oils of bergamot, chamomile, elemi, eucalyptus, geranium, juniper, lavender, melissa, myrrh, neroli, rose, and tea tree are soothing and help to quiet flare-ups of eczema. You can add a few drops of one or two of the oils to your tepid bath, a warm compress, or a small quantity of jojoba oil to make a healing body oil. Never apply the essential oil directly to your skin, as it can be irritating.

▪ Eucalyptus oil is useful for washing bedding to eliminate dust mites. University of Sydney researchers found that 99 percent of dust mites on wool blankets were killed when soaked for one hour in a solution of 6 tablespoons eucalyptus oil, 1¼ tablespoons liquid laundry detergent, and 13 gallons of water, then rinsed.

HOMEOPATHY

▪ *Graphites* 6c is used for moist, itchy eczema with a honey-like discharge and a tendency to become infected. The areas of the body most likely to be affected are the scalp, the palms of the hands, the webs between the fingers, the corners of the mouth, the corners of the eyes, and the areas behind the ears and behind the knees. Take one dose four times a day for two weeks.

■ *Sulfur* 6c is best for dry eczema that is rough, red, hot, itchy, and aggravated by water and heat. Scratching generally causes soreness, burning, and chronic skin changes. Take one dose four times a day for two weeks.

■ *Petroleum* 6c is the remedy of choice for eczema of the hands, fingertips, and genital areas that crack, bleed, and are covered with thick, pus-filled scabs. The itching of these lesions is generally much worse at night. Take one dose four times a day for two weeks.

■ Remedies commonly used for other specific manifestations of eczema are described below and should be used twice a day until improvement is noted:

- *Anacardium* 6c is helpful for eczema with violent itching that is accompanied by irritability. Take one dose twice a day until you notice an improvement.
- *Calcarea carbonica* 6c is best for white, itchy crusts on the scalp that extend to the face. Take one dose twice a day until you notice an improvement.
- *Kali muriaticum* 6c is helpful for moist, chronic, scalp eczema. Take one dose twice a day until you notice an improvement.
- *Mezereum* 6c is best for blistering, infected, oozing eczema on the scalp that is made worse by warmth and occlusion. Take one dose twice a day until you notice an improvement.
- *Natrum muriaticum* 6c is good for eczema that is moist, greasy, and raw, especially around the hairline. Take one dose twice a day until you notice an improvement.
- *Psorinum* 6c is best for eczema on the cheeks and ears that looks dirty, greasy, and unwashed, or for eczema that is worse on the legs. Take one dose twice a day until you notice an improvement.
- *Rhus toxicodendron* 6c is useful for eczema with multiple small, itchy blisters that flare up at night and with damp weather. People who like warmth do best with this remedy. Take one dose twice a day until you notice an improvement.
- Topically, homeopathic *Calendula* cream is helpful, especially if the skin is cracked, wet, and weeping, or scratched raw.

- Applying Rescue Remedy topically helps to relieve the symptoms of eczema and speed healing.
- *Urtica urens* lotion helps the itching, stinging, and burning of eczema, especially if it is dry and scaly.

▪ In addition to this large choice of single remedies, a homeopathic practitioner may prescribe a constitutional remedy to help with an underlying problem associated with the onset of the eczema.

▪ Combination homeopathic remedies can be helpful. Biological Homeopathic Industries (BHI) produces BHI Allergy, Hair and Skin, Injury, and Skin preparations that are useful for different forms of eczema. Heel Pharmaceuticals also makes at least five different combinations, each one best for a different manifestation of atopic eczema.

ACUPUNCTURE

▪ Acupuncturists view atopic dermatitis as linked to exposure to the traditional Chinese elements of heat, cold, wind, and dampness. They also view it as a failure of the physical and emotional elimination processes of the body. This results in a buildup of toxins and suppressed emotions that are then expressed in an unhealthy way through the skin. Chinese research has shown acupuncture to be successful in treating eczema, with an over 50 percent improvement for more than 80 percent of patients claimed. Consult a qualified acupuncturist if you are interested in trying this type of treatment.

ACUPRESSURE

Acupressure is also said to be very helpful for allergic and stress-related problems such as atopic dermatitis. Using the hands instead of needles to achieve similar effects at the acupuncture points, acupressure was probably an early massage-like forerunner of acupuncture. However, results may take longer to attain than with acupuncture. Subvarieties of acupressure used for eczema include do-in, jin shen, shen tao, and shiatsu, which is the most popular variant, originally developed in Japan. See Acupressure Points in Part Three for the locations of these points on the body.

- Press the Bladder 23 and Bladder 47 points for three minutes three times a day to relieve itching. These points are located in the lower back between the second and third lumbar (lower back) vertebrae, two to four finger-widths away from the spine at waist level.
- Acupressure on Large Intestine 4 relieves itching and helps to purify the blood. The Large Intestine 4 points are located in the center of the triangle between the thumb and the index finger. Apply pressure with the thumb of the opposite hand, angled slightly toward the wrist. Repeat using the other hand, and then twice a day.
- Pressing Conception Vessel 12 can relieve eczema symptoms due to food allergies. This point is located on the midline of the abdomen, halfway between the navel and the edge of the breastbone. Press deeply perpendicularly on this point using your second or third fingers.
- Pressure on the Stomach 36 points improves the body's use of nutrients.
- Press on the Bladder 18 points to strengthen the liver and help to purify the blood and detoxify the body and skin. These acupoints are located two finger-widths on either side of the spine, level with the ninth thoracic (chest) vertebra, about two-thirds of the way down the back. Press at the Bladder 18 acupoints using your knuckles or two tennis balls placed under your back as you lie on the floor.
- Apply pressure to the Spleen 10 points to help regulate the circulation and relieve the skin irritation of eczema. The Spleen 10 points are located on the inside edges of the top of the knees. Use your thumbs to apply acupressure perpendicularly into the points, with your fingers resting on the outside of your knees.
- Pressure on Liver 3 helps to relax the nervous system, indirectly improving flare-ups of eczema.

OTHER THERAPIES

- Kinesiology is a diagnostic system used by some naturopaths to identify specific allergens or nutritional imbalances that cause flare-ups of eczema and also cause weakness of specific muscles. This practice is based on measuring energy flow throughout the body. Your arm is held steady against gentle pressure. You are then retested while you hold suspected allergens in the other hand. A loss of strength in your arm suggests sensitivity or allergy to the specific food. An increase in energy may reveal a deficiency state.

Treatment can then be instituted by using homeopathic remedies or electrotherapy to balance your energy system while the offending allergen is in your energy field.

▩ Specialized testing used by clinical ecologists include not only the standard skin and blood tests for allergens, but also pulse tests and electrical, or Vega, testing. After eating a food to which you are allergic, the pulse rate increases by ten beats or more per minute. This helps to diagnose specific food allergies.

▩ Electrical testing involves the use of specialized electrical measuring devices over certain acupuncture points. Changes in the electrical charges over the acupuncture points are noted when suspected food allergens are introduced. Great changes signal the presence of a food to which you are allergic.

▩ Electrotherapy may be useful for eczema. In 1987, Norwegian researchers H. Bjorna and B. Kaada published work showing that low-frequency transcutaneous nerve stimulation (TNS) may successfully treat atopic eczema. It is believed to work by inhibiting the sympathetic nervous system, resulting in the dilatation of the small blood vessels of the skin, allowing an increased supply of nutritients to the skin and increased elimination of toxins out of the skin. In this study, TNS was reported to increase blood levels of ACTH, cortisol, and vasoactive intestinal polypeptides, hormones, and enzymes that can aid in healing of the skin.

▩ Reflexology is a Chinese system of foot massage. It may be even older than acupuncture, and is thought to have been practiced by many ancient cultures. The feet are seen as mirrors of the body, with different areas of the feet corresponding to specific organs and systems of the body. Reflexologists see disease as arising from blockage of energy channels. Precise foot massage is used to stimulate energy, increase blood and lymph flow, detoxify the body, and reduce stress. For atopic dermatitis, massage would be given to the areas of the feet related to the digestive system, liver, kidneys, thyroid, adrenals, pituitary, and the affected skin.

▩ Eczema, as much as any skin disease, is closely interconnected with the individual's emotional and mental state. Practitioners of mind-body medicine feel that certain personalities and reactions to stress are typical of those who develop eczema. In turn, having eczema may have very poor consequences for a person's self-esteem, work, hobbies, social life, and relationships. A vicious spiral may develop in which a worsening skin condition causes deteriorating mental health, which in turn causes the eczema to worsen. A randomized, controlled trial out of the University of Oxford compared a combination of relaxation therapy, dermatologic education, and cognitive-behavioral treatment with standard medical care for eczema. After one year, the subjects treated with psychological techniques were significantly more improved and needed much less medication to control their eczema than did those treated with standard medical care only.

▥ Some researchers have linked eczema to an unsatisfied hunger for love and affection as an infant or child. Investigators have found that atopic children often have anxious, undemonstrative, overprotective mothers who do not provide the holding and cuddling that infants need to thrive. Breast-fed babies have a lower rate of eczema, perhaps due to the skin contact that is part of nursing. Other researchers think that along with love hunger, atopic people often must deal with much unconscious anger. Many people with atopic eczema are intensely active, compulsively driven, bright people. Some researchers postulate that their striving for control and success, like the eczema itself, represents a reaction to the insecurity of feeling unwanted and unloved. In turn, the psychological impact of atopic dermatitis can be emotionally debilitating. It interferes with the stroking a baby needs to build a strong sense of self. The pleasure and pain of scratching can become the focus of the child's life, and a substitute for fully dealing with the ups and downs of normal relationships with friends, family, and others.

▥ Decreasing their stress helps many patients to avoid flare-ups of eczema. The brain and the skin develop from the same cells in the embryo. Thus, the autonomic nervous system, which is involved in stress, also regulates unconscious flushing, sweating, and pricking up of hairs in the skin. It may be that chronic stress with overstimulation of these nerves leads to the various skin manifestations of atopic eczema. Many types of psychological techniques have been used with documented success. Biofeedback, counseling, guided imagery, hypnotherapy, relaxation techniques, massage, meditation, positive affirmation, and visualization are all very helpful in keeping eczema under control.

GENERAL RECOMMENDATIONS

▥ Simple lifestyle changes such as being out of doors as much as possible, getting regular exercise, sleeping enough, keeping harmonious relationships, developing a satisfying social life, getting involved in community activities, keeping a healthy level of reality in your life, taking time off, and cultivating a purpose in life can be very useful in keeping eczema under control.

▪ Nails should be trimmed to decrease trauma from scratching. Avoid scratching as much as possible to prevent secondary infection of the skin and to break the itch–scratch–rash cycle. Cover affected skin with bandages or clothing to minimize the temptation to scratch. Or apply soothing creams or cool, wet compresses instead of scratching.

▪ Gentle exposure to sunlight may help, but avoid extremes of temperature. Sweating can also cause flare-ups. Humidifiers and any dampness or rapid temperature changes around the house should be avoided.

Hair Loss

Everyone normally loses at least 100 of his or her 100,000 scalp hairs each day. So you shouldn't be alarmed if this is the case with you. Usually, the lost hair is replaced by a new hair from the same hair follicle, located just below the scalp's surface. But we are all familiar with male pattern baldness, the most common cause of hair loss. As men age, their thick hairs begin to thin and recede back from the forehead, from the crown, and from the temples. They are often replaced by a fine, downy type of hair. Male pattern baldness is linked to high levels of testosterone and a person's heredity. Men may be able to see what their hair may look like in time by looking at their mothers' grandfathers' hair.

Women also lose more hair as they age. Many experience a generalized thinning of the hair or a "widened part" in the center of the scalp after menopause. This is called female pattern baldness. As with male pattern baldness, hormonal changes and genetic predisposition are to blame. Although they do not usually lose as much hair as men do, women are also constantly searching for a cure for this distressing problem. All in all, more than two-thirds of all men and women have some type of hair loss or thinning during their lifetime.

Premature hair loss or thinning can also be due to a wide variety of other causes. Most women lose quite a bit of hair in the two to three months after they deliver a baby, and this can continue for up to six months. One and a half to three months after severe stress, operation, infection, or high fever, a person may also lose a lot of hair. Likewise, two to three months after crash dieting with insufficient protein intake, hair may come out in handfuls.

Many prescription drugs can cause reversible hair loss. Cancer patients treated with certain chemotherapeutic drugs may lose up to 90 percent of their scalp hair, but it eventually returns after their treatment is finished. Birth control pills that contain high levels of progestin also can cause hair loss. Other possible causes of hair loss include trauma; syphilis; tumors; thyroid disease; connective tissue diseases; bacterial, fungal, or herpes infections of the scalp; improper hair care with tight hairstyles, overbrushing, or overuse of dyes and permanents; and, in women, too-high levels of male hormones.

Many different nutrient deficiencies result in hair loss, including deficiencies of vitamins A, B$_6$, B$_{12}$, folic acid, biotin, vitamin C, copper, iron, and zinc. Hair loss can be a sign of vitamin A toxicity as well as deficiency. Vitamins B$_6$, B$_{12}$, folic acid, copper, and iron are necessary for the normal formation of red blood cells that supply oxygen to the hair shaft. Copper also functions in the formation of hair pigmentation, so copper deficiency can also cause color changes in the hair. With vitamin-C deficiency, the hair splits and breaks easily, resulting in dry, kinky, tangled hair. Silica also is important for hair growth and strength. Vitamin E is also necessary for good scalp and hair follicle health.

There is also an immune problem known as *alopecia areata,* in which the hair suddenly comes out in totally smooth, round patches. This condition can cause a lot of pyschological stress. A person with alopecia areata can also lose hair from his or her eyelashes, eyebrows, beard, and the other hairy areas of the body.

Because a full head of hair is associated with virility, youth, and attractiveness, hair loss and thinning can have a huge negative psychological impact on a person. If you start losing more hair than normal, a dermatologist will try to identify the cause by taking a complete history, doing blood tests, and examining your hair visually, under the microscope, with hair analysis, and, perhaps, with a scalp biopsy.

CONVENTIONAL TREATMENT

■ Minoxidil (Rogaine) can be prescribed for hair loss in both men and women. This medication is normally applied twice a day to the areas of hair loss on the scalp. Unfortunately, it provides only modest improvement.

■ Finasteride (Propecia) is the first prescription oral drug for mild to moderate male pattern hair loss. It is a type of synthetic steroid that stops the activity of an enzyme responsible for breaking down testosterone into a related compound, dihydrotestosterone, which causes hair follicles to shrivel up and hair loss to be accelerated. Propecia is for use by men only, and should not even be handled by pregnant women or children, as it can cause abnormalities of the genitalia in a male fetus. Otherwise, it is relatively safe, with possible side effects including rash, decreased sex drive, and breast tenderness. Taking just one pill a day, most men can see slowing of hair loss over the top and front of the scalp after three months. There is visible regrowth of hair in these areas after six months.

■ Hair transplants have recently become much more popular. This is due in part to the fact that the transplanted "microplugs" have become smaller, consisting of only a few hairs, and the results look more natural. In this technique, plugs of healthy hair are taken from areas of thick hair growth and transplanted into areas of the scalp that have lost hair and from which smaller skin plugs have been removed to make room for the new ones containing thick hair and hair follicles. Multiple doctor visits spaced weeks apart are usually necessary to complete the hair transplant if large areas are involved. In general, men over the age of fifty with light-colored hair and skin and more advanced stages of balding benefit the most from hair transplants. If the blood flow to the scalp is still good, as it is in most cases of nonscarring alopecia, this may provide an excellent solution to the hair loss problem.

■ Scalp reduction is another surgical option. In this procedure, bald areas of the scalp are removed and the remaining hairy areas of the scalp are pulled and stitched together. The appearance of more hair is given, especially if the hair is still thick on the sides of the head. This procedure is often combined with hair transplantation.

■ Wigs or hair weaves are always an option if hair loss is extreme or very bothersome.

■ More aggressive treatments such as steroid shots or pills are sometimes used for alopecia areata, as large areas of hair loss can sometimes develop.

DIETARY MEASURES

■ Hair is made up mostly of protein. Therefore, it is necessary for everyone to eat enough protein to maintain normal hair production. Good sources of protein include meat, chicken, fish, eggs, milk, cheese, soy beans, tofu, grains, and nuts.

■ Eat a well-balanced diet, with lots of mineral-rich vegetables, grains, legumes, nuts, seeds, and sea vegetables for healthy hair.

NUTRITIONAL SUPPLEMENTS

■ Vitamin and mineral deficiencies need to be evaluated and any deficient nutrients replaced. In general, a good supplementation would include the following:

- A high-potency multivitamin and multimineral daily.
- Beta-carotene. Take 25,000 international units daily.
- Vitamin-B complex. Take a supplement containing 100 milligrams of most of the major B vitamins. Also take an additional 50 milligrams of biotin daily.
- Vitamin C. Take 1,000 milligrams twice a day.
- Vitamin E. Take 400 international units daily, with 100 micrograms of selenium to aid its absorption.
- Iron. Take 50 milligrams daily.
- Zinc. Take 50 milligrams daily, with food and with 2 milligrams of copper.
- Silica. Take 250 milligrams twice a day.
- Free-form amino acid complex. Take 2 grams (2,000 milligrams) three times a day, before or after meals.

■ In addition to correcting any vitamin deficiencies, women whose hair loss is due to physical trauma, crash diets, or heavy menstrual periods can benefit from supplementation with a high-potency multivitamin and 50 milligrams of iron, together with 1,000 milligrams of vitamin C to boost iron absorption.

■ Thinning hair can be a sign of poor nutrient absorption, which in turn can be due to an insufficient supply of stomach acid or bacterial overgrowth in the stomach. Taking one tablet of hydrochloric acid (HCl) and one digestive enzyme capsule after starting each meal, plus ½ teaspoon of powdered acidophilus dissolved in 2 ounces of water twice a day between meals, can aid in nutrient absorption.

■ Inositol with choline has been found to stimulate hair regrowth in some people with nonscarring alopecia. Take 200 milligrams twice a day.

HERBAL TREATMENT

■ Saw palmetto is the first choice of many herbalists for male pattern baldness. Saw palmetto blocks the formation of dihydrotestosterone, a hormone thought to kill off hair follicles and lead to androgenic alopecia. Take 160 milligrams twice a day.

■ Some people have had success using aloe. It is suggested that you apply the gel to the scalp every night before bed, and also take 2 tablespoons of aloe juice orally each day.

■ Arnica can be applied to the scalp twice a day in the form of a cream, ointment, or hair rinse made from arnica tincture diluted with warm water. Arnica increases local blood circulation, and may thereby help promote hair growth.

■ Jojoba oil may help with hair loss when applied to the scalp.

■ Emu oil, or kalaya oil, is recommended as a moisturizer and hair-root stimulant to promote hair growth.

■ Licorice also contains a chemical that prevents testosterone from being changed to dihydrotestosterone. You can add licorice tincture or extract to your favorite shampoo.

■ Rosemary has long been believed to keep hair healthy and lush. Add one part rosemary oil to two parts almond oil and massage the mixture into your scalp for twenty minutes a day.

■ Sage has been believed for centuries to help prevent hair loss. Like licorice, sage extract can be added to your favorite shampoo. Or you can use double-strength sage tea daily as a hair rinse to encourage hair growth.

■ Safflower is considered to be a good vasodilator. Massage your scalp with safflower oil for twenty minutes a day to increase local blood flow and stimulate hair growth.

AROMATHERAPY

■ Essential oils of bay and lavender can be used to make a scalp treatment. Add 6 drops of each to ½ cup warm almond, soy, or sesame oil. Massage the mixture into the scalp for twenty minutes daily, then wash it out with shampoo to which 3 drops of bay oil has been added. The scalp massage itself increases local blood flow and stimulates hair regrowth.

■ Rosemary and cayenne oils can also help with hair regrowth. Add 1 to 2 drops of cayenne oil to each ounce of rosemary oil in a clean, small bottle. Massage your entire scalp with this mixture for at least twenty minutes daily. Rinse the oil out of your hair using shampoo to which 5 drops of essential oil of rosemary has been added per ounce of shampoo.

HOMEOPATHY

■ *Alumina* 200x or 200c is good for hair loss that is accompanied by dry, itchy skin, scalp, and mucous membranes, as well as constipation and throbbing headache. Take one dose three times a week for one week, stop for two weeks, then repeat.

■ *Carbo vegetabilis* is helpful for hair loss caused by an acute illness. Take it as directed by the manufacturer.

■ *Lachesis* is recommended for hair loss caused by pregnancy. Take it as directed by the manufacturer.

■ Use *Lycopodium* or *Sulfur* for hair loss caused by childbirth. Take it as directed by the manufacturer.

■ *Natrum muriaticum* 200x or 200c is for hair loss accompanied by terrible morning headaches, craving for salt, or heavy, irregular menstrual periods. Take one dose twice a week for one week, stop for one week, then repeat.

■ *Phosphoric acid* 30x or 15c is good for hair loss caused by grief or accompanied by fatigue. Take one dose three times a day for three days, stop for two weeks, then repeat.

■ *Phosphorus* is appropriate if hair comes out in handfuls after an acute illness. Take it as directed by the manufacturer.

■ *Sepia* is helpful if hair loss is caused by menopause. Take it as directed by the manufacturer.

ACUPRESSURE

■ Tap over the areas of the balding scalp or the entire scalp with a fine-toothed metal comb. A plum-blossom hammer, which has seven small needle tips, can also be used. These are available through acupuncture supply shops. Do this until the scalp reddens in color, meaning that the flow of blood to the scalp has increased. Repeat once or twice daily.

Hives

Hives, or *urticaria,* are very itchy swellings of the skin and/or deeper tissues caused by the release of histamine. Pea-sized red or white bumps or large patterns of raised red patches covering an entire side of the body may develop, depending on the intensity of the reaction. Hives can be minimal and last only a few hours in acute cases, or they can be extensive, and life threatening if internal organs or the windpipe becomes swollen. By definition, acute hives last less than six weeks, while chronic urticaria persists for longer than six weeks. This is a very common problem, affecting about 20 percent of the population at some time in their lives.

Many things can cause acute cases of hives, including foods such as nuts, shellfish, eggs, milk, chocolate, tomatoes, and berries. Drugs, most commonly aspirin, penicillin, sulfa drugs, codeine, or nonprescription antacids, vitamins, and laxatives, are also common causes of urticaria. Insect bites, a change in the environment, or bacterial, viral, or yeast infections can also trigger hives. Other causes of hives include allergens such as pollens and dander, chemicals, heat, cold, pressure, water, vibration, exercise, collagen vascular diseases, cancer, emotional stress, and pregnancy. Foods, food additives, and infection are the most common causes of hives in children. Reactions to medication are the most frequent things leading to hives in adults. A complete physical examination, lab work, urinalysis, chest x-ray, sinus series, and a strep test may be done by your physician to rule out underlying disease in severe and chronic cases of hives.

CONVENTIONAL TREATMENT

- Try to determine and eliminate the cause(s) as soon as possible.
- Discontinue all nonessential drugs.
- Avoid any foods or substances you suspect of being aggravating.
- Taking an antihistamine such as diphenhydramine (Benadryl, Diphenhist, and others), hydroxyzine (Atarax, Hyzine-50, Vistaril), cyproheptadine (Periactin), or chlorpheniramine (Chlor-Trimeton, Teldrin, and others) every four to six hours can be helpful for the swelling and itching. Some of these drugs are available only by prescription, others over the

counter. Nonsedating antihistamines such as cetirizine (Zyrtec) and loratadine (Claritin) may also be prescribed.

■ If you have trouble breathing, or have a large amount of swelling of any body part, especially the lips, mouth, or genital area, go to the nearest hospital emergency room immediately. You may need an injection of epinephrine if there is acute swelling of the throat or tongue.

■ In acute, severe cases, oral prednisone may be necessary, but is usually withheld as it may obscure the cause of the hives or worsen any underlying infection.

■ In chronic cases of hives, oral prednisone may be necessary to control the outbreak, once the possibility of underlying infection has been evaluated and ruled out.

■ In chronic cases, ultraviolet light therapy is often helpful as well.

DIETARY MEASURES

■ Allergenic foods most commonly associated with hives are eggs, dairy products, yeast, chocolate, soy, beef, pork, citrus fruits, tomatoes, strawberries, onions, shellfish, peanuts, food colorings, and preservatives. Try eliminating these foods from your diet for several weeks, and then add them back one by one after the hives clear.

■ Eat a varied diet without eating the same food twice for several days in a row.

NUTRITIONAL SUPPLEMENTS

■ Take a high-potency hypoallergenic multivitamin supplement daily to ensure an adequate supply of all basic nutrients.

■ Take a vitamin-B complex supplying 100 milligrams of most of the major B vitamins four times a day during an outbreak, then twice a day for a week.

■ Vitamin C is an antioxidant with anti-inflammatory properties. Take 1,000 milligrams of vitamin C with bioflavonoids three times a day.

■ Vitamin E aids in healing and helps to regulate the immune response. Take 200 to 400 international units daily.

■ Pantothenic acid supports the adrenal glands, which helps to normalize the body's immune response. Take 1 to 2 grams (1,000 to 2,000 milligrams) daily.

■ Bromelain is an enzyme that acts as an anti-inflammatory. Take a bromelain supplement as directed by the manufacturer three times a day, between meals.

■ Evening primrose and flaxseed oils provide essential fatty acids that are anti-inflammatories and promote healthy skin. Take 1 tablespoon or 1,000 milligrams of either one daily.

■ Quercetin is also an anti-inflammatory that reduces itching and swelling. Take 200 to 400 milligrams, five minutes before meals, four times a day.

■ Naturopathic physicians sometimes use a treatment called a Meyer's cocktail for severe cases of hives. This is a mixture of calcium, magnesium, vitamin C, and the B-vitamin complex plus additional vitamins B_6, and B_{12} and pantothenic acid, administered intravenously.

■ Liquid beta-carotene can be mixed with calamine lotion and applied directly to the hives. Another topical remedy involves squeezing out the contents of a vitamin A capsule, mixing it with an equal amount of zinc-oxide ointment, and applying the mixture to your hives.

HERBAL TREATMENT

■ Bilberry extract calms hives by decreasing capillary permeability and, therefore, swelling. Take 60 milligrams three times a day.

■ Jewelweed, or impatiens, contains a compound known as lawsone, which is great for hives, especially if they are caused by contact with stinging nettle. Jewelweed is a perennial wildflower that should be available at herb shops and through herbalists. It is not the same plant as the flowering annual called impatiens that is commonly sold in nurseries and garden centers.

■ Stinging nettle—a plant that will cause hives if you brush up against it—helps to clear hives when taken in capsule form every two to four hours until the problem clears.

■ An herbal tea made from two parts each of agrimony and chamomile plus one part each of stinging nettle and heart's-ease can be taken three times a day as an aid to clearing the hives. In addition to drinking the tea, dip a clean cloth into it and apply it as a compress to the hives for five minutes as needed. Other herbs that contain natural antihistamine compounds and from which you can make a combination tea include basil, fennel, ginkgo, oregano, tarragon, tea, thyme, and yarrow.

■ A cabbage leaf, cabbage juice, sliced onions, heart's-ease, chamomile cream, feverfew, comfrey ointment, goldenseal, or stinging nettle can each be applied directly to the hives in the hope that their anti-inflammatory properties will help resolve the hives.

AROMATHERAPY

■ Diluted essential oils of chamomile, lavender, and rosemary are soothing and relaxing, and help ease itching. You can add up to 10 drops of any of these oils (or a combination) to a tubful of water to make an aromatherapy bath, or you can dilute them in a carrier oil such as jojoba oil and apply the mixture to the hives with a compress.

HOMEOPATHY

There are many possible remedies that can be used for hives, depending on the cause and symptoms. The following are the ones most commonly used.

■ *Apis mellifica* 30c is good if fever and sweating accompany the hives, or if they are worse at night. Take one dose every hour for a total of up to ten doses.

■ Use *Dulcamara* 6c if the hives are lumpy, caused by getting cold, or are worse with heat or after scratching. Take one dose three times a day.

■ *Rhus toxicodendron* 30x or 15c is recommended for hives that are burning, stinging, and itching, and are accompanied by joint pain or fever, or are caused by getting wet or cold, or are worse with the cold or with scratching. Take one dose four times a day, up to a total of eight doses.

■ *Urtica urens* 6c is a good choice if the hives are burning, stinging, and itching, or are caused by insects or stinging nettle. This remedy is also appropriate if the hives improve with rubbing, or are worse at night, with heat, or with exercise. Take one dose every hour for a total of up to ten doses.

ACUPUNCTURE

■ Acupuncture has been used for centuries to treat hives in Asia. According to Drs. Chung-Jen Chen and H.S. Yu of Kaohsiung Medical College in Taiwan, acute hives can be cleared by stimulating Large Intestine 11 and Spleen 6, 10, and 36. Moreover, ear acupuncture combined with ordinary acupuncture has been effective in curing chronic hives, as have acupuncture-point injections of vitamin B_1 (thiamine). Consult a qualified acupuncturist if you are interested in trying this type of treatment.

ACUPRESSURE

See Acupressure Points in Part Three for the locations of these points on the body.

■ Press the Spleen 7 points for three to five minutes to relieve itching, and press Spleen 10 to detoxify the blood and remove the excess histamine. Then press the Large Intestine 4 points, which relieves itching and helps to purify the blood. Repeat twice a day, as needed.
■ Pressing the Bladder 18 points also strengthens the liver and aids in detoxification. Repeat twice a day, as needed.
■ Applying pressure to Conception Vessel 12 can relieve digestive sensitivity and skin reactions due to food allergies. Repeat twice a day, as needed.

GENERAL RECOMMENDATIONS

■ Use only unscented hypoallergenic skin-care and laundry products.
■ Apply cold compresses locally to hives. Avoid hot water, which tends to make the problem worse.
■ Making a bath with baking soda, cornstarch, or oatmeal can soothe the itch of hives.

Itching

Itching, or pruritus, is the most common symptom in dermatology. It is something we have all experienced many times. If itching is persistent and severe, it's maddening. If it is bad enough, it interferes with sleep and a permanent state of fatigue follows. This can lead to trouble with work and family and personal relationships. Severe, continuous itching can take over and change a person's life if not controlled or cured.

Itching is a superficial sensation in the skin, probably originating at the border between the epidermis and the dermis. Histamine, a body chemical released in response to contact with an irritant of some kind, is thought to be one of the most common triggers for itching, although there are other chemical mediators in the skin and blood.

There are many causes of itching. Common causes of acute itching include allergies to plants, pollens, cats, dogs, feathers, perfumes, cosmetics, cleaning solutions, other chemicals, and smoke. Short-lived skin problems such as very dry skin, fungal infection, lice, scabies, and sunburn are also frequent reasons for itching. Pregnancy can sometimes produce itching and related skin problems.

Itching that does not rapidly go away may be due to a dermatologic disease such as eczema, seborrheic dermatitis, or psoriasis. It can also be due to a drug reaction, such as a reaction to aspirin, penicillin, sulfa drugs, codeine, or over-the counter laxatives or antacids. An internal medical problem involving the hormones, thyroid, kidney, liver, brain, or blood can trigger severe itching. Thus, itching may be a sign of underlying diabetes, parasites, hepatitis, leukemia, or cancer in the rare patient. After ruling out other causes, mental or emotional disorders have to be considered. These might cause a person to take out frustrations on his or her skin, or focus more attention on itching than most people would.

CONVENTIONAL TREATMENT

■ In long-standing cases of itching without an obvious cause, blood tests, a chest x-ray, stool exam, and urinalysis are usually done to rule out internal disease. Allergens causing itching on contact may be found with the use of patch testing.

■ If known, any underlying cause or causes of itching should be immediately prevented and/or treated. Appropriate treatment depends on the cause of the itching.

■ Topical combinations of ¼ to ½ percent menthol and phenol, such as Sarna lotion, are soothing.

■ Calamine lotion is available over the counter to calm itching.

■ Topical formulas containing pramoxine, such as Pramagel, also help to control itching.

■ Short-term, topical steroids are often used if there is an accompanying rash.

■ Oral antihistamines such as Atarax or Benadryl help to relieve the itching and promote sleep. Nonsedating antihistamines such as cetirizine (Zyrtec) and loratadine (Claritin) are also often prescribed.

■ Activated charcoal capsules, up to 6 grams daily for eight weeks, are a good solution for severe itch as well. They are available over the counter.

■ Ultraviolet-B (UVB) light therapy three times a week often helps relieve the itching, especially in cases of itching caused by underlying internal medical problems.

DIET AND NUTRITION

■ A whole-foods-based, balanced diet helps to prevent nutritional deficiencies that can make itching worse. A healthy diet will also help to keep your immune system strong to fight the causes of itching.

NUTRITIONAL SUPPLEMENTS

■ Take a multivitamin and multimineral supplement daily to ensure an adequate supply of all basic nutrients.

■ A paste made from aloe vera gel and green clay soothes the skin.

■ Chamomile cream, calendula lotion, or comfrey ointment can be applied directly to the itchy areas as often as needed. They have anti-inflammatory properties that help to relieve your discomfort.

■ Jewelweed, otherwise known as impatiens, can be boiled in a gallon of water, strained and cooled. The liquid stops itching extremely well. In fact, in clinical trials, it worked just as well as prescription cortisone creams. Jewelweed is a perennial wildflower that should be available at herb shops and through herbalists. It is not the same plant as the flowering annual called impatiens that is commonly sold in nurseries and garden centers.

■ An herbal tea made from two parts each of agrimony and chamomile and one part each of stinging nettle and heart's-ease can be taken three times a day as an aid to soothing the itching. In addition to drinking the tea, dip a clean cloth into it and apply it as a compress to the affected areas for five minutes every half hour, as needed. Other plants containing naturally antihistaminic compounds from which you can make a combination tea include basil, fennel, ginkgo, oregano, tarragon, tea, thyme, and yarrow. These teas should be used to compress the affected areas of itchy skin, as well as drunk three times a day.

AROMATHERAPY

■ Diluted chamomile, lavender, and rosemary essential oils are soothing and relaxing, and help ease itching. You can add up to 10 drops of any of these oils (or a combination) to a tubful of water to make an aromatherapy bath, or you can dilute them in a carrier oil such as jojoba oil and apply it to the hives with a compress.

HOMEOPATHY

■ *Rhus toxicodendron* 30x or 15c is recommended for itching, especially if it is accompanied by joint pain or fever, or if discomfort is worse with the cold or scratching. Take one dose four times a day, up to a total of eight doses.

■ *Urtica urens* 6c is a good choice for itching, especially if the itch is caused by insects or stinging nettle. This remedy is also appropriate if the itching improves with rubbing, or becomes worse at night, with heat, or with exercise. Take one dose every hour for a total of up to ten doses.

ACUPUNCTURE

■ Dr. T. Lundeberg and colleagues at the Karolinska Institute in Stockholm, Sweden, reported in the *British Journal of Dermatology* in 1987 that acupuncture and electroacupuncture performed close to the itchy area for five minutes after the onset of itching decreased the intensity of the itch to a significant degree. However, the time over which the itching occurred was not significantly decreased. Consult a qualified acupuncturist if you are interested in trying this type of treatment.

ACUPRESSURE

See Acupressure Points in Part Three for the locations of these points on the body.

■ Applying pressure to the Large Intestine 4 and 11 points for three minutes three times a day helps to relieve itching. Large Intestine 4 is located in the webbing between your thumb and index finger, at the highest spot of the muscle. Large Intestine 11 is located on the top, outer end of the elbow crease.

Caution: Do not use the Large Intestine 4 acupoint if you are pregnant, as it may cause premature contractions.

OTHER THERAPIES

■ Electrotherapy can be helpful for chronic itching. In 1993, Dr. B.E. Monk of the Department of Dermatology at Bedford Hospital in England published results of trials with transcutaneous electric nerve stimulation (TENS) therapy for generalized itching in the journal of *Clinical and Experimental Dermatology.* He described TENS therapy as very helpful in relieving severe chronic itch in two patients who were suffering despite having tried many other treatments. In 1996, Dr. L. Ward and colleagues at St. Thomas' Hospital Medical School in London, England, published work in the journal *Pain,* finding that experimentally induced itch in healthy human volunteers can be controlled by mild electrical stimulation for up to one-half hour after the current is applied. They concluded that the electrotherapy might be useful for severe itching associated with underlying disease or skin disorders.

■ An electronic device called the Itch Stopper is FDA-approved for relief of itching. The manufacturer claims that a one-minute treatment can stop itching for up to twenty-four hours, and that it is safe for children. They also claim that there are no side effects such as allergy or steroid dependence. This device is thought to be more effective than pharmaceuticals, as it penetrates the skin barrier more readily. One model is designed for the itch of a rash, and one for itching of normal-appearing skin.

GENERAL RECOMMENDATIONS

■ Cut your fingernails short so they cannot be as destructive.
■ Regardless of the cause, applying cool water and ice locally can usually provide immediate relief from itching.
■ Baths prepared by adding oatmeal or baking soda can also temporarily calm an itch.

Lupus

Systemic lupus erythematosus (SLE) is a chronic autoimmune disease in which the body's immune system attacks its own connective tissue. This causes inflammation and damage to the skin and other organs, and leads to more and more varied infections. SLE is most frequently a disease of women in their thirties and forties. Genetic factors play a role. In a predisposed person, environmental factors such as a latent viral infection, the use of certain drugs, exposure to ultraviolet light, or bodily injury can provoke the onset of the disease.

Chronic cutaneous lupus erythematosus, or discoid lupus erythematosus (DLE), is a form of the condition in which only the skin is involved. DLE is generally much less severe than SLE, which can affect not only the skin, but also the kidneys, blood vessels, eyes, lungs, nerves, and joints. Another form of the disease, subacute cutaneous lupus erythematosus (SCLE), is midway in severity between DLE and SLE. People with SCLE have a psoriasis-like skin rash and may also have joint pains and some blood-count abnormalities. However, they do not have the very serious problems that SLE sufferers can develop.

Typical lesions of DLE are sharply defined red, scaly patches across the cheeks, nose, and outer ear canals. Other small red, scaly patches may also be seen on sun-exposed sites, such as the arms, legs, scalp, and upper body. Often there are also prominent blood vessels and large follicular openings in these patches. The lesions expand, become white and slightly sunken in the center, and heal with scarring and darkened or lightened pigmentation. The rash is more common in the summer months, as it tends to flare up in response to sun exposure. Other factors that can make the rash worse include local trauma, menstruation, fatigue, and illness. Persons with DLE may also suffer from oral and nasal ulcers and permanent hair loss.

The skin rash of SCLE may look like psoriasis, with large scaly, red raised plaques that heal with dark hyperpigmentation of the involved skin. The sun-exposed areas such as the arms, upper back, and trunk are most affected.

Approximately 10 percent of people who have DLE later develop SLE. The skin lesions of DLE and SLE can look the same. People with SLE often also have a so-called butterfly rash, a red rash with very fine scaling continuous over the upper cheeks and bridge of the nose. Redness of the fingertips and palms is also common, as are oral and nasal ulcers. Almost half of all people with SLE are photosensitive, breaking out in a red rash with sun exposure. In addition, people with SLE can have fever and joint aches, and severe problems with their kidneys, heart, lungs, blood, and/or central nervous system.

The rashes of DLE, SCLE, and SLE are usually diagnosed by how they look and by skin biopsy. If you develop a rash typical of DLE or SCLE, your doctor will do blood tests to check for signs of SLE. You may need to consult a rheumatologist.

In this section, we will look at what can be done for the skin problems typical of the various forms of lupus. Mild cases often respond well to natural therapies. Even serious cases of lupus can benefit from some alternative-therapy techniques.

CONVENTIONAL TREATMENT

▓ Avoid the sun. Use a sunscreen with a sun protection factor (SPF) of 15 or higher that shields against both UVA and UVB rays, and reapply it frequently. Sunscreens that contain zinc oxide or titanium dioxide are especially helpful. A total sun block (a product with an SPF of 60) together with six antioxidants and cover-up protective liquid makeup is marketed under the brand name Total Block. It can cover and protect the hyper- or hypopigmented or reddened skin of lupus. Be very careful about which sunscreen you choose. You need one that is hypoallergenic and for sensitive skin.

▓ Wear long, sun-protective clothing, a hat, and gloves when going outside. There is a very good line of sun-protective clothing with an SPF of over 30 called Solumbra, made by Sun Precautions of Everett, Washington. (See the Resources section at the end of this book.)

▓ Use only hypoallergenic makeup and unscented, hypoallergenic shampoos.

▓ Do not use birth control pills, but do avoid becoming pregnant, both of which can cause flare-ups of the disease.

▓ Evaluate all of your medicines to be sure they are not causing or exacerbating lupus.

▓ Dermatologists often prescribe steroid creams and injections directly into the rash. However, since these lesions already have a tendency to thin, caution has to be used with these treatments, which can cause thinning of the skin.

■ Antimalarial medications such as hydroxychloroquine (Plaquenil) or, less commonly, chloroquine (Aralen) are prescribed for the rashes, hair loss, and mucous-membrane involvement of DLE, SCLE, and SLE. Vision changes need to be watched for with these drugs.

■ Azathioprine (Immuran) and cyclophosphamide (Cytoxan, Neosar) are drugs that suppress immune function. They may be needed in addition to prednisone for severe cases of SLE.

■ Plasmapheresis may also be used in extremely serious cases of SLE. In this procedure, blood is removed from the body and centrifuged to separate the cellular elements from the plasma. The plasma is then reinfused into the patient.

DIETARY MEASURES

■ A low-calorie, low-fat diet, with only limited amounts of beef and dairy products that are high in saturated fat, is recommended.

■ Have plenty of green raw and steamed vegetables, chicken, and fish. Eating oily fish such as salmon or sardines packed in sardine oil three times a week helps to fight inflammation and heal the skin manifestations of lupus.

■ Drink eight glasses of pure water every day.

■ Look for any food sensitivities that may be worsening the disease, and eliminate those foods from the diet. Sensitivities to wheat and chocolate are often involved in causing flare-ups.

■ Avoid alfalfa, alfalfa seeds, and alfalfa sprouts. These foods contain an immune-stimulating compound, l-canavanine, and also interfere with protein metabolism. Researchers at the Oregon Health Sciences University first found that monkeys eating alfalfa or alfalfa sprouts became sick with a lupus-like infection within six months, the effects of which were partially reversible with the elimination of alfalfa products from their diet. L-canavanine fed directly to monkeys also caused lupus-like symptoms. These same results have been seen in individuals who eat large quantities of alfalfa products.

■ Avoid plants in the nightshade family, including tomatoes, eggplant, and peppers. These can also make the symptoms of lupus worse.

■ Eliminate from your diet animal fats and oils high in omega-6 oils, such as corn, safflower, and sunflower oils. These promote inflammation.

■ Take a high-potency multivitamin and multimineral daily to ensure an adequate supply of all basic nutrients.

■ Beta-carotene is converted into vitamin A, which is needed to keep your immune system and adrenal glands functioning well. It is also an antioxidant and fights inflammation. Take 25,000 international units of beta-carotene daily.

■ Vitamin B_{12} injections help to increase energy. Ask your physician to give you a 1-milligram dose twice a week.

■ Vitamin C is an antioxidant that decreases inflammation. It also strengthens collagen. Take 1,000 milligrams of vitamin C with bioflavonoids three times a day.

■ Vitamin E fights free radicals, fights inflammation, and promotes healing. In two studies of people with DLE, those who took between 900 and 1,600 international units of vitamin E a day had more rapid clearing of inflamed skin. Take 400 international units of a vitamin-E supplement containing mixed tocopherols once or twice a day.

■ Zinc is needed for healthy immune function. Take 15 milligrams three times a day, with meals and with 0.5 milligram of copper.

■ Selenium is an antioxidant that works with vitamin E. Take 50 micrograms a day.

■ Dehydroepiandrosterone (DHEA) is a hormone that stimulates the adrenal glands, whose function is depressed in lupus. In a small, uncontrolled study of ten patients with SLE, both the patients and their physicians agreed that symptoms were improved after three to six months of DHEA therapy. Start by taking 25 milligrams of DHEA a day, then increase or decrease as symptoms make it necessary.

■ Essential fatty acids such as those found in evening primrose oil, flaxseed oil, fish oil, and black currant seed oil reduce inflammation and benefit the skin. A recent British study of twenty-five people with lupus over an eight-month period found that those taking fish oil capsules improved significantly as opposed to those who took a placebo, whose lupus symptoms worsened or stayed the same. Take 1 to 2 tablespoons of evening primrose, flaxseed, fish, or black currant seed oil each day.

■ Taking oral steroids causes a loss of bone mass that can lead to osteoporosis. If you must take these drugs, also take 1,000 milligrams of calcium and 400 international units of vitamin D daily. These nutrients are necessary for bone formation.

▨ Green food supplements provide a wide range of trace elements and phytochemicals. Take them as directed by the manufacturer.

HERBAL TREATMENT

▨ Anti-inflammatory herbs that can help to calm the inflammation of lupus include the following:
- Pine bark extract. Take 50 milligrams twice a day.
- Grapeseed extract. Take 50 milligrams twice a day.
- Turmeric. Take 300 milligrams three times a day.

▨ Reishi mushroom extract enhances immune function. Take 1 gram (1,000 milligrams) three times a day.

▨ *Avoid* the herb echinacea. It stimulates the immune system, and should not be used in an autoimmune disease such as lupus.

HOMEOPATHY

▨ *Natrum muriaticum* 30x or 15c can be taken as needed for mouth sores. For more severe mouth sores, *Mercurius solubilis* 30x or 15c can be taken as needed.

▨ *Psorinum* 30x or 15c may be helpful for rash on the cheeks. Take it as directed by the manufacturer.

▨ *Sulfur* 30x or 15c is recommended for the butterfly rash of lupus. Take it as directed by the manufacturer.

Nail Problems

Many different problems can cause nails to be weakened, to split, to change color, or to change shape. The nails may grow slowly, become brittle, or have horizontal or vertical ridges. Nail growth becomes abnormal if anything reduces the body's absorption and use of proteins for tissue repair. This includes allergies to nail cosmetics, insufficient stomach acid or digestive enzymes, poor protein intake, nutritional deficiencies, repetitive nail trauma due to water or chemicals, allergies, and drug reactions.

The condition of our nails often gives good clues as to what is going on inside the body. A deficiency of protein, omega-3 fatty acids, vitamins A or D, biotin, calcium, or trace minerals such as silica can cause the nails to become brittle and break easily. This may be due to insufficient intake of these nutrients, or food allergies or low levels of digestive enzymes, either of which can lead to poor absorption in the gastrointestinal tract. Calcium deficiency can also show up as white half-moons on the nails. Red skin around the cuticles may also be caused by poor metabolism of essential fatty acids. Iron deficiency causes spoon-shaped nails. Brittle, ridged, and curved nails can be a sign of anemia due to iron deficiency. Vitamin A deficiency can cause ridging or peeling of the nails. Zinc or vitamin B_6 deficiencies cause white spots to develop in the nails as well as poor nail growth. Darkening of the entire nail bed may be a sign of vitamin B_{12} deficiency. Any severe stress on the body will produce horizontal lines on the nails. Poor absorption of nutrients can cause vertical ridges in the nails, as will the normal aging process. Thickened and curved nails most often are seen in the big toes of older adults.

Other causes of nail problems include acute or chronic health problems, such as thyroid disease, cardiovascular disease, liver or kidney disease, respiratory problems, arthritis, anemia, and nail-biting associated with anxiety. Your doctor may want to do blood tests for iron or other nutritional deficiencies, or for abnormal thyroid function. Fungal or bacterial infection of the nails, acute nail injury, or a primary problem of the skin, such as alopecia areata, psoriasis, lupus, eczema, warts, tumors, and malignant melanoma can also cause nail changes.

Now let's take a look at the many therapies traditional and alternative medicine have to offer us if your nails should split, become brittle or ridged, or change color.

CONVENTIONAL TREATMENT

■ If a secondary infection develops in the nail, treatment with oral antibiotics may be necessary.

■ Psoralens plus ultraviolet light (PUVA) therapy may be recommended for severe nail changes associated with psoriasis or eczema.

■ Strong steroid creams under occlusive dressings are used for severe nail changes associated with psoriasis or eczema.

■ Shots of steroid may be put into the nail plate for severe changes associated with psoriasis or eczema.

DIETARY MEASURES

■ Eat a diet high in iron, lean protein, whole grains, seeds, and nuts for healthy nails. Eggs are a great source of quality protein and sulfur, both of which are important for nails to grow well.

■ Avoid excessive sugar, coffee, and alcohol consumption.

■ Fresh carrot juice containing lots of calcium and phosphorus is great for strengthening the nails.

■ Include in your diet foods high in biotin, a B vitamin essential for strong and healthy nails, skin, and hair. Good sources of biotin include egg yolks, soybean flour, cereals, yeast, cauliflower, lentils, milk, and peanut butter.

NUTRITIONAL SUPPLEMENTS

■ Brittle nails can also be associated with deficiencies of protein, vitamins A, B_6, B_{12}, and D, biotin, calcium, zinc, iron, essential fatty acids, silica, and other trace minerals. In general, to have healthy nails, augment your diet with the following:

- A multivitamin and multimineral supplement including vitamins A and D. Take this daily.
- Vitamin-B complex. Take this daily.
- Biotin. Take 2,500 micrograms daily.
- Calcium. Take 1,200 milligrams daily.
- Iron. Take 30 milligrams daily.
- Methylsulfonylmethane (MSM). Take 500 milligrams three times a day,

with meals. This is is a good source of sulfur, which is needed for healthy nails.

- Zinc. Take 15 milligrams three times a day, with meals and with ½ milligram of copper.

Other nutrients may be necessary as well, depending on the shape and color of your nails and the results of blood testing.

▨ Brittle nails can be a visible sign of poor digestion and poor protein absorption. Take 1 or 2 capsules of a digestive-enzyme formula with betaine hydrochloride after each meal for at least three months.

▨ Brittle nails often respond to biotin, in doses of 2,500 micrograms daily. Before being applied to human nail problems, biotin was found to harden horse hooves. Biotin, which is part of the B-complex, is absorbed into the nail matrix, where new nail cells are generated. Dermatologists have found that biotin supplements help patients with frail nails in about two-thirds of cases. In a recent Swiss study, subjects who had a normal intake of biotin (28 to 42 micrograms a day) but still had thin, frail, and split nails were given a biotin supplement of 2,500 micrograms a day, and overall had a 25 percent increase in the thickness of their nails.

▨ Collagen and vitamin E in horse-hoof moisturizing formulas also strengthen human nails and help to prevent brittle, split nails.

HERBAL TREATMENT

▨ Onymyrrh is a nail-growth accelerator derived from the myrrh plant. Myrrh has been used for decades by horse trainers to toughen and condition their horses' hooves. This lotion claims to improve the user's nail thickness, strength, and flexibility.

▨ Nettle and horsetail are good sources of silica, an important mineral for nails and skin. Drink an infusion made from equal parts of nettle and horsetail three times a day.

▨ If a nail injury, hangnail, ingrown toenail, or other nail problem begins to look infected, apply a goldenseal poultice locally for fifteen minutes twice a day to help draw out the infection. Also, take 500 milligrams of echinacea and 300 milligrams of goldenseal three times a day for five days to aid with any early signs of infection. If the problem does not appear to be resolving within a couple of days, seek the advice of your physician.

HOMEOPATHY

- *Antimonium crudum* 9c is used for injured or crushed fingernails that grow in splits. Take one dose three times a day for three months.
- *Antimonium tartaricum* 12x or 6c is helpful for thick or brittle nails. Take one dose three times a day, three days per week, for three weeks.
- *Graphites* 6c or 12x can be used for all sorts of nail problems, including thickening, cracking, roughness, inflammation, and brittleness. Take one dose three times a day, three days a week, for three weeks.
- *Hepar sulfuris* 6c or 12x will help to clear any minor inflammation or infection following a nail injury. Take one dose three times a day for up to three days.
- *Silica* 15c or 30x is helpful for weak nails that split and peel easily. It also helps to heal white spots on the nails. Take one dose three times a day, three days a week, for three weeks.
- *Zincum metallicum* is also used for white spots on the nails. Take it as directed by the manufacturer.

GENERAL RECOMMENDATIONS

- In general, avoid exposing your nails to strong chemicals, trauma, and too much water. Less is better—do not overmanicure your nails either.
- Trim nails back, but do not cut cuticles back. Instead, push them back gently.
- To prevent and treat dry, brittle, and splitting nails, keep your nails well moisturized with rich creams or plain olive oil after soaking them in warm water.
- Use cotton-lined vinyl gloves whenever working with your hands, especially in water.

Oily Skin

Oily skin is the result of overproduction of sebum by the sebaceous glands. The sebum travels through the pores of the sebaceous glands to the surface of the hair and skin, producing shiny spots on the face and greasy hair on the scalp.

Oily skin is usually hereditary. If you have this condition, you may not see its advantages. However, your skin does stay well moisturized and is smooth, and wrinkles are less noticeable as you get older.

If you have oily skin, you also know that it can often break out in acne, especially in the teenage and early adult years. The extra sebum can mix with the skin cells that line your pores and make them stick together. This plugs up the pores, causing them to stretch and break as more sebum flows into them. This leads to the bumps and nodules we know as acne.

CONVENTIONAL TREATMENT

- Use cleansers that also contain toners to remove excess oil and tighten the pores. The ingredients in toners may make your pores appear smaller temporarily. Do not use lipid-rich or moisturizing soaps. On the other hand, also avoid excessively drying cleansers. These can create a rebound oily effect.
- Do not use abrasive or medicated soaps, and resist the temptation to overscrub your face. Do not use very hot water, but only tepid water. Gently blot your skin dry after washing. In general, do not irritate your skin. This will only make your skin look and feel worse.
- Use mild, alcohol-free toners twice a week to remove excess oil from your face.
- After cleansing, use a small amount of a light, oil-free moisturizer if necessary. Too much moisturizer can clog your pores and give your face a greasy appearance.
- Use only oil-free cosmetics. You can find "oil-control" foundations and powders which actually have oil-absorbing ingredients.
- Use only noncomedogenic sunscreens with a sun protection factor (SPF) of 15 or greater.

DIETARY MEASURES

 ▓ Eat lots of foods that are high in vitamin B_2 (riboflavin), including wheat germ, organ meats, grains, beans, nuts, and yeast. A deficiency of this vitamin can cause oily skin.

 ▓ Avoid fatty foods, such as fried foods, fatty meats, and chocolate.

HERBAL TREATMENT

 ▓ Grind a cup of almonds into a fine powder in a blender. Splash water on your face and rub on a handful of almond powder to cleanse. Work it *gently* into a foam before rinsing with warm, then cool water and blotting dry. Store the almond powder in an airtight container between uses.

 ▓ Rub oily areas with diluted apple-cider vinegar daily.

 ▓ Puree ½ cup of fresh mint leaves and three ice cubes in the blender. Strain and apply the liquid to your face, allowing it to dry. You can use this several times during the day, but you should rinse it off before bedtime.

 ▓ Rub your cleansed face and neck with a papaya slice, and reapply papaya juice over a thirty-minute period. Remove with warm followed by cool water, and blot dry.

 ▓ Parsley is good for oily, acne-prone skin. Boil ½ cup of fresh parsley in 1 cup of water. Steep until lukewarm, then strain. Soak a washcloth in the parsley solution and apply as a compress to your face for fifteen minutes a day.

 ▓ Another aid for oily skin is to rub a raw potato slice directly on your face and neck to cleanse. Rinse with cool water, then blot dry.

 ▓ Simmer ½ cup of fresh sage leaves in 1 cup of water for two minutes. Steep, then chill in the refrigerator. Apply the liquid freely as a cleanser when it has cooled.

 ▓ Make a shampoo by blending together 1 tablespoon lemon juice, 1 ounce pure castile soap, ½ teaspoon vinegar, and 1 egg . Massage the shampoo into wet hair and rinse it out.

AROMATHERAPY

 ▓ Aromatherapy offers many essential oils to include in cleansers, toners, oils, and shampoos for oily skin. In general, geranium, jasmine, juniper, lemon, neroli, orange, peppermint, rosemary, rosewood, tea tree, and thyme oils can improve the condition of oily skin. Add 4 or 5 drops of any of these oils to a cup of water to make a toning lotion, or add a couple of drops to your favorite cleanser or shampoo.

■ Make a lemongrass facial oil by adding 2 drops of lemongrass essential oil to ½ ounce apricot or hazelnut oil. Apply a few drops to the face after every cleansing. Lemongrass is antibacterial and degreasing, and the essential oil formulation is light and quickly absorbed.

HOMEOPATHY

■ *Natrum muriaticum* 6c is good if your face is oily and shiny, and if the hairy parts of the body are very oily. It is also a good choice if you are constipated. Use it as directed by the manufacturer.

Poison Ivy, Oak, and Sumac

Many of us, unfortunately, have had firsthand experience with the itchy red rash of poison ivy, oak, or sumac. These plants produce more cases of allergic contact dermatitis—medically termed *rhus dermatitis*—in the United States than all other substances combined. The rash develops from a sensitivity to urushiol, a chemical compound found in the resin in all of the parts of the *Rhus* plants. You can also acquire the rash if you come into contact with the resin carried on clothing or pets. A severe case of poison ivy, oak, or sumac can also be produced by coming into contact with the smoke from burning plants. In the United States, rhus dermatitis is most common in the spring, when the plants are growing most abundantly, but the rash can also be contracted through contact with the roots or stems in the fall and winter.

Contact with the plant's resin results in the formation of red, very itchy pimples. The pimples may then change into itchy blisters. Weeping and crusting of the lesions then develops. The pattern of the rash depends on where contact with the plant is made and where on the skin the oleoresin is streaked by scratching. The characteristic linear lesions of poison ivy occur when part of the plant is drawn across the skin as one goes through undergrowth. The appearance of the rash is the same whether poison ivy, oak, or sumac is the culprit. It takes between four hours and ten days for the rash to develop. It can then spread rapidly during the next three days, especially with scratching. However, contrary to popular belief, the blister fluid does not contain the resin and is not contagious. Rhus dermatitis can last from one to four weeks. The severity of the rash is a function of how much resin one comes in contact with and how sensitive one is to the urushiol in the resin.

The best way to prevent getting rhus dermatitis is to learn how to recognize and avoid poison ivy, oak, and sumac. Poison ivy grows as a vine or a shrub up to seven feet tall in wooded and partly wooded areas everywhere in the United States. Its leaves turn from a bright green in summer to a bronze-red in the fall. Most important to remember, its leaves always occur in groups of three, with the end leaflet pointed and on a slightly longer stalk. Poison oak is similar to poison ivy in appearance, except that it always grows as a shrub and its trio of leaves are shaped more like oak leaves. Poison sumac, although much more toxic than poison ivy or oak, is much less common. The poison sumac plant is usually found in swampy, partly wooded areas of the eastern United States. It grows as a small tree or shrub. Seven to thirteen smooth-edged leaflets make up each leaf. During the fall and winter, whitish berries in clusters also form on the poison sumac plants.

Now let's take a look at what we can do to provide relief from the itchy rashes of poison ivy, oak, and sumac if you are unfortunate enough to get them.

CONVENTIONAL TREATMENT

- Apply cool water compresses for fifteen minutes every few hours over blisters and crusts to soothe. Adding 1 tablespoon of sea salt per pint of water is even more calming. Or you can add Domboro's tablets to the water to make Burow's solution, which is astringent and antiseptic. Cool oatmeal or salt water baths can also help relieve the itching.
- Use a blow-dryer over the lesions to dry up blisters and help relieve itching.
- Calamine lotion, Rhulicream, and Rhuligel are products available over the counter to calm itching.
- An antihistamine such as diphenhydramine (Benadryl, Diphenhist, and others) or chlorpheniramine (Chlor-Trimeton, Teldrin, and others), which are available over the counter, can be taken to help relieve the itching and swelling. For daytime use, your doctor may prescribe a nonsedating antihistamine such as cetirizine (Zyrtec).
- If your rash is very extensive or you have pain and swelling of your face or genitals, seek the help of your dermatologist immediately. Your physician may use topical steroid creams or, if your rash is severe, a short course of oral prednisone or a steroid injection to speed recovery and help relieve swelling, itching, and pain.

DIETARY MEASURES

- A diet rich in sea vegetables will provide lots of immune-boosting minerals.
- Avoid sugar, fried foods, and fats.

NUTRITIONAL SUPPLEMENTS

■ The following supplements are recommended to help boost the immune response and speed healing:
- Beta-carotene. Take 20 milligrams a day.
- Vitamin C with bioflavonoids. Take 1,000 milligrams three times a day.
- Calcium. Take 2 to 5 grams (2,000 to 5,000 milligrams) three times a day.
- Zinc. Take 50 milligrams a day.

HERBAL TREATMENT

■ Aloe vera gel soothes and dries poison ivy lesions immediately.

■ Calendula lotion is very useful to reduce itching, limit the spread of the rash, and aid in healing.

■ A detoxification tea can be made from any or all of the following: burdock, nettle, red clover, and yellow dock. Drink a cup three or four times a day.

■ Jewelweed, also known as impatiens, is a bushy plant with salmon-colored leaves that often grows near poison ivy, oak, and sumac. It contains the active ingredient lawsone, which is thought to beat urushiol to the binding sites on the skin, locking it out. You can slit the stem of the fresh plant and rub the juice on your rash. Jewelweed can also be boiled in a gallon of water, strained, and cooled. Rinsing with jewelweed juice stops the itching and spread of poison ivy extremely well. In fact, in clinical trials, it worked just as well as prescription cortisone creams. Jewelweed is a perennial wildflower that should be available at herb shops and through herbalists. It is not the same plant as the flowering annual called impatiens that is commonly sold in nurseries and garden centers.

■ The Chinese herb lycium root, in a dosage of 9 to 15 grams daily, can be used for poison ivy.

■ Cool oatmeal or diluted vinegar baths soothe irritated skin.

■ Plantain leaves made into poultices can help control the itching of poison ivy as well.

AROMATHERAPY

■ Many essential oils can help soothe inflamed skin, reduce itching, and relieve anxiety. They include benzoin, cedarwood, chamomile, everlasting, geranium, jasmine, juniper, lavender, neroli, orange, patchouli, peppermint, rose, rosemary, rosewood, sandalwood, tea tree, thyme, and ylang ylang. To get some relief from your rash, use any of these oils (or a combination) in baths, compresses, and body oil.

■ Topically, *Rhus toxicodendron* 6c in 75 percent alcohol is useful to limit the rash. *Rhus toxicodendron* 6c taken can also be taken orally three to four times a day.

■ A variety of other oral homeopathic remedies may be taken depending on the location and symptoms of the lesions:

- *Anacardium,* if primarily the face is affected by the rash.
- *Anagallis,* if blisters are found only on the palms.
- *Apis mellifica,* if the face is involved, especially if the eyelids are swollen.
- *Croton tiglium,* if mostly the genitalia and/or scalp is involved.
- *Grindelia,* if the skin is purplish and swollen, and asthmatic symptoms are also present.
- *Sulfur,* if the itch has a burning quality.

ACUPUNCTURE

■ Stimulating acupuncture points along the spleen and nervous-system channels relaxes and detoxifies the body. In 1988, Dr. S.J. Liao of New York University reported moderate success with acupuncture for four cases of unbearably itchy poison ivy. In three milder cases, the patients' itching was greatly reduced in a few hours and the rashes were healed within two days after a single treatment. In a very severe case, three acupuncture treatments were necessary for the itch to resolve and most of the lesions to heal. Itching lasted about two days, and the skin lesions lasted about four days. Dr. Liao concluded that the acupuncture may have stimulated the body's production of natural steroids. Consult a qualified acupuncturist if you are interested in trying this type of treatment.

ACUPRESSURE

See Acupressure Points in Part Three for the locations of these points on the body.

■ Press the Spleen 7 points at least three times a day to relieve the itching and heat from the rash. The Spleen 7 points are located halfway up the inner aspects of the calves, just slightly to the front of the body.

■ If you have recurrent poison ivy, press the Liver 3 points on each side of the body three times a day to strengthen the liver, which helps to filter toxins from the body. The Liver 3 points are on the backs of the feet, about one finger-breadth up from the toe joints, between the first and second toes.

GENERAL RECOMMENDATIONS

■ To avoid getting poison ivy, wear a long-sleeved shirt, long pants, and socks if you will be spending time in the woods and areas known to have *Rhus* plants growing in them. Learn how to identify these plants, and use that knowledge to avoid them.

■ If you come into contact with any of these plants, immediately wash thoroughly. If you can wash the resin off within fifteen minutes of contact, you may inactivate it and avoid the rash. Also change clothes immediately, and wash the contaminated clothes in hot water with a strong detergent and bleach.

■ Trim your nails to limit scratching and spread of the rash.

Psoriasis

Psoriasis is among the most common and most difficult to control of all skin diseases, affecting about 2 percent of the population. It affects men and women equally, and usually appears between the ages of fifteen and thirty. It generally follows a chronic course of acute flare-ups alternating with periods of remission.

The word *psoriasis* is derived from the Greek *psora,* which means "to itch." Salmon-red bumps with a silvery scale appear on the skin, get bigger, and grow together to form large plaques. Lesions of psoriasis vary in size from fractions of an inch in diameter to large plaques covering most of the body and requiring hospitalization. Places on the body most commonly affected by psoriasis include the elbows, knees, scalp, and sacral areas. The nails are involved in about one-half of cases, with pitting, breaking, thickening under the nail, or thickening of the nail itself. In addition, between 10 and 30 percent of people with psoriasis also suffer from psoriatic arthritis, which can be quite painful. Because of the chronic, difficult nature of psoriasis, professional help is needed in all but the least severe cases.

There appear to be many reasons why some people develop psoriasis and others do not. It has a tendency to be inherited—about one-third of those who have it have another family member with psoriasis. Several studies have documented the relationship between specific stresses and the start and flare-ups of psoriasis. Almost half of all people with psoriasis report that a specific stressful event occurred within one month before the first episode of psoriasis, according to a study of 132 patients reported by Dr. R.H. Seville in the *Journal of the American Academy of Dermatology*. Stress has also been shown to precipitate flare-ups in up to 70 percent of people whose psoriasis had previously cleared. This may be because the health of the skin depends on proper blood circulation to the dermis that nourishes the cells of the epidermis above it. Stress, researchers theorize, may cause the body to shunt blood away from the upper layer of the skin, and this in turn may result in psoriasis. The dermis of the skin also causes changes in the top layer of the skin by bringing many stimulated inflammatory cells into the epidermis of the psoriasis lesions.

Some experts have viewed an abnormal intestinal tract as the main underlying problem causing psoriasis, believing that psoriasis is really an external manifestation of a problem that begins internally. According to this view, thin, porous, intestinal walls allow toxic elements to seep through and make their way through the lymphatic channels to the bloodstream. This problem is known as "leaky gut syndrome." When the liver, the major detoxifying gland of the body, gets overloaded, the skin aids in the elimination of these toxins. Also, the gut no longer works as well to make immunoglobulins, or antibodies, which are the first line of defense against infection. According to this theory, an improper diet with too many acid-forming foods, failure to drink enough pure water, misaligned vertebrae, negative emotions, and hereditary factors cause the intestinal walls to become thin and porous. Thus, a proper diet, adequate eliminations, spinal adjustments, and positive thinking make up a major part of the psoriasis solution.

Psoriasis has since been determined to be an autoimmune disease, a disorder in which the immune system works against the body's own tissues by creating abnormal levels of immunoglobulins and immune complexes. Dr. W.H. Reeves and associates at Rockefeller University, in 1986, and Dr. R.M. Fine of the Emory University School of Medicine, in 1988, published works citing clinical evidence of this link between psoriasis and autoimmunity.

Recent research indicates that deficiencies of sulfur and essential fatty acids are also responsible for psoriasis. Metabolically, there are abnormalities in psoriasis, with skin cells moving from the bottom to the top of the epidermis in one-seventh the normal time, causing the thick scales to pile up and form lesions on the skin. Abnormal energy metabolism leads to an increase in the size of skin cells, an increased number of skin cells due to too-rapid turnover, and changes in the body's inflammatory response.

Inadequate intestinal absorption of amino acids, together with bacterial degradation in the colon, produces certain types of compounds called polyamines that are toxic. Other toxic products that are formed inhibit the production of cyclic adenosine monophosphate (cAMP), another type of polyamine that acts as a biochemical messenger and plays a role in cellular reproduction. Still other gut-derived toxins lead to increased skin-cell levels of a form of stored energy called cyclic guanosine monophosphate (cyclic GMP or cGMP). These increased cGMP and imbalanced cGMP/cAMP levels in turn increase the rate at which skin cells proliferate, and can lead to flare-ups of psoriasis. Endotoxins (toxins produced by bacteria) can also magnify the problem by inhibiting the liver's ability to filter out other toxins, thereby further initiating inflammation and new, large cells in the skin.

Conventional treatments are very important in trying to control psoriasis. Professional help should always be sought for all but the most minor forms of psoriasis. However, as psoriasis is so difficult to eradicate, the use of alternative methods can enhance the effectiveness of conventional Western therapies. In the last decade, more and more psoriasis sufferers have turned to alternative medicine for relief. In a 1990 study, Norwegian researcher Dr. P. Jensen found that almost half of Norwegian psoriasis patients had previously used or currently were using at least one type of alternative medical therapy. A 1992 Canadian study found that a total of one-fifth of psoriasis patients had used herbal, dietary, and vitamin therapies to try to improve their psoriasis. A September 1996 study published in *Cutis* by Dr. A.B. Fleischer, Jr., and colleagues from the Bowman Gray Department of Dermatology at the Bowman Gray School of Medicine at Wake Forest University found that half of more than 300 university dermatology patients used alternative medical therapies on their own for their psoriasis. Those with the most severe cases of psoriasis were more likely to have tried herbal remedies, vitamin therapy, and dietary manipulations. It is very likely that all of these statistics have jumped dramatically in the last decade, as there has been a tremendous upsurge of interest in complementary medicine.

Psoriasis is rarely really dangerous, but it can diminish self-esteem and quality of life, as well as drain one financially and psychologically. The purpose of this section is to give not only information, but hope. With patience and persistence, and the use of both natural alternatives and conventional treatments, there really can be a striking improvement and remission of even the most severe cases of psoriasis.

CONVENTIONAL TREATMENT

■ The simplest forms of treatment for psoriasis are tried first: topical moisturizers, ointments, and corticosteroids. Various topical preparations have been found to be very helpful in diminishing the size and thickness of the plaques. Often, one topical treatment works better for a given individual than does another. Patience with trial and error is required to find the most helpful topical treatment for your skin chemistry.

■ A good moisturizer is most important to prevent further dryness, which can lead to more cracking and bleeding of the skin. Some of my favorite moisturizers include Moisturel and Neutrogena, but there are many other good ones. Plain olive oil, vegetable shortening (Crisco), or clear petroleum jelly (Vaseline) can also be spread on the skin. The important thing is to put the moisturizer on the skin immediately after washing and bathing, at least twice a day.

■ Zinc-oxide ointment is also good at preventing cracking of the skin, and helps to heal cracks that are already present. Some people have found A&D ointment to be very helpful for controlling outbreaks and itchiness.

■ Infections that may provoke psoriasis need to be ruled out or treated.

■ Topical steroid preparations have long been the mainstay of psoriasis therapy. The strength of the cream prescribed generally depends on the severity and location of the psoriasis. However, the long-term side effect of thinning of the skin with excessive topical steroid use limits its usefulness.

■ Anthralin (Drithocreme, Micanol) is a cream or ointment that is often highly effective. It works by inhibiting skin-cell proliferation. However, it is irritating to the skin and causes discoloration of clothes and skin, so it is not usually the first topical agent to be prescribed.

■ A retinoid gel called tazarotene (Tazorac) may be prescribed to help clear stable plaque psoriasis that covers up to one-fifth of the body. This medication is used nightly, and a steroid cream such as mometasone (Elocon) is used in the morning to reduce irritation and photosensitivity. Good results on psoriatic plaques have been seen as soon as two weeks after starting treatment. Because tazarotene can cause birth defects, it is not to be used by pregnant women or women who are planning to become pregnant.

■ A topical vitamin D_3 derivative, calcipotriene (Donovex) ointment, can be very helpful in the treatment of psoriasis. It slows the growth of the skin cells to a closer to normal rate, decreases itching, and decreases inflammation in the skin. Studies have shown that people with psoriasis have low levels of vitamin D, but that their skin cells have receptors for activated vitamin D. When the activated vitamin D attaches to the receptors in psoriatic skin cells, it prevents these cells from growing and shedding too rapidly. There is reportedly a greater than 50-percent (and up to 60-percent) improvement in psoriatic lesions after two or three weeks of Donovex ointment treatment.

■ Topical coal-tar preparations, although effective against psoriasis, have never been very popular because they were bad-smelling and stained clothes and bedsheets a grayish-brown. A newer coal-tar product, Exorex, has been developed that is clear, greaseless, nonstaining, and odorless. It has been found to be as effective as Donovex in the treatment of psoriasis of the body or scalp. Like other coal-tar products, it decreases the speed at which the skin cells turn over.

■ Although messy, carbolated Vaseline and Baker's P&S, applied with a cotton swab, are very helpful for psoriasis along the hairline. A tar shampoo such as T-Gel is scrubbed in and left on for ten minutes under a shower cap before rinsing out. To relieve scalp itching, diluted Lavoris, Listerine, and Glyco-Thymoline mouthwashes are very helpful when used as scalp rinses.

■ For more severe cases of psoriasis, oral medications are often prescribed. The vitamin A derivatives isotretinoin (Accutane), etretinate (Tegison), and acitretin (Soriatane) have proved very useful to quiet severe cases of psoriasis. However, women cannot get pregnant while on these medications or for a time afterward, because these medications can cause serious birth defects. Also, lab work has to be done regularly to make sure that the liver enzymes and blood lipids don't rise too high while a person is on any of these medications.

■ Methotrexate (Folex, Rheumatrex) is the most effective treatment for severe disabling psoriasis, especially when it is associated with severe psoriatic arthritis. It works by decreasing DNA synthesis in the epidermis and interfering with rapid skin-cell proliferation. It is an extremely toxic drug, however, so it is reserved for unresponsive, widespread cases and its use must be closely monitored. A topical cream for use by people with psoriasis is currently under development.

■ Cyclosporines, which are drugs developed to suppress the immune system in transplant patients, are also useful in treating this autoimmune disorder. This treatment too is saved for only the most severe, unresponsive cases, due to the risk of side effects. A topical form is currently being studied for use in psoriasis.

DIETARY MEASURES

■ Diet is thought to be key to controlling psoriasis, both in terms of the many suspected sensitivities that may keep the skin reacting, and as a major factor in determining the alkalinity of the blood. In general, a whole-foods diet with lots of fresh yellow and green vegetables, soybeans, chickpeas, lentils, black beans, sesame seeds, lean proteins, and low-fat fish is recommended.

▪ Food sensitivities need to be assessed and treated, either by professional testing or by elimination and then careful reintroduction of one food at a time, noting any flare-ups of symptoms on the way. Usually, if you itch, it is something eaten earlier in the day or, more often, the previous day, that your skin cannot tolerate and is reacting to. Suspects to test for possible allergy or sensitivity to include wheat, milk, eggs, meat, dairy products, shellfish, aromatic spices, citrus fruits and juices, and nuts. In a study published in the *California Medicine Journal* in 1980, an elimination diet was shown to significantly help patients' psoriasis.

▪ Limit your intake of protein. As far back as the early 1900s, Dr. L. Duncan Bulkley reported in a speech to the Section of Dermatology of the American Medical Association that a low-protein, mainly vegetarian diet is best for people with psoriasis. In 1932, Dr. Jay Schamberg, a highly respected professor of dermatology at the University of Pennsylvania, wrote in the *Journal of the American Medical Association* that in his patients with psoriasis, "a low-protein diet, without any other internal or external treatment, causes a disappearance of the greater part of the eruptions. . . ." The growth of skin cells can also be curbed by fasting. Reducing caloric intake is always helpful, and many people with psoriasis have noted improvement on a fasting and vegetarian regime. Overeating intensifies the buildup of toxins in the body.

▪ Many natural-medicine experts recommend that the blood be kept slightly alkaline, with a pH of 7.3 to 7.5, in order to maintain the optimal internal chemical milieu for good health, strong immunity, efficient removal of toxins, and clearing of skin lesions. The daily diet should consist of 80 percent alkaline-forming foods and 20 percent acid-forming foods. Fruits, vegetables, and fiber form the core of the diet. The exceptions to this are the citrus fruits, and vegetables of the nightshade family. Citrus fruits, citrus juices, strawberries, tomatoes, tobacco, eggplant, white potatoes, peppers, paprika, and hot, spicy foods should be eliminated from the diet.

▪ Eat a high-fiber diet to aid in moving toxins out of the bowel.

▪ Proteins, starches, sugars, fats, and oils should be limited. Fish, poultry, and lamb are the more readily digestible forms of animal protein, and are recommended over red meat. Red meat and dairy products also contain arachidonic acid, which increases the inflammation in psoriasis. These foods are best avoided during flare-ups.

■ Fish like salmon, sardines, mackerel, herring, and tuna are especially suggested. They are high in omega-3 essential fatty acids, which can help reduce itchiness and inflammation. Free fatty acid levels are abnormal in psoriatic skin. One tablespoon of olive oil, cod liver oil, flaxseed oil, or canola oil should be added to food each day to increase the intake of oils with beneficial omega-3 fatty acids.

■ If you consume dairy products, choose nonfat or low-fat varieties.

■ Choose whole-grain products over white bread and foods made with white flour. In studies, people intermittently following a strict rice diet found that their psoriasis cleared significantly. Cravings for sweets should be satisfied as much as possible with fresh fruits, or foods sweetened with honey or pure maple syrup. Sugar, tea, animal fats, food additives, vinegar, and carbonated beverages increase the body's acidity, and should also be limited as much as possible.

■ Increase your consumption of fresh vegetable juices, particularly beet, carrot, cucumber, lettuce, parsley, and spinach. Suggested combinations include apple and carrot, cucumber and grape, and beet, carrot, and garlic juice mixed together. Citrus juices should be avoided.

■ Coffee, caffeine, and alcohol impair liver function and should be avoided, if possible.

■ Drink six to eight glasses of pure, filtered water every day in addition to any other liquids. This is particularly important in aiding elimination and acidity problems. As a substitute for soft drinks that are filled with sugar or artificial sweeteners, preservatives, and artificial flavorings and colorings, you can enjoy naturally carbonated water such as Perrier or Saratoga water (or just plain seltzer water).

NUTRITIONAL SUPPLEMENTS

Although it is best to get as many vitamins and minerals in the fresh foods one eats, supplemental vitamin therapy is highly recommended for people with psoriasis.

■ Take a high-potency multivitamin and multimineral supplement daily to ensure an adequate supply of all basic nutrients.

■ Beta-carotene is an antioxidant and is healing for the skin. Antioxidants decrease levels of cGMP, which helps to limit psoriasis. Beta-carotene is also converted into vitamin A in the body. Vitamin A inhibits the synthesis of body chemicals called polyamines, which are responsible for regulating the size and number of skin cells. People with psoriasis have higher than normal levels of polyamines. Take 50,000 international units of beta-carotene daily for two months, then cut back to 25,000 international units a day. Also take 150,000 to 300,000 international units of a liquid combination carotenoid supplement daily.

▩ The B vitamins are helpful in the repair and healing of skin cells. Take a complex containing 100 milligrams of most major B vitamins daily. Also take an additional 500 micrograms of folic acid daily. People with psoriasis lose greater than normal amounts of folic acid through their skin.

▩ Vitamin E is an antioxidant and promotes healing. Take 400 international units daily.

▩ Selenium is an antioxidant and increases the effect of vitamin E. Take 200 micrograms daily.

▩ People with psoriasis lose greater than normal amounts of zinc through their skin. Zinc is necessary for the absorption of linoleic acid, a crucial omega-3 fatty acid. Take 25 milligrams of zinc picolinate daily.

▩ Lecithin is an excellent alkaline aid to digestion, and is also a helpful laxative. Take 1 tablespoon twice a day, with meals, for one month.

▩ Quercetin is a phytochemical that has antipsoriatic properties. Take ¼ teaspoon four times a day.

▩ Glutathione is an amino acid that slows the growth of skin cells in psoriasis. Take 500 milligrams twice a day, between meals.

▩ Omega-3 and omega-6 esential fatty acids (EFAs) can improve psoriasis, and are abundant in fish oil, black currant seed oil, borage oil, evening primrose oil, and flaxseed oil. These EFAs interfere with the inflammation caused by another fatty acid, arachidonic acid, in the body. Take 4 capsules of evening primrose or flaxseed oil three times a day or 1,000 milligrams of black currant seed oil daily.

▩ Limit your intake of vitamin C to 1,000 milligrams a day, and biotin to 50 micrograms a day. These nutrients stimulate cGMP, which can make psoriasis worse.

Herbal liver tonics, together with tissue and blood cleansers, or alteratives, form the most important initial part of herbal treatment for psoriasis. Slightly less important are nerve tonics, or nervines, which soothe the nerves and lessen the itching of psoriasis.

- Applying aloe vera gel to the lesions can help. Dr. Andrew Weil reported that 83 percent of psoriasis patients who applied aloe-vera cream three times a day for up to four weeks noted an improvement. Dr. Weil recommends using pure aloe vera gel instead of an aloe vera cream that contains other ingredients.

- Apple-cider vinegar diluted in water can be used to temporarily help relieve itching and scaling. Apple cider vinegar or white vinegar can also be diluted in three to four times as much lukewarm water and poured over the head, rubbed in, left for one minute, and then rinsed out. Or you can add ½ cup of cider vinegar to a tubful of bath water to help restore acidity to the skin.

- Banana peel is a key ingredient in Exorex. This is a lotion concocted from coal tar and a specific essential fatty acid from banana peel that is associated with the immune system. Reportedly, the idea was derived from Zulu folklore, in which banana peels have been used for a variety of skin ailments for years.

- Burdock root can help improve flare-ups of psoriasis. Take 20 to 40 drops of tincture three times a day.

- Chamomile is widely used in Europe for treating psoriasis. It contains anti-inflammatory flavonoid compounds. If you have ragweed allergies, however, do not use chamomile, as it is a member of the ragweed family.

- Castor oil is particularly helpful when left overnight on thick, small, well-circumscribed lesions. If cold-pressed castor oil is mixed with baking soda, it has been found to greatly improve thick, scaly heel skin, as long as the skin isn't cracked.

- Cayenne pepper has anti-inflammatory properties and helps with healing. Two clinical trials reviewed in the November 1998 issue of *Archives of Dermatology* reported that 0.025 percent capsaicin cream, made from hot peppers, works to reduce the redness and scaling in psoriasis. Capsaicin cream is available over the counter as Capzasin-P or Zostrix. It should be used over a six-week period. Care should be taken not to apply it to broken skin.

■ Common figwort helps to clear psoriatic plaques. The recommended dose is 2 milliliters of tincture, taken twice a day.

■ Dandelion tincture is useful for stimulating bile flow and clearing toxins out of the system. It is frequently combined with yellow dock (see below) for this purpose. The recommended dose is 30 to 60 drops twice a day.

■ Echinacea tincture is occasionally used for psoriasis. It boosts the immune system, and so may decrease the incidence of colds, which can lead to flare-ups in some individuals. The recommended dose is 20 to 30 drops three times a day for up to ten days. Stop for two weeks, then repeat.

■ Emu oil contains essential fatty acids and may be helpful for psoriasis. Apply it to the lesions as directed by the manufacturer.

■ Flaxseed oil is chemically similar to fish oil and helps treat psoriasis. Adding flaxseed oil to salad dressing is a good way to get this helpful supplement into your diet. Take 1½ tablespoons of flaxseed oil daily.

■ Fumitory contains fumaric acid, which has been found to be very helpful for psoriasis. Make a strong tea from fumitory and apply it to the affected areas with a cotton ball twice a day.

■ Garlic is detoxifying and includes a number of sulfur-containing compounds. Sulfur deficiency may contribute to psoriasis. Take three to six garlic capsules daily.

■ Goldenseal tincture helps to clear the body of toxins that lead to flare-ups. Take 20 to 30 drops twice a day for up to ten days at a time.

■ Gotu kola extract reduces inflammation and speeds skin healing. In India, it has been used for psoriasis for hundreds of years. Take 200 milligrams three times a day for one month.

■ Liquid licorice extract, applied directly to the affected areas with a cotton ball, is felt by some naturopaths to work as well as corticosteroid creams.

■ Flaxseed oil, applied to affected areas twice a day, is said to help heal psoriasis. Avocado, garlic, and walnut oils, applied topically twice a day to the psoriatic patches, are equally helpful for moisturizing and healing.

■ Milk thistle cleanses and protects the liver, increases bile flow, and helps in blood purification. It also helps to correct the abnormal cell replication present in psoriasis. Take 300 milligrams of milk-thistle extract three times a day.

■ Neem-seed oil, an Ayurvedic herbal remedy, is highly recommended by some psoriasis sufferers. It was introduced to the United States in 1994 from India and Pakistan. Neem lotions are usually found in East Indian markets and in health food stores. Use these products as directed by the manufacturer.

■ Nettle is used as a cleanser. Ideally, it should be taken as a juice or infusion two or three times a day. To increase the effect, it can be combined with cleavers.

■ Red clover is a blood-cleansing herb that can help with psoriasis. Take 30 drops of red clover tincture twice a day. You can also apply a red clover cream to the plaques twice a day to speed healing.

■ Saffron tea, best taken in the evening, acts on the stomach and intestines to help them to function more normally, and thus calm psoriatic flare-ups.

■ Sarsaparilla is very important in botanical therapy for psoriasis. It is generally taken as ¼ teaspoon of solid extract twice a day or 25 to 30 drops of tincture three times a day. You can also brew a strong sarsaparilla tea and apply it to the affected areas twice a day with a cotton ball or clean cloth. Sarsaparilla is thought to both normalize fat metabolism and bind toxins in the skin cells.

■ Slippery-elm bark, best taken in the morning, is thought to form a protective coating along the inner lining of the intestinal tract, preventing seepage of toxins and speeding healing of the intestinal walls. This in turn improves psoriasis.

■ Yellow dock tincture helps to remove toxins from the blood and thereby improve psoriasis. Take 30 drops twice a day.

■ Combination herbal detoxification formulas can be helpful. A mixture of equal parts of burdock, cleavers, sarsaparilla, and yellow dock tinctures, taken in a dose of 1 teaspoon three times a day (or drunk in tea form), may be used to improve psoriatic plaques. There are also combination detoxification teas, capsules, and liquids for psoriasis that are sold over the counter in health food stores and over the Internet. Most consist of various combinations of burdock, dandelion, milk thistle, red clover, sarsaparilla, yellow dock, and/or other cleansing herbs.

■ Herbal teas that help to reduce stress can be very helpful. These include chamomile, lavender, lemon balm, and lime blossom.

AROMATHERAPY

■ Debrae A. Walsh of the Homerton School of Health Studies in Cambridge, England, reported in 1996 that aromatherapy can produce both physiological and psychological benefits in the management of psoriasis. Essential oils can be used topically to decrease inflammation and irritability of the skin, or can be added to the bath as a stress-reliever. Essential oils that can soothe the skin and decrease irritation and inflammation include chamomile, everlasting, lavender, and myrrh. Neroli, rose, tea tree, and ylang ylang oils may also be helpful.

A combination of calendula and lavender essential oils is recommended for decreasing local inflammation of the skin. Add 2 drops of calendula oil and 1 drop of lavender to 2 tablespoons of almond oil and massage the mixture into the affected skin at least twice a day.

An electrical heat cap, mitts, and boots can be used in conjuction with various oils to increase their effectiveness on psoriatic plaques of the scalp, hands, and feet.

HOMEOPATHY

Homeopathy is useful for psoriasis primarily in conjunction with diet and relaxation therapy, and as a short-term aid for flare-ups.

Arsenicum album 30x or 15c is helpful for dry, roughened, red, hot skin that may have a burning sensation. Take it as directed by the manufacturer.

Graphites 12x or 6c is useful if itchy psoriatic skin dries out and cracks and bleeds. It is also good for psoriasis behind the ears, with honey-colored pus. Take it as directed by the manufacturer.

Kali arsenicosum 12x or 6c is good for intense itching that becomes worse with heat. Take it as directed by the manufacturer.

Psorinum 30c is sometimes used to tone down psoriasis. Take a dose once a week.

Sulfur 6c is used for hot, dry, itchy skin that is made worse by heat. Scratching gives very temporary relief, but then causes soreness and burning. Take one dose twice a day.

ACUPUNCTURE

Case reports on using acupuncture in the treatment of psoriasis in the professional literature provide conflicting results. In general, acupuncture is occasionally recommended in conjunction with diet and elimination techniques to tone down symptoms. In 1992, Drs. S.J. and T.A. Liao of the New York University Dental College published an article in *Acupuncture and Electro-Therapeutics Research* in which they reported treating sixty-one cases of psoriasis with acupuncture. None of the subjects had responded to conventional Western medical management of extensive psoriasis. The average duration of their battles with psoriasis was about sixteen years. They received an average of nine acupuncture sessions each. The Drs. Liao found that about one-half of the subjects experienced total or almost total clearing of the skin lesions, and one-quarter had approximately two-thirds clearance of the skin lesions. Only about one-seventh failed to have any improvement. The Drs. Liao concluded that acupuncture was an effective type of therapy for psoriasis, particularly for severe cases where conventional treatment had been unsuccessful. However, a controlled study of acupuncture compared with placebo reported by Dr. B. Jerner and colleagues at Linköping University in Sweden in 1997 found no convincing effect of acupuncture therapy in psoriasis. In this study, fifty-six subjects with longstanding plaque psoriasis received either electro-stimulation by needles plus ear acupuncture or "minimal placebo acupuncture" twice a week for ten weeks. Thus, the professional literature provides conflicting evidence for the use of acupuncture in the treatment of psoriasis, and it is not widely employed for this purpose. If you are interested in trying this type of treatment, however, consult a qualified acupuncturist.

ACUPRESSURE

There are many acupressure points that can be useful for psoriasis. Apply pressure to the acupoints you choose on both sides of the body for three minutes three times a day. See Acupressure Points in Part Three for the locations of these points on the body.

- If your psoriasis itches, press the Spleen 7 acupoint for three to ten minutes, as needed during the day to relieve the itch.
- Pressing the Spleen 6 and 10, and Bladder 18 points cleanses the blood.
- The following points govern general skin health: Large Intestine 1, 4, 5, and 20, and Lung 2, 7, and 9. Press at least two of these points for three to five minutes on a daily basis.

   Caution: Do not use Large Intestine 4 and Lung 7 if you are pregnant.

- Pressing Conception Vessel 12 and the Stomach 36 points can help relieve psoriasis if it is due to food allergies and digestive sensitivity.
- Pressing the Four Gates combination relaxes the nervous system, thus helping psoriasis that flares up in response to stress.

OTHER THERAPIES

- Internal cleansing, with clearing out toxins in bowels and kidneys, can be crucial for the treatment of psoriasis. Opening up the normal channels of elimination relieves backup pressure on the liver and intestine, allowing the liver cells to filter out and purify the blood and lymph. Thus the skin is then prevented from taking over eliminative functions. The skin is viewed by some experts as a sort of "third kidney," with the sweat glands in the skin approximating the eliminative capacity of one kidney. Also, it has been found that metabolic patterns in the skin's sweat ducts are similar to those in kidney tissue, and that they respond to the hormone aldosterone, which is also very important in the exchange of fluids and salts in the kidney. Several high-colonic irrigations or enemas, properly administered by a good technician, can be extremely helpful, clearing accumulated waste around the inner lining of the colon, and helping with chronic constipation. Home enemas usually clean out only the last foot of intestine, while high colonics clean out the entire large intestine, about five feet in most people. However, home enemas are private, convenient, inexpensive, and can be done more frequently. In order to ensure the optimal benefit from the colonics or enemas, they may be preceded by a fasting diet of apples, grapes, or fresh fruits only. Laxatives can also be used to help in the eliminative process.
- External massage over the intestines and liver with an olive oil/peanut oil mixture, olive oil/myrrh mixture, or warm castor oil packs is helpful in achieving a healthy gut.
- Small-intestine enzyme supplements can aid in digestion and, thus, elimination. Take two capsules after the start of each meal.
- Acidophilus and bifidus, which encourage the growth of helpful intestinal bacteria, can aid digestion and elimination. Stir ½ teaspoon of acidophilus or bifidus powder into a few ounces of warm water and take this twice a day between meals.

■ Glyco-Thymoline is an alkaline intestinal antiseptic that is sold as a mouthwash but requires a prescription for internal use. Taking 4 to 5 drops in a glass of water before bed five days a week is said to be very beneficial for psoriasis.

■ Clearing toxins from the kidneys is also important. It has been noted that some people with psoriasis who have had to undergo dialysis for other reasons have found that their lesions have cleared. For most people, keeping the kidneys free of accumulated waste is accomplished primarily by drinking six to eight glasses of pure water daily.

■ Eliminating toxins from the lungs is important as well. The following steps are recommended:

- Avoid exposure to chemical fumes and automotive exhaust.
- Do deep breathing exercises daily.
- Get aerobic exercise such as walking, jogging, bicycling, or swimming for thirty minutes three times a week. This aids in deep breathing and also causes you to work up a good sweat, both of which help to cleanse the system.

■ Toxins are also eliminated from the body through sweating. Sitting in a sauna is one way to work up a good sweat. Start with only two minutes a day, and increase slowly up to thirty minutes a day. Be sure to drink two glasses of water before and after each treatment to avoid dehydration and encourage the elimination of toxins.

■ To increase circulation and thereby help to cleanse the body, alternating hot and cold showers are also suggested.

■ It is well known that emotional factors have a strong correlation with the onset and flare-ups of psoriasis. It is thought that stress affects the autonomic (involuntary) nervous system and the immune system, which then influences the course of psoriasis. In a cyclical interaction, the emotions affect the skin and the condition of the skin affects the emotions. Relaxation techniques and suggestion also affect the autonomic nervous system and the immune system. They may therefore affect the severity of psoriasis. Drs. M.L. Price, I. Mottahedin, and P.R. Mayo of the Brighton Health Authority in Sussex, England, found that people with psoriasis tended to be very anxious, with tenser, more insular personalities than the population as a whole. They did a study in which subjects with psoriasis were taught relaxation techniques and given the opportunity to discuss problems associated with the psoriasis. At the end of the study, the people in this group were significantly more relaxed and also showed a slight physical improvement. A control group showed no positive psychological or dermatologic improvements. Similarly, Dr. Zachariae and colleagues at Aarhus University in Risskov, Denmark, published findings in 1996 suggesting that stress management, guided imagery, and relaxation techniques have a beneficial effect on psoriasis. In this randomized study, subjects in the treatment group, who participated in seven individual psychotherapy sessions over twelve weeks, experienced significant changes in the number and severity of psoriatic lesions.

▓ Meditation may have some role in managing psoriasis. Dr. Jon Kabat-Zinn and colleagues at the Stress Reduction Clinic of the University of Massachusetts have reported that listening to tapes combining mindful meditation and visualization during ultraviolet-light or PUVA therapy increased the rate at which lesions cleared by 3.8 times.

▓ Reflexology may provide symptomatic relief of itching and scaling and redness. The points for the thyroid, adrenals, liver, diaphragm, kidneys, intestines, and all glands are stimulated on both the hands and feet to effect a response.

▓ According to the understanding of mind-body medicine, our personal reactions to a situation determine the effect that the situation has on us, making us partially responsible for our own happiness and misery. Dr. John Pagano, an advocate of natural healing, goes so far as to maintain that negative, destructive thoughts in themselves produce harmful toxins, while frequently repeating positive affirmations such as "I am Healthy!" eventually enter one's subconscious mind and manifest themselves physically. He recommends smiling, being kind and gentle with oneself and others, appreciating oneself in a healthy, assertive way, and helping others as much as possible. He is also a proponent of using positive imagery, visualizing one's skin as pure and clear often during the day, with the expectation that the body will follow the mind's imagination.

▓ Psychotherapy to deal with unresolved psychological issues can be very important. A number of case studies have shown improvement of psoriasis using a variety of psychological techniques.

▓ Hypnotherapy with imagery may be helpful for some people. There have been reports that imagery used in hypnosis may alter skin temperature. Integrative medicine advocate Dr. Andrew Weil recommends seeing a hypnotherapist if psoriasis is severe. Several case studies have documented successful treatment of psoriasis with hypnosis and biofeedback. There have also been reports of success with thermal biofeedback. Researchers postulated that biofeedback helps psoriatic skin to heal by having a positive psychoneuroimmunologic effect in restoring and maintaining a balanced and calm central nervous system and brain.

■ Chiropractic physician and psoriasis expert Dr. John Pagano feels that the spine can be important in the genesis of psoriasis. He recommends manual adjustments of the spine as an integral part of therapy. The upper intestinal tract is supplied by nerve impulses from the spinal cord at the level of the mid-back, while the skin receives sympathetic nerve impulses from the area of the spinal cord at the level of the upper back and lower chest. If these nerves are pinched by injury or by abnormal shape or movement of the spine, the normal blood circulation to portions of the intestinal tract may be reduced, increasing any malfunctioning and resulting level of toxins in the blood. Also, sympathetic nerve stimulation to the dermis may be interrupted if these nerves are pinched at the spinal level. Chiropractic spinal manipulation is therefore recommended to help maintain the very important functions of the nervous system that keep the gut and skin healthy. Dr. Pagano also suggests employing a muscle stimulator, a device to be used by a licensed chiropractor only, to the areas of the spine directly involved in psoriasis. This sends small electrical impulses to stimulate the nerve roots coming from between these vertebrae, increasing nerve-impulse flow to the organs thought to be involved.

GENERAL RECOMMENDATIONS

■ Avoid using harsh soaps at the sites of psoriasis. They can dry out the plaques and flare the symptoms.

■ To increase the sloughing of old skin cells, rub the thickened skin with moistened finely ground oatmeal. Aveeno is a commercially available product that has an oatmeal base and is added to the bath. Epsom-salts baths can also be used to cleanse and soothe, but should not be used if the skin is very cracked or sensitive. One to two pounds of baking soda added to a hot bath can also help to relieve the itching of psoriasis.

■ Exposing the skin to sunlight for about thirty minutes (without burning) on a daily basis is recommended for many people with psoriasis, especially those who have found that the problem improves with summer sun. On normal areas of skin, always use a sunscreen with a sun protection factor (SPF) of 15 or higher one-half hour before sun exposure to prevent sunburn, which can make the psoriasis worse. Approximately 80 percent of people with psoriasis find improvement within three to six weeks with this simple sunlight therapy.

▪ If you live in a cold climate where sun exposure is difficult, topical coal tar and ultraviolet-B light therapy is another option, as is topical psoralen with ultraviolet-A light (PUVA) therapy. Both treatments work by inhibiting DNA synthesis in the epidermis, or top layer of skin, and selectively applying a "metabolic brake" to the rapidly proliferating skin cells in psoriasis.

▪ Whirlpool or Jacuzzi bath treatments, which can be done at home, are very helpful to remove scales and cleanse the skin.

▪ Dissolve 1 to 2 pounds of Dead Sea salts in a tubful of warm water at least three times a week, and soak in the bath for at least forty-five minutes each time. Do this for a period of at least six weeks. If you can, you might want to consider a trip to the Dead Sea itself for treatment. The unique environment there, and the concentration of various salts in the water and mud from the sea, combine to provide an effective alternative treatment for psoriasis. Dr. D.J. Abels and colleagues at the Dead Sea Psoriasis Clinic in Israel published an article in 1995 in which they reported observing clearing of about 90 percent of psoriatic lesions in 88 percent of nearly 1,500 patients. Almost 60 percent of the patients had complete clearing. Interestingly, patients from overseas responded better than Israelis did. Researchers speculated that this might be due to the added psychological benefit of relaxation in a vacationlike setting, far away from the pressures of home and work. Similar treatment at the Copahue Thermal Basin Complex in Argentina has also been reported to yield improvement. Admittedly, such treatment is not a choice for everyone. But salts and mud that simulate conditions at the Dead Sea are available for purchase.

▪ Seek out sources of support, such as the National Psoriasis Foundation. It can help to realize that the disease is not contagious and that psoriasis is actually quite common.

▪ To treat severe hand and/or foot lesions of psoriasis, first whirlpool the areas with hot Epsom salts, then massage warm peanut oil in. Follow this by applying a pastelike mixture of baking soda and castor oil. Cover the hands and/or feet with white cotton socks and leave the mixture on for at least one-half hour, and overnight if possible.

■ Using a humidifier in the winter can help to prevent increased drying and painful cracking of the skin.

■ A filter to remove chlorine from bath and shower water is very helpful. Most municipal water supplies have chlorine added to kill bacteria. The chlorine further dries out the skin, making psoriasis worse.

■ Avoid stress as much as possible, as this provokes and worsens flare-ups of psoriasis.

Ringworm

Ringworm, or *tinea,* is a fungal infection growing on the outer layers of the skin, scalp, and/or nails. Athlete's foot and "jock itch" are actually localized forms of ringworm. Other favored sites of fungal infection are the palms and soles, nails, scalp, beard, and trunk.

Fungal infections are rapidly spread from one person to another or even from the family pet to the family. They recur often, and when they do, they have to be treated again.

Fungal infections on the body usually start as itchy, slightly scaly, round red spots on the skin. As the lesions grow, they heal from the inside of the round circle out, giving the rash its characteristic ringlike appearance. The infection often spreads from one area of the body to another. If your groin is involved, there is usually a diffuse red, scaling rash that is very itchy. If you have tinea of your palms or feet, they often scale and are red and may blister, but do not usually form separate small spots. Nail infections appear as areas of yellowish or whitish discoloration and crumbling. Scalp infection with ringworm produces red, itchy scaling and, later, hair loss and breakage.

Doctors confirm a diagnosis of tinea by looking at some of the skin scales under a microscope to see if fungal bodies are present. Generally, treatment is very effective and relatively quick, and there are many good options. Therapy takes longer if the fungi have been invading the scalp, fingernails, or toenails for some time.

CONVENTIONAL TREATMENT

- Over-the-counter clotrimazole (Lotrimin), undecylenic acid (Cruex, Desenex, and others) or miconazole (Micatin) cream or powder is effective for early, very mild cases.
- If over-the-counter medications fail, prescription creams containing ketoconazole (Nizoral), miconazole (Monistat-Derm), itraconazole (Sporanox), or fluconazole (Diflucan) are very effective, although expensive.
- Oral griseofulvin (Fulvicin, Grifulvin, Grisactin, Gris-PEG) is used in more widespread cases that do not respond to topical treatments. However,

this drug can cause side effects, including gastrointestinal upset and, rarely, liver toxicity, so caution needs to be used.

■ Oral ketaconazole (Nizoral), itraconazole (Sporanox), fluconazole (Diflucan), and terbinafine (Lamisil) are newer drugs in the dermatologist's arsenal against fungal infections. They are very effective, but also expensive. However, they may be necessary if the nails or scalp are involved.

DIETARY MEASURES

■ Eat a balanced diet with lots of vegetables, yogurt, and acidophilus-containing foods.

■ Avoid coffee, cola, tea, and chocolate. These foods increase the alkalinity of the skin, making it more desirable for fungi.

■ Avoid sugary foods, including honey and fruit juices. Fungi thrive on sugar.

■ Avoid yeasty foods, such as beer and breads made with yeast.

NUTRITIONAL SUPPLEMENTS

■ Acidophilus supplements replenish beneficial intestinal bacteria that inhibit the growth of pathogens such as fungi. Take 1 teaspoon of powdered acidophilus in water or two acidophilus capsules on an empty stomach twice a day.

■ Garlic aids in the destruction of fungi. Take two garlic tablets three times a day.

■ Take a multivitamin supplement that includes vitamin A, the B complex, and vitamin E daily.

■ Vitamin C increases immunity to fungi. Take 3,000 milligrams of vitamin C with bioflavonoids daily.

■ Zinc increases immunity and inhibits fungi. Take 50 milligrams of zinc daily.

■ Methylsulfonylmethane (MSM) is a good source of sulfur, which is thought to fight fungi. It is now available in cream or spray forms to apply topically to the involved areas of skin. Use it as directed by the manufacturer.

■ Calendula cream, ointment, or tincture diluted in warm water has anti-fungal, astringent, and healing properties, and can be used two to three times a day as an aid in fighting fungal infections of the body.

■ Chamomile tea, taken three times a day, should help clear ringworm. It can also be applied directly to the affected areas with a cotton ball three times a day.

■ Garlic is one of the best herbal antifungals. Its antifungal properties have been documented by clinical studies showing that the blood of people taking garlic has significant antifungal activity. Take 6 teaspoons of garlic extract daily. In addition, you can put raw garlic in a blender and apply the resulting paste to areas of ringworm with a clean cotton ball three times a day.

■ Ginger tea, made by simmering 2 ounces of fresh ginger root simmered in 8 ounces of water for twenty minutes, contains more than twenty antifungal compounds. Drink the tea three times a day and also apply a compress consisting of cotton soaked with the ginger tea to the affected areas for five minutes three times a day.

■ Goldenseal is another good antifungal agent. Add 5 drops of the tincture to juice and drink it three times a day. Or simmer 6 teaspoons of the dried herb for twenty minutes to make a tea, strain out the herbal matter, and apply the tea to your areas of tinea three times a day with a fresh cotton ball. You can also dust your feet, socks, and shoes with goldenseal powder twice a day.

■ Take a cup of lemongrass tea three times a day. While you drink the tea, apply the used tea bags to the affected areas. This should help ringworm to clear faster.

■ Licorice contains at least twenty-five fungicidal substances. Add 6 teaspoons of powdered licorice root to a cup of boiling water and simmer for twenty minutes. Strain out the herbal matter, and apply the tea to the areas of ringworm three times a day using a fresh cotton ball.

■ Myrrh is a good antifungal. Make a paste by mixing equal parts of myrrh and goldenseal powder with a little water, and apply it to the areas of rash three times a day.

■ Olive-leaf extract has antifungal properties and helps to fortify the immune system. Take 250 milligrams three times a day.

■ Pau d'arco increases the body's immunity and enhances lymphatic drainage. Sip a cup of pau d'arco tea three times a day.

■ Turmeric oil, diluted with two parts water to one part turmeric oil, can be put on areas of ringworm three times a day using fresh cotton balls to speed healing of a fungal infection. Additionally, you can take 300 milligrams of turmeric extract orally three times a day.

■ Some commercial antifungal lotions combine herbs with pharmaceuticals, using the best of both. Also, it has been found that mixtures of antifungal herbs work synergistically, or much better than single herbs. One such product combines tolnaftate, myrrh, tea tree oil, aloe vera, calendula, rosemary, and thyme.

AROMATHERAPY

■ Tea tree oil is one of the strongest known antifungals. Tea tree oil is a very potent antifungal. Apply a few drops of the oil directly to your areas of ringworm three times a day. If you find this irritating, dilute it with an equal amount of vegetable oil. Remember never to drink this oil.

HOMEOPATHY

■ A few drops of *Thuja* 6c can be rubbed directly on the affected areas twice a day. You can also take a dose by mouth three times a day for ten days.

GENERAL RECOMMENDATIONS

■ Always practice careful hand-washing, so as not to spread your fungal infection to others.

■ Keep your skin cool and dry, as fungi love to live in warm, moist places.

■ To avoid reinfection or spreading the infection to other household members, wash your clothing after each wearing.

■ As fungal infections are contagious, do not share your clothing, combs, hats, socks, pillows, or sheets with other people.

■ Avoid contact with animals that have the telltale red, round patches with hair loss. Take any pets you suspect may be infected to a veterinarian for treatment immediately.

Rosacea

Rosacea is a vascular inflammatory skin disease of the small blood vessels of the face. Although it is sometimes called acne rosacea, it is not associated with a previous history of acne. It affects about 5 percent of the population, mostly women who are menopausal and in their forties, especially those who are fair-skinned and of Celtic ancestry. The face, especially the nose and central face, is affected with a symmetrical red rash, with or without prominent fine blood vessels, or telangiectasia. Papules (small, solid bumps), pustules (inflamed, pus-filled bumps) and firm red nodules that look like acne lesions are often scattered over the cheeks and nose as well. However, unlike acne, rosacea is not characterized by the formation of blackheads or whiteheads. In some cases, a bulbous red nose, or *rhinophyma,* may develop slowly if the condition is left untreated.

Many experts believe that the cause of rosacea is infectious—a result of infection with skin mites, the yeast *Pityrosporum ovale,* which is normally present in hair follicles, or with as-yet-unidentified bacteria or fungi. Others think that psychological factors, genetics, and/or connective tissue problems in the skin are the likely cause. Probably a combination of these factors, and possibly others, is responsible.

Many people with rosacea experience blushing or flushing of the face, especially in hot weather, with sun exposure, and after consuming spicy foods, alcohol, hot drinks or soup, coffee, or tea. These factors, which dilate local facial blood vessels, also worsen the acne-like lesions. Food intolerances, inadequate stomach-acid production, and a deficiency of the B vitamins, especially vitamin B_{12}, are also thought to worsen the chronic symptoms of rosacea.

CONVENTIONAL TREATMENT

- A cream containing 3 percent precipitated sulfur cream and 1 percent hydrocortisone, applied twice a day, may be prescribed to lessen the redness of the rash.
- Metronidazole gel (Metrogel) is a prescription gel that many dermatologists favor to reduce the redness, visible blood vessels, and bumps of rosacea.

■ Applying ketoconazole (Nizoral) cream locally twice a day has been found to be very helpful in diminishing flare-ups of rosacea.

■ Topical antibiotics such as topical tetracycline (Achromycin, Topicycline), erythromycin (Emgel, Erygel, Erythra-Derm, and others), and clindamycin (Cleocin T) are often prescribed. They are usually applied twice a day to the affected areas.

■ Oral tetracycline (Achromycin V), erythromycin (ERYC, Ilotycin, and others), ampicillin (Omnipen, Polycillin, and others), metronidazole (Flagyl, Metromidol, Protostat), dapsone, or other oral antibiotics can control the outbreaks of acnelike bumps.

■ Prominent blood vessels can be epilated using electric current (applying an electric needle to coagulate the blood-vessel walls) to make them far less noticeable.

■ Isotretinoin (Accutane), a strong derivative of vitamin A, is reserved for difficult cases of rosacea with lots of papules and pustules, especially in women past childbearing age. It is very effective, but has many potentially serious side effects, including severe birth defects, liver toxicity, arthritis, elevation of blood fats, and drying out of the skin and mucous membranes.

■ The argon, carbon dioxide, and pulsed dye lasers are helpful in getting rid of unsightly facial blood vessels and reducing the size of an enlarged nose, which may be part of the rosacea picture. Plastic surgery also can markedly improve the appearance of a large, bulbous red nose.

DIETARY MEASURES

■ Investigate the possibility of food allergies and sensitivities that may be causing flare-ups.

■ Eat a well-balanced diet filled with vegetables, fruits, whole grains, and lean sources of protein.

■ Eat plenty of dark-green vegetables, which are rich in vitamin B_{12}.

■ Drink at least eight glasses of filtered water daily.

■ Avoid alcohol, spicy foods, hot drinks, coffee, and tea. These usually aggravate rosacea.

■ Avoid animal and hydrogenated fats, which promote inflammation. That means eliminating dairy products, red meat, fried foods, and margarine.

■ Avoid junk food, refined sugars, and artificial flavorings and preservatives, all of which are toxic for your body and skin.

NUTRITIONAL SUPPLEMENTS

■ Take a multivitamin and mineral supplement daily to ensure an adequate supply of all basic nutrients.

■ Beta-carotene, which the body uses to make vitamin A, helps to strengthen capillaries and is healing for the skin. Take 25,000 international units twice daily.

■ The B vitamins, especially vitamin B_2 (riboflavin), are necessary for healthy skin, hair, and nails. Take a vitamin-B complex containing 100 milligrams of most of the major B vitamins daily.

■ Vitamin C raises immunity, promotes healing, and strengthens connective tissue. Bioflavonoids are anti-inflammatory and help to strengthen blood vessels, and work with vitamin C. Take 500 milligrams of vitamin C with bioflavonoids three times a day.

■ Zinc also helps to heal the skin. Take 25 milligrams twice a day, with meals and with 1 milligram of copper.

■ Flaxseed oil supplies essential fatty acids that help to reduce inflammation. Take 1,000 milligrams or 1 teaspoon three times a day.

■ Acidophilus and bifidus help to restore "friendly" bacteria. If you are taking antibiotics, take either of these supplements as directed by the manufacturer.

■ Betaine and hydrochloric acid promote healthy digestion. If you suspect your stomach-acid levels are not high enough, take this supplement as directed by the manufacturer.

HERBAL TREATMENT

■ Cat's-claw extract helps to reduce food sensitivities by reestablishing a healthy intestinal environment. Take 500 milligrams three times a day.

  Caution: Do not take this herb if you are pregnant, nursing, or on blood thinners, or if you are an organ transplant recipient.

■ Gotu kola extract promotes healing of the skin. Take 100 milligrams three times a day.

■ Grapeseed extract is an anti-inflammatory and antioxidant, and helps in collagen formation. Take 50 milligrams three times a day.

■ Some people with rosacea report that horse-chestnut cream or rose-wax cream is helpful. Either of these products can be applied to the affected areas twice a day.

■ Jigucao is a Chinese herbal patent medicine that may be very effective. Take 500 milligrams three times a day.

AROMATHERAPY

■ Essential oils recommended for treating visible blood vessels in the skin include borage oil, cypress oil, lemon oil, neroli oil, and rose oil. Add a few drops of any of these, or a combination, to jojoba oil, rose hip seed oil, and/or evening primrose oil, and apply sparingly to the affected area once or twice a day. Be careful not to use too much essential oil in the mixture, or it may be irritating. If irritation does occur, either increase the dilution or discontinue use.

■ Chamomile and lavender are calming oils. A few drops of either or both of these can be added to a relaxing warm (not hot) bath.

HOMEOPATHY

■ *Arsenicum album* 30x or 15c is best if the rash is dry, burning, flaky, and scaly. Take one dose three times a day for three days.

■ *Carbo animalis* 9c is especially effective for older adults with rosacea who also chill easily. Take one dose three times a day.

■ *Lachesis* 12c is best if primarily the nose is involved. Take one dose twice a day.

■ *Rhus toxicodendron* 12x or 6c is appropriate if rosacea is swollen, itchy, painful, and red, and flares up in cold or wet weather. Take one dose three times a day for three days.

■ *Sanguinaria* 12x or 6c is especially useful if the rash of rosacea burns and stings and is made worse by heat. Take one dose three times a day for three days.

■ *Sulfur* 30x or 15c is best if the rosacea flares up with heat or a hot bath. Take one dose three times a day for three days.

ACUPUNCTURE

■ There is not a great deal of evidence to support the use of acupuncture for rosacea, but there is some. In 1990, Dr. Xu Yihou of Wuhan Municipal Hospital of Traditional Chinese Medicine in China reported treating a group of patients who had rosacea with acupuncture, and 50 percent experienced a clinical cure. All of those who were cured were in the early, reddened stage of the problem. There have also been anecdotal reports of acupuncture being effective for resistant rosacea. Consult a qualified acupuncturist if you are interested in trying this type of treatment.

ACUPRESSURE

See Acupressure Points in Part Three for the locations of these points on the body.

■ Pressure to the Third Eye Point and to the Small Intestine 18, Gallbladder 20, Large Intestine 4, Stomach 2, and Stomach 3 points for three minutes three times a day helps lesions of the head and face. The Third Eye Point is located directly between the eyebrows, where the bridge of the nose meets the middle of the forehead. The Small Intestine 18 points are situated directly beneath the outer corner of each eye, immediately underneath the cheekbone. The Gallbladder 20 points are at the back of the head, in the depression between the neck muscles and the bottom of the skull. The Large Intestine 4 points are at the center of the triangle made between the small bones of the thumb and index finger. The Stomach 3 points are located on the cheeks, directly below the pupil and level with the outside edge of each nostril.

OTHER THERAPIES

■ Practice deep breathing, relaxation techniques, and meditation to reduce stress, which can contribute to flare-ups of rosacea.
■ Guided imagery of a quiet, serene place can help you to relax and can augment other therapies.

■ As much as possible, avoid anything that you know causes your rosacea to flare up.

■ Wear a sunscreen with a sun protection factor (SPF) of at least 15 every day, even if you are indoors. Wear a hat when outdoors.

■ Avoid extremes of heat, humidity, cold, and dryness. Do not go in hot baths or showers, hot tubs, steam rooms, or saunas.

■ Get regular low-intensity exercise, but take care not to become over-heated or flushed, or to sweat profusely.

■ Use a mild soap like Purpose or Cetaphil and lukewarm water to wash your face. Do not scrub or irritate your skin.

■ Use a water-based, noncomedogenic moisturizer daily in cold, dry weather.

■ Use only fragrance-free, hypoallergenic, water-based cosmetics.

■ Do not repeatedly touch or pick at your skin lesions, as this will only make them worse.

Scars and Keloids

When the boundary of the skin is crossed or cut, it heals with a scar. New scars are thick and full of blood vessels, but over a period of several months they become flatter and the blood supply decreases. Scars that remain thick and wide but are confined to the area of the original injury are called *hypertrophic scars.* Hypertrophic (overgrown) scars are usually flesh-colored, pink, or red, and are dome-shaped. They can have areas with many prominent, tiny red blood vessels or areas that are flat and shiny within the raised, broad scar.

Scars that become inappropriately large, in which the scarring process has gone out of control, are known as keloids. Keloids grow not only on the site of the original injury but also outside it, often with clawlike extensions. In fact, keloids can continue to grow slowly for years. They are most common among dark-skinned people, and they have a tendency to run in families. Keloids usually appear in areas of trauma, such as sites of previous acne, burns, cuts, ear piercings, insect bites, or vaccinations. However, some keloids develop spontaneously, especially on the upper chest in the area of the breastbone. They are typically very smooth, shiny, thick, and large. Keloids usually cause no symptoms, but they may be itchy or tender to touch, especially early in their formation. They can also be distressing from a cosmetic point of view.

Making scars and keloids smaller and less obvious is a common dermatologic concern. Let's now take a look at what both traditional and alternative medicine have to offer us for help with this problem.

CONVENTIONAL TREATMENT

■ Apply a sunscreen with a sun protection factor (SPF) of 15 or higher to the area of any healing scar every morning to keep sun exposure from further darkening the scar.

■ Topical hydroquinone solution (Melanex) is a very useful lightening agent that may be prescribed. It is usually applied directly to the scar twice a day with a toothpick or cotton swab.

■ ReJuveness is a product that helps to soften, smooth, and flatten scars;

relieve burning and itching; and restore normal skin color to scars. It is a silicone sheeting material that is taped over the scar. It is available over the counter. However, it is quite expensive.

■ High-potency cortisone cream or local injections of the steroid triamcinolone aid in lightening and flattening raised scars. The injections are painful, however, and generally require several visits unless the scar is small.

■ Deep phenol peels are often done for diffuse acne scarring of the face, chest, or back. However, this is quite a significant procedure, and is not without risk of further scarring, burning, and pain.

■ Liquid nitrogen is often used to freeze hypertrophic scars and keloids, thus reducing their volume. More than one treatment may be necessary. Liquid nitrogen spraying, followed fifteen minutes later by injection of triamcinolone directly into the lesion, is very effective for thick scars and keloids. After freezing, the scar becomes swollen and is much softer and easier to inject.

■ Injection of recombinant interferon alfa-2b (Intron-A) has shown some promise for local, difficult scars that have not responded to other treatments.

■ Keloids can be surgically removed but, of course, they can re-form in the surgical scar. The possibility of this happening can be reduced by injecting the steroid triamcinolone into the incision site at the time of surgery. However, this is likely to prolong the time it takes the wound to heal.

NUTRITIONAL SUPPLEMENTS

■ Vitamin E cream, applied to the area twice a day, is helpful in softening scars.

HERBAL TREATMENT

■ Mederma, a topical gel containing a proprietary botanical extract made from onion and allantoin, can by applied to a scar three or four times a day. An improvement in the color, texture, appearance, and flexibility of the scar should be noted sometime between eight weeks and six months of treatment. This product is available over the counter. It works best on newer scars.

■ Applying calendula gel or cream to a scar twice a day reduces inflammation and increases healing in an early scar.

■ An ointment containing 10 percent mustard-seed oil, applied to a scar three times a day for several weeks, is said to aid in improving the appearance of the scar.

AROMATHERAPY

■ Mix 1 ounce each of rose hip seed oil and essential oils of rose and everlasting and apply daily to the scar after bathing. This should help to improve the appearance of the scar. Store the mixture in a dark glass bottle.
■ Lavender oil has skin-cell-rejuvenating properties and reportedly helps with all forms of scarring. Apply it to the scar or keloid several times a day.

HOMEOPATHY

■ *Thiosinaminum* 5c, applied externally to a scar or keloid twice a day, reduces the swelling of a lumpy, bumpy scar. However, it must be used within three months of the scar's formation to have any effect.

OTHER THERAPIES

■ Massage can help to soften scars. Roll stiff scars several times daily to break down scar tissue and soften the scars.
■ Studies show that pulsed electrotherapy greatly reduces the growth of hypertrophic scars and keloids.

GENERAL RECOMMENDATIONS

■ Don't pick at any healing wound, as this will increase scarring.
■ If you are prone to forming keloids or thick scars, avoid cosmetic or elective surgical procedures if possible. If surgery is necessary, discuss your concern about scarring with your surgeon. Triamcinolone acetonide, a steroid, can be injected into the incision site to reduce the risk of hypertrophic scarring and keloid formation. However, this may slow healing of the wound as well.

Scleroderma

Scleroderma is an autoimmune disorder involving abnormal excessive collagen formation and immune-system-induced damage to the tiny capillaries throughout the body. There are various forms of scleroderma, including linear scleroderma, progressive systemic scleroderma, localized morphea, and generalized morphea.

Linear scleroderma appears as a linear area of thick, hard, darker-colored skin, usually on the lower legs. Females are more likely than males to be affected. An unusual form of linear scleroderma called *coup de sabre* ("cut of the sword") begins in childhood, with the formation of a groove of thick, hairless skin across the forehead, and down the face and back of the scalp. This can be very disfiguring and traumatic.

Progressive systemic scleroderma (PSS) also involves thickening of the skin, but other symptoms are present as well. The skin becomes taut and shiny. Often, the face develops a smooth, waxy, masklike quality, and chewing and speaking become difficult. People with PSS can become almost encased in thick scars, especially of the trunk, face, and arms. Skin folds on the fingers often disappear, and the skin of the fingers often becomes very tight and bound down. This is termed *sclerodactyly.* Small ulcers that are difficult to heal often form on the fingertips. Prominent, visible tiny blood vessels, or telangiectasia, develop on the skin of the face, chest, and fingertips. Calcium deposits form under the skin over bony areas and on the fingertips, a condition known as *calcinosis cutis.* Often, Raynaud's syndrome develops as well. This is a condition characterized by painful constriction of the blood vessels of the hands and feet in response to the cold. Some hair loss is usual.

In addition to the skin changes in progressive systemic sclerosis, pain and stiffness of the joints, especially those of the hands and knees, is common. At least one-half of people with this disorder also have esophageal, intestinal, kidney, heart, and/or lung problems, which can be life-threatening. Often, the esophagus gradually becomes narrowed, and severe heartburn and blockage of food develops. Many people have intestinal involvement, with diarrhea, constipation, and difficulty with nutrient absorption, especially with the fat-soluble vitamins A, D, E, and K. If thickening of lung tissue occurs, breathing difficulty develops. Hardening of the heart muscle can produce heart blocks and arrhythmias. Kidney failure is the most common dangerous effect of the disease. The usual natural course of the disease is a slow, relentless progression of skin and/or organ tissue thickening. However, the ten-year survival rate is greater than 50 percent.

The *CREST syndrome* is a variant of PSS with calcinosis cutis, Raynaud's syndrome, esophageal dysfunction, sclerodactyly, and telangiectasia. It generally progresses more slowly and has a better prognosis than other forms of systemic sclerosis.

Morphea is believed to be a localized form of scleroderma, and is the most common form of the disease. Localized morphea begins as a small, slightly pink, dime-sized area, most frequently on the trunk, where the deeper tissues become hard and thickened. The top layer of skin is not hardened, but as the involved area enlarges, it loses pigmentation and becomes very white. Usually only a single spot is involved, but the spot may grow to be quite large, and may be itchy. In generalized morphea there are many involved areas all over the body. Fortunately, morphea commonly resolves on its own.

Unfortunately, treatment of scleroderma is often difficult and helps only to slow the progression of the disease, not to reverse it. Let's take a look at what traditional and alternative medicine can offer for those who suffer with this problem.

CONVENTIONAL TREATMENT

■ Topical 1-percent nitroglycerin ointment, applied three times a day, increases local dilation of blood vessels.

■ Aminobenzoate potassium (Potaba), an antifibrotic agent, is very effective in softening involved skin. It must be used for at least three months to be effective.

■ Topical or oral corticosteroids are often given to help control the symptoms of scleroderma. If only a few areas of skin are involved, strong topical steroids applied under plastic wrap or an occlusive wound dressing may help the most.

■ Penicillamine (Cuprimine, Depen) interferes with collagen bonding and slows the disease progression. However, blood counts may be affected and need to be monitored closely.

■ Antimalarial drugs such as hydroxychloroquine (Plaquenil) are commonly prescribed to reduce skin thickening and slow the progression of the disease.

■ Colchicine, a medication primarily used to control gout, is also often frequently tried.

■ Isotretinoin (Accutane) has been helpful in some cases.

■ If the blood vessels are involved to a great extent, as with Raynaud's syndrome, blood-pressure drugs can be very effective.

■ Oral immunosuppressive and cancer drugs, such as cyclosporine (Neoral, Sandimmune, SangCya), cyclophosphamide (Cytoxan, Neosar), chlorambucil (Leukeran), and azathioprine (Imuran) are used in very severe cases.

■ Photopheresis is a new therapy being tried for PSS. In this technique, blood is removed from the body, irradiated with ultraviolet light, and then reinfused. It is believed that this treatment restores chemical balance and reduces the effect of toxins in the blood.

■ Interferon-gamma is also being tested clinically for systemic sclerosis.

NUTRITIONAL SUPPLEMENTS

■ In general, the following supplementation regimen is recommended for people with scleroderma:

- A high-potency multivitamin and mineral supplement. Take this daily.
- Beta-carotene. Take 25,000 international units daily.
- Vitamin B_6 (pyridoxine). If you are on penicillamine therapy, take 200 milligrams a day.
- Vitamin B_{12}. Take 1 milligram (1,000 micrograms) daily.
- Vitamin D. Take 200 to 600 international units daily. If intestinal absorption is diminished, also take 100 micrograms of vitamin K daily.
- Vitamin E. Take 1,000 international units a day. Several studies have confirmed the usefulness of vitamin E for the problems of scleroderma. One study with laboratory animals showed that vitamin E helped prevent calcium deposits in the soft tissues of the animals. Another study of three scleroderma patients who took 800 to 1,200 international units of vitamin E daily had decreased stiffness of the hands and decreased calcium deposits in their soft tissues.
- Selenium. Take 50 micrograms daily.
- Zinc. Take 15 milligrams a day.
- Flaxseed or fish oil. Take 1 to 2 teaspoons a day.
- Dehydroepiandrosterone (DHEA). Start by taking 25 milligrams daily,

and gradually increase or decrease as necessary to achieve the maximum benefit.

▨ *Do not* take supplemental vitamin C. Vitamin C promotes collagen production, which is one of the problems present in scleroderma.

HERBAL TREATMENT

▨ Avocado oil, used in massage creams and oils, helps to soften the hard, inelastic skin of people with scleroderma if it is used long-term, on a daily basis.
▨ Capsaicin ointment is very helpful for increasing local dilation of the capillaries in the areas where it is applied.
▨ Gotu kola has been found to be helpful for symptomatic relief of the pain and bound-down feeling of scleroderma. Take 60 to 120 milligrams a day.

HOMEOPATHY

▨ Many homeopathic remedies have been used for scleroderma. The exact remedy is best chosen by a qualified homeopath, as this is a complex, multisystem disease. The homeopathic remedies most often prescribed for people with scleroderma include *Alum, Antimonium crudum, Arsenicum album, Berberis vulgaris, Calcarea fluorica, Causticum, Cuprum metallicum, Dulcamara, Graphites, Lachesis, Lycopodium, Mercuricus, Pulsatilla, Rhus toxicodendron, Sepia,* and *Sulfur.*

ACUPUNCTURE

▨ Japanese dermatologist M. Maeda and colleagues at Gifu Prefectural Hospital in Japan have reported finding dilation of blood vessels and elevation of the skin's surface temperature in patients with scleroderma treated with electrical acupuncture. This was not seen in normal controls. Consult a qualified acupuncturist if you are interested in trying this type of treatment.

OTHER THERAPIES

■ Electrotherapy may be helpful. Polish researcher M. Kruk and colleagues found that after superficial electric stimulation in patients with Raynaud's syndrome, a component of scleroderma, a significant increase of blood flow through the stimulated region was seen. Dr. N. Francaviglia and colleagues at the University of Genoa Medical School in Italy published a report of the successful treatment of symptoms of scleroderma with spinal-cord stimulation in the *British Journal of Neurosurgery* in 1994. Over a five-year period, fifteen patients with this debilitating disease were treated with electrical stimulation of the spinal cord. The pain, ulcers, thickening of the blood vessels, limited hand function, and severity of Raynaud episodes was improved with this therapy, whereas many other therapies had failed.

GENERAL RECOMMENDATIONS

■ Keep your the skin well moisturized. This helps to prevent painful fissuring and cracking.
■ Avoid exposure to cold weather, which further constricts blood vessels.
■ If you smoke, you must stop. Smoking further constricts blood vessels. Also avoid secondhand smoke.
■ Warm paraffin baths for the hands increase dexterity and decrease pain.

Seborrhea

Seborrhea, or seborrheic dermatitis, is one of the most common skin problems. It is characterized by dry, itchy, reddish or greasy scales on the scalp and face. It affects almost 5 percent of the population and usually recurs throughout a person's lifetime. It is seen in all age groups, more often in men than in women. It is made worse by dry climate, scratching, nutritional deficiencies, stress, immune dysfunction, and neurological disorders. Therefore, it is often seen in people with HIV/AIDS and Parkinson's disease.

The appearance of seborrheic dermatitis varies, depending on the person's age. In infants, usually only the scalp is affected. This condition is also known as *cradle cap*. In adults and teens, the flaking of dandruff is accompanied by inflammatory itching, scaling, and redness of the scalp and/or skin of the face. The eyebrows, eyelids, and the areas behind the ears, inside the ears, and the sides of the nose are commonly affected. The front of the chest, groin, underarms, and sides of the neck can be involved in more widespread disease. In more severe cases, the scales may become thickened, oozing, crusting, and yellow to orange in color.

It is thought that seborrheic dermatitis occurs when the sebaceous (oil) glands make too much sebum. It then dries into flakes and obstructs the ducts through which the sebum is delivered from the glands to the surface of the skin. In turn, the sebaceous glands produce even more sebum in an attempt to force out the obstructions and clear passageways to the skin's surface. As a result, itchy, greasy flakes of dried sebum and dead skin cells are sloughed off from the scalp and other areas rich in sebaceous glands. It is thought that the overgrowth of yeast organisms such as *Pityrosporum ovale* also contributes to seborrheic dermatitis.

CONVENTIONAL THERAPY

■ A zinc pyrithione (ZNP) shampoo such as Sebulon, Zincon, or others can be massaged into the scalp and affected face for at least five minutes a day before rinsing out.

■ An anti-dandruff shampoo containing selenium sulfide, menthol, or salicylic acid as its active ingredient may be more effective for some people. You can switch back and forth between shampoos if one loses its effectiveness.

■ Coal-tar shampoos such as Ionil T or Polytar are stronger, but also have a strong smell and can darken light-colored hair. They also should be massaged into the scalp for at least five minutes before rinsing out.

■ Ketoconazole (Nizoral) shampoo and 2-percent topical ketoconazole cream or lotion are newer therapies for seborrhea. They are directed against the yeast *Pityrosporum ovale,* which may overgrow and contribute to the problem. The shampoo, cream, or lotion is applied to the affected areas of the face and body

■ Hydrocortisone creams and lotions are often prescribed to control the itching and redness on the scalp, face, and body. Milder formulations are used on the face and areas where skin contacts skin, rather than on the chest or back.

DIETARY MEASURES

■ Eat a high-fiber, whole-foods-based diet.

■ Eat plenty of lean protein foods that are free of chemicals and preservatives.

■ Include soybeans and soy foods in your diet. Soy is a rich source of biotin, a B vitamin important for healthy skin and hair.

■ Avoid saturated and hydrogenated fats, refined sugars, and processed foods.

NUTRITIONAL SUPPLEMENTS

■ Take a multivitamin and mineral supplement daily to ensure a good supply of all your basic nutrients.

■ Biotin is most important for preventing and treating dandruff. Take 6 milligrams (6,000 micrograms) daily.

■ Vitamin A and beta-carotene are important for healthy skin and help to clear dandruff. Take 10,000 international units of vitamin A with 25,000 international units of beta-carotene daily for two weeks.

Caution: If you are pregnant, do not take such high doses of these nutrients. Consult with your doctor before taking any supplemental vitamin A or beta-carotene.

■ Vitamin B_{12} has been found to be helpful in clearing dandruff. Take 1,000 micrograms a day.

■ Vitamin E helps to speed skin-tissue healing. Take 400 international units daily. Vitamin E oil can also be used topically to help soften the scalp. Massage it into the scalp for at least thirty minutes, then shampoo out.

■ Essential fatty acids (EFAs) reduce the skin's dryness. Flaxseed oil is a good source of EFAs. Take 1,000 milligrams of flaxseed oil twice a day.

■ Selenium is an antioxidant that works together with vitamin E to reduce dandruff. Take 100 micrograms twice a day.

■ Kelp provides the iodine and trace nutrients your scalp needs to be healthy. Take two kelp tablets in the morning and another at lunch.

■ Probiotics such as *Lactobacillus acidophilus* and *Bifidobacterium bifidum* help to create an internal environment conducive to healthy bacteria and help to fight yeast infection. Take a probiotic supplement as directed by the manufacturer.

■ Zinc helps to both heal and prevent dandruff. Take 50 milligrams a day, with food and with 1 milligram of copper.

HERBAL TREATMENT

■ Use a mild calendula or chamomile soap to clean the affected areas of the face and body gently.

■ A popular folk-medicine treatment for dandruff and seborrhea of the scalp entails applying a warm mixture of two parts apple-cider vinegar and one part pure water to your scalp. Cover with a towel for thirty minutes, then wash out.

■ A thyme scalp rinse can be made by boiling 2 tablespoons of dried thyme in 1 cup of water for ten minutes. Strain and cool before pouring the mixture over clean, damp hair. Massage in gently, and do not rinse out.

■ Rosemary has astringent and antiseptic properties, and increases circulation locally. You can make a rosemary scalp rinse by boiling 2 tablespoons of dried rosemary in 1 cup of water for ten minutes. Strain and cool before using.

■ Massaging burdock-root oil into the scalp helps to reduce seborrhea and dandruff. You can mix it with an equal amount of calendula oil to soothe the scalp if it is very irritated and red.

■ Pine-tar shampoos are available commercially for help with dandruff.

■ To make a warm conditioning oil that also lessens itching, heat either al-mond, calendula, vitamin-E, or sesame oil, and apply it to the affected area. To use it on the scalp, gently comb the oil into your hair, wrap a towel around your head, and leave the oil on for at least fifteen minutes before shampooing and rinsing out. Then, using a fine-toothed comb, gently comb away any loosened scales.

AROMATHERAPY

■ Essential oils that have been recommended for treating seborrhea include cedarwood, clary sage, geranium, juniper, pine, rosemary, and tea tree. You can add up to 10 drops of any of these oils, or a combination, to 1 ounce of a vegetable carrier oil, and apply to the affected area once or twice daily. You can also add up to 8 drops of essential oil to an ounce of your favorite shampoo and use it to shampoo your hair daily.

HOMEOPATHY

■ *Mezereum* 12x or 6c is good if your skin and/or scalp is very itchy, with thick, leathery crusts. Take one dose three times a day for three to five days.
■ *Psorinum* 200x or 200c is useful for oily, greasy, very itchy seborrhea. This is particularly helpful if you are extremely sensitive to the cold and think that you will never get rid of your seborrheic dermatitis. Take one dose once weekly for three weeks.
■ *Sulfur* 30x or 15c, taken three times a day for up to four days, helps to improve seborrhea. You can repeat this treatment after one month if it is helpful. It is especially useful if you are a person who is usually hot, restless, forgetful, and irritable.

ACUPRESSURE

See Acupressure Points in Part Three for the locations of these points on the body.

■ Acupressure to the Gallbladder 20 points improves circulation to the head. These points are located at the back of the head, in the depressions between the bottom of the skull and the neck muscles, three finger-widths on either side of the spine. Using your thumbs, apply acupressure to these points, angling upward under the edge of the skull.

■ Pressing the Large Intestine 4 points works on the head, skin, and face. These are located in the centers of the triangles between the small bones of the index finger and thumbs. Press these points gently with the thumb of the opposite hand for one minute. Repeat on the other hand. Do this three times a day.

■ Pressing the Large Intestine 11 acupoints helps to relieve itching and to tone the skin. The points are found in the depressions at the end of the skin creases towards the outside of the elbows when the elbows are bent. Press with the thumbs for three minutes on each side three times a day.

GENERAL RECOMMENDATIONS

■ Do not pick or scratch your scalp or affected skin.
■ Use a mild hypoallergenic cleanser, not harsh soaps.

Shingles

Shingles, or herpes zoster, is a very painful reactivation of varicella zoster, the virus that causes chickenpox. After a chickenpox infection, the virus does not go away, but lies dormant in a single or group of sensory nerve roots. Even many years later, it can come out to wreak havoc. Shingles is most frequently experienced by people who are over fifty years old, who are immunosuppressed for one reason or another, or who have a triggering factor such as a severe physical or emotional stress that temporarily lowers the immune response.

Three to four days before blisters appear, you may have chills, fever, malaise, and gastrointestinal symptoms. Locally, a red band, pain, and burning develop along the site of the future rash. Finally, one-sided, burning, extremely painful patches or groups of blisters appear on reddened skin for three to five days. The blisters are infectious for up to a week. After five days, the blisters dry out and scab over, and the lesions are usually totally gone within two weeks. However, very severe pain, called postherpetic neuralgia, may persist in the area where the rash was for months or even years. The pain is so extreme that it drives some people to have surgery to sever the sensory nerves.

Let's take a look at what conventional and alternative medicine have to offer to relieve the pain and rash of herpes zoster.

CONVENTIONAL TREATMENT

■ Oral antivirals such as acyclovir (Zovirax), famcyclovir (Famvir), and valcyclovir (Valtrex) are the cornerstone of conventional medical therapy for shingles. Treatment with valcyclovir requires taking three pills a day for seven days.

■ Shingles is particularly dangerous for people with suppressed immune systems, in whom the infection can spread all over the body. For such individuals, treatment with intravenous acyclovir and recombinant interferon alpha-2a is generally recommended.

■ Warm compresses made with Burow's solution are soothing. Apply compresses to the affected areas for fifteen minutes four times a day until the blisters have cleared. Calamine lotion can also be soothing.

- To relieve pain, acetaminophen (in Tylenol and other products) or acetaminophen with codeine is usually needed.
- Topical lidocaine (Alphacaine, Anestacon, Lidoderm, Xylocaine, and others) or lidocaine with procaine (EMLA) cream often relieves the pain temporarily. Injections of lidocaine or lidocaine plus triamcinolone into the most painful sites may also be used. This usually provides good relief of pain. If the pain is very severe, a nerve block with lidocaine is sometimes done.
- A topical antihistamine such as doxepin (Zonalon) and oral antidepressants such as amitriptyline (Elavil, Endep) and fluphenazine (Prolixin) can provide good pain relief.
- For people over fifty, a short course of oral steroids can reduce the pain of shingles and postherpetic neuralgia.
- If the pain of postherpetic neuralgia is excruciating, a transcutaneous electric nerve stimulation (TENS) unit, which provides electrical stimulation to the nerves, may be tried for pain relief.
- If shingles occurs near the eyes or on the tip of the nose, you should consult an ophthalmologist immediately to prevent spread of the disease to the eyes.
- If shingles lasts for more than two weeks or spreads to other areas, you should consult an internist to treat the infection more aggressively and to rule out a possible underlying disease.
- Immunization with the varicella-zoster virus vaccine can decrease the incidence of shingles by as much as 80 percent. If you have had chickenpox at some point in your life (and most people have) you may wish to discuss the possibility of immunization with your doctor.

DIETARY MEASURES

- As early as the 1950s, it was found that adding the amino acid lysine stopped the growth of herpes viruses in cells, whereas adding the amino acid arginine made the herpes cells grow very rapidly. Many experts therefore recommend a diet for herpes infections in which the lysine is very high as compared with the amount of arginine. Dairy foods, fish, seafood, chicken, turkey, eggs, black beans, lentils, soybeans, brewer's yeast, potatoes, and other foods very rich in lysine should be the mainstay of the diet. Foods high in arginine, like most cereal grains, seeds, nuts, peanut butter, chocolate, coconut, beer, raisins, and gelatin should be avoided.

- Drink fresh carrot, celery, parsley, spinach, and beet juices.
- If you like spicy foods, eat foods seasoned with cayenne pepper. This can be helpful for pain relief.
- Avoid immune-weakening foods such as sweets, alcohol, coffee, tea, and junk food.

NUTRITIONAL SUPPLEMENTS

- Take a high-potency multivitamin and mineral supplement daily to ensure an adequate supply of all basic nutrients.
- Beta-carotene is an antioxidant that helps to repair and protect against free-radical damage to the nerves. It is also healing for the skin. Take 10,000 international units daily.
- The B vitamins, especially vitamin B_{12}, are important for healthy nerves. Take a vitamin-B complex containing 100 milligrams of most of the major B vitamins daily, plus an additional 1,000 milligrams of vitamin B_{12} each day.
- Vitamin C is an important antioxidant and also helps to improve immune function. Take 1,000 to 2,000 milligrams of vitamin C with bioflavonoids three times a day. Also take an additional 1,000 milligrams of quercetin, a potent bioflavonoid, each day.
- Vitamin E is another vitamin antioxidant, and benefits the skin. Take 400 international units daily. Vitamin-E oil can also be applied topically. Squeeze the oil from a capsule of vitamin E and apply it to the rash three times a day.
- Lysine is an amino acid that fights herpes viruses directly. Take 500 milligrams of supplemental L-lysine three times daily for two weeks. Lysine is also available in a cream form that can be applied directly to the blisters every few hours.
- Alpha-lipoic acid is an antioxidant that helps to protect nerve cells. Take 100 milligrams twice a day.
- Coenzyme Q_{10} is another powerful antioxidant. Take 60 milligrams twice a day.
- Zinc is an antioxidant that also boosts immune-system function. Take 25 to 50 milligrams twice a day, with food and with 1 to 2 milligrams of copper. Zinc can also be used topically, in the form of zinc oxide ointment applied directly to the sores.

Flaxseed oil supplies essential fatty acids that are important for a healthy nervous system and for healthy skin. Take 1 tablespoon twice a day.

Selenium is an antioxidant that works synergistically with vitamin E. Take 100 micrograms a day.

Acidophilus is important in maintaining the health of the digestive tract by encouraging the growth of "friendly" bacteria that maintain the strength and integrity of the intestinal wall. Take ½ teaspoon of acidophilus powder dissolved in 2 ounces of warm water twice a day, between meals.

HERBAL TREATMENT

Capsaicin, a natural compound derived from cayenne or chili pepper, can be used topically for pain relief. It is available in ointment form as Zostrix, and can be applied four to five times daily for pain relief. It works by blocking pain signals from nerves just under the skin, and is very effective in reducing the pain of herpes zoster.

Cat's-claw extract has anti-inflammatory and antiviral actions. Take 1,000 milligrams three times a day.

Caution: Do not take this herb if you are pregnant.

The combination of echinacea and goldenseal is antiviral, immune-stimulating, and detoxifying, and is helpful in the treatment of herpes. Take ¼ teaspoon of tincture in tea or juice three times a day. Or combine equal parts of tinctures of echinacea, goldenseal, nettle, and Siberian ginseng, and take ½ teaspoon of this mixture three times a day to strengthen your immune system and make it less vulnerable to infection.

Garlic has antiviral properties. Take 2 capsules of garlic extract twice a day for a week. Or just add a few minced garlic cloves to food such as pasta or salad every day for as long as you have shingles.

Lemon balm, also known as melissa, contains compounds known as polyphenols that have anti-herpes properties, and is felt by some to be a first-choice herbal treatment. Use topical applications of lemon-balm tea, which you can make by steeping 2 to 4 teaspoons of herb per cup of boiling water. Apply the tea to the blisters with a cotton ball four times a day. In Europe, an ointment containing 700 milligrams of dried lemon-balm leaf per gram is widely used.

■ Lemon balm is only one of the herbs in the mint family that are effective anti-herpes agents and contain at least four antiviral compounds that target herpes. Other members of this botanical family include hyssop, oregano, rosemary, sage, and thyme.

■ Licorice contains several antiviral and immune-boosting compounds. You can apply a licorice ointment locally, drink a weak licorice tea, and/or apply a strong tea directly to the rash three times a day.

■ Oat-straw extract calms the nervous system. Take 500 milligrams three times a day.

■ Reishi mushroom extract stimulates the immune system to fight infections such as herpes. Take 500 milligrams three times a day.

■ St. John's wort extract has antiviral properties. Take 300 milligrams three times a day.

■ A combination of equal parts of oat straw, St. John's wort, and skullcap can be mixed and one teaspoon taken four times a day.

■ Diluted tinctures of calendula, licorice, myrrh, St. John's wort, and slippery elm can be used topically to aid in healing. You can brew a strong tea from any of these herbs and dab it on your blisters with cotton balls after it cools.

AROMATHERAPY

■ At the first signs of an outbreak, a few drops of chamomile, clary sage, eucalyptus, geranium, lavender, lemon, myrrh, rose, or tea tree oil can be added to olive oil and applied directly to the blisters using cotton balls. Or add a few drops of one or more of these oils to a warm bath and soak for at least thirty minutes. This will speed healing and reduce the severity of the outbreak. Always be careful not to swallow essential oils.

■ Tea tree oil can also be used topically to aid in healing. If it is too irritating, dilute it in water or vegetable oil, such as olive oil.

HOMEOPATHY

■ Different remedies are useful for the pain of shingles and to limit the course of the rash. Unless otherwise indicated, use them as directed by the manufacturer.

- *Mezereum* 12x or 6c is helpful for the severe pain and burning. Take one dose four times a day for three days.
- *Ranunculus bulbosus* 6c is useful for the pain of shingles.
- *Rhus toxicodendron* 30x or 15c is best if the rash is red and swollen. Take one dose four times a day for three days.
- *Staphylococcinium* 30c helps to shorten the course of the outbreak.
- *Sulfur* 12c decreases the risk of postherpetic neuralgia.

ACUPUNCTURE

▣ There have been anecdotal reports of acupuncture relieving residual pain from shingles. Consult a qualified acupuncturist if you are interested in trying this type of treatment.

ACUPRESSURE

See Acupressure Points in Part Three for the locations of these points on the body.

▣ Press the Spleen 7 points for three minutes three times a day to decrease the itching from shingles. The Spleen 7 points are on the inner ankles, just above the ankle bone.

OTHER THERAPIES

▣ Breathing exercises, meditation, and yoga are helpful in preventing stressors from reactivating the virus, and for dealing with the pain during and after the rash.
▣ Reflexology, working the diaphragm, spine, and all the gland reflex points on the feet and/or hands, has been found to be helpful for shingles.
▣ Ultrasound treatments to the affected nerves have helped some people with the pain of shingles.

GENERAL RECOMMENDATIONS

■ A heating pad can be helpful for local pain relief.

■ Turn a blow-dryer on over the blisters to help dry them up.

■ Take measures to prevent others, especially pregnant women, from coming into contact with the blisters.

Skin Cancer

It is an alarming fact that one in six Americans will develop skin cancer. This is the most common cancer in the world today, and it is increasing at an epidemic rate. The good news is that the most common forms of skin cancer are not life-threatening, and all forms are curable if treated early.

Cancer is a group of diseases in which cells reproduce in an unrestrained fashion and not in the best interests of the body as a whole. The most common types of skin cancers are basal cell carcinomas, squamous cell carcinomas, and malignant melanomas. Their names reflect the fact that each starts in a different part of the epidermis. Basal cells are just under the outermost surface of the skin. Squamous cells are in the middle of the epidermis. Melanocytes are the pigment-producing cells located near the bottom of the epidermis, where it meets the dermis.

Basal cell carcinomas (BCCs) make up almost 75 percent of all skin cancers, affecting nearly 1 million Americans each year. They are often raised, translucent, pearly nodules that may crust, ulcerate, and, sometimes, bleed. Other signs of a BCC are a persistent sore that does not heal; a reddish patch on the trunk, arm, or leg; a smooth growth with an elevated, rolled border and an indentation in the center; or a scarlike area with poorly defined borders. Fortunately, basal cell carcinomas rarely spread, or metastasize, to vital organs, but they can destroy surrounding tissue if left untreated, even destroying a nearby eye, ear, or nose if left for many years.

Squamous cell carcinomas (SCCs) are less common than basal cell carcinomas, but more serious because they involve deeper tissues and are somewhat more likely to spread. This is the second most common skin cancer, affecting more than 100,000 people each year. They are usually raised, pink, opaque nodules or patches, and they frequently ulcerate in the center. An SCC can also take the form of a wartlike growth or an open sore that persists for weeks. It is particularly important to treat SCCs, as in a small percentage of cases—usually those that arise on chronically inflamed skin, on the lips, or mucous membranes—it spreads to distant tissues and can be life-threatening.

Malignant melanoma (MM) is a very serious type of skin cancer that arises in moles or in the pigment-producing cells of the skin. If caught early, it is not very dangerous, but in later stages it is far more likely than other types of skin cancer to spread to other parts of the body and become life-threatening. People at increased risk for malignant melanoma include the following:

- Those with a personal or family history of MM.
- Those with unusual, dysplastic (abnormal) moles that are larger than one-quarter inch in size, irregular in shape, and multicolored.
- Those with fair skin, light hair, and light-colored eyes, and a tendency to sunburn easily.
- Those with large brown moles that have been present from birth.
- Those with a history of painful or blistering sunburns.
- Those who have a history of lots of outdoor exposure, especially while living in sunny regions.

Malignant melanomas are usually brown-black or multicolored patches, plaques, or nodules with irregular outlines, larger than one-quarter inch. They may crust on the surface or bleed. Anyone who has moles (which is most people) should inspect them every three months, alert for the ABCD's of melanoma: *a*symmetry, irregular *b*order, uneven *c*olor, and *d*iameter larger than a pencil eraser. Warning signs that malignant melanoma may be developing include changes in size, color, shape, elevation, surface, surrounding skin sensation, and/or consistency of a new or existing pigmented area of the skin.

Another important type of cancer in the skin is *mycosis fungoides*. This is actually a relatively rare type of lymphoma that starts in the skin and later invades the lymphatic tissue, spleen, liver, blood, and other internal organs. The skin lesions may appear as red, scaling plaques, or as nodules, larger tumors, or ulcers, and may last for months to years.

Exposure to the sun's ultraviolet (UV) rays is responsible for more than 90 percent of all skin cancers. How warm and bright the weather is not a good indication of how damaging the sun is on any given day. Clouds and haze block as little as 20 percent of the harmful UV radiation. The closer to the equator you go, the more potent the sun's rays are because they hit the earth more directly for a greater part of the year. UV radiation also increases by 4 to 5 percent for every 1,000 feet you go above sea level. The sun's rays are damaging even if they do not strike you directly. Sand, concrete, and snow are highly reflective surfaces, bouncing back as much as 90 percent of the rays that hit them upward and sideways and increasing the amount of UV exposure we receive. Other, less important causes of skin cancers include radiation treatments, arsenic exposure, chronic scarring, and immune suppression, whether by the use of certain drugs or the presence of cancer or other serious diseases.

Many skin cancers are preceded by the formation of sun spots, or *actinic keratoses*. An actinic keratosis (AK) is a scaly or crusty, rough bump that arises on the skin's surface and slowly grows in size from one-eighth to one-quarter inch. One often sees the development of several actinic keratoses at a time, usually on the sun-exposed areas of the face, ears, scalp, neck, backs of the hands, forearms, and lips. If untreated, a small number of these lesions take the next step and progress to become cancerous.

Many natural-medicine practitioners believe that cancer is the end result of a long period of degeneration resulting from poor circulation of blood, lymph, and chi in the involved area. This is thought to be a result of the stagnation of body, mind, and spirit. Unhealthy foods, exposure to chemicals, and lack of exercise and flexibility create poor circulation. Negative or stressful thoughts and fears create muscle tension and worsen poor circulation. Unresolved grief or anger, or a feeling of disconnectedness from others, sabotages the immune system and the body's detoxifying and eliminative functions. Thus, alternative approaches to treating cancer from a total body-mind-spirit perspective involve measures to increase the blood, lymphatic, and chi flow to the whole body, and especially to the area of the tumor.

In 1997, Dr. W. Sollner and colleagues at Leopold Franzens University in Innsbruck, Austria, published work compiling the results of questionnaires filled out by 215 melanoma patients at their clinic. They found that over half of the patients reported interest in nonconventional therapy. However, only one in seven admitted to actually using such methods. As a group, these tended to be the people with more advanced cancer. Those interested in alternative methods had faith in their physicians' conventional therapies and were just as likely as other patients to adhere to them. However, they felt that they were receiving insufficient emotional support from their physicians, and were turning to alternative methods in part in the hope of getting more psychological support. Dr. Sollner concluded that physicians should receive more intense education to help them to understand their patients' psychological situations and to provide more emotional support.

■ Treatment options for sun spots, or actinic keratoses, include the following:

- Liquid nitrogen or cryosurgery to the actinic keratoses to freeze them. This causes a separation of the area of the epidermis containing the actinic keratosis from the underlying dermis. This is a good alternative for people with light complexions. In people with dark complexions, light spots may develop in the treated areas, so this is not the best treatment for them.

- Applying 5-fluorouracil (Efudex, Fluoroplex) cream each night to areas of sun damage for four weeks. This drug is incorporated into rapidly dividing cells, resulting in the cells' death. Thus, cancer cells are affected much more than are normal skin cells, which remain unchanged. A mild topical steroid cream should be used once in the morning to decrease any inflammation, pain, and redness from the fluorouracil treatment. If the cream produces severe burning or erosions, treatment should be discontinued and you should consult with your dermatologist to determine whether to alter the dosage or try a different kind of treatment.

- Tretinoin (Retin-A), used either alone or with topical 5-fluorouracil. This is a good treatment if the actinic damage is mild. Many doctors start by recommending the application of tretinoin cream nightly to areas of actinic keratoses.

- Shaving and biopsy by a dermatopathologist. This may be recommended for thicker actinic keratoses to determine whether or not they have become cancerous.

■ Treatment options for basal cell carcinomas include electrodesiccation and curettage. In this technique, cancerous tissue is scraped from the skin and then an electric needle is used to burn the scraped area and a safety margin of normal skin around the base. The treatment is repeated three times in rapid succession. It is the most common treatment for basal cell carcinomas.

■ Treatment options for basal cell carcinomas and squamous cell carcinomas include the following:

- Surgical removal, or excision, of the entire growth and an additional safety margin of normal skin around it.

- Cryosurgery, in which the tumor tissue is destroyed by freezing it with liquid nitrogen.

- Radiation therapy directly to the malignant cells. This is usually done several times a week for a few weeks. It is used if excision of the lesion is not possible because of the an individual's age or health, or if the cancer is on a surgically difficult area of the head or neck.

- Moh's surgery. In this technique, the dermatologist removes very thin layers of the malignant growth, checking each layer under a microscope until the site is tumor-free. It is especially useful for skin cancers that return or skin cancers on the face, where it is cosmetically important to take the least amount of normal skin possible.
- Laser surgery to either cut out the tumor or destroy it by vaporization.

■ Treatment for malignant melanoma includes:
- Wide excision (surgical removal) of the primary cancer.
- Evaluation of lymph nodes. This is done to determine whether or not the cancer may have spread to other sites in the body. It can be done clinically, by lymphoscintigraphy (a test utilizing a radioactive tracer and imaging technology), and by biopsy. If lymph nodes are involved or enlarged, they will likely be removed.
- Blood tests and a chest x-ray to look for possible spread of the tumor.
- If the melanoma has metastasized, chemotherapy with drugs such as dacarbazine (DTIC-Dome) may be prescribed.
- Interferon and interleukin-2 are promising treatments for metastatic disease.

■ Treatment for mycosis fungoides includes a combination of the following, depending on the stage of the cancer:
- Blood tests, a chest x-ray, and a lymph-node biopsy to determine the stage of the disease.
- Topical treatment with nitrogen mustard (mechlorethamine). This is a chemotherapeutic lotion applied to the lesions.
- Psoralens plus ultraviolet light (PUVA) therapy. In this technique, a precise amount of ultraviolet-A (UVA) exposure is administered in a light box after taking oral psoralen to accentuate the effect of the light therapy.
- Electron-beam therapy, in which electron beams are focused at the tumors to destroy them.
- Chemotherapy.
- Bexarotene (Targretin), a type of retinoid. This may be used to treat mycosis fungoides that has not responded to at least one prior oral or intravenous medication.
- Photophoresis, a technique in which a portion of the blood is removed from the body, irradiated, and then returned to the bloodstream.

■ In the future, it may be possible to use genetic research to identify susceptible people before cancer develops. This is important because the earlier cancer is detected, the more curable it is. Ultrasound technology is showing promise in aiding doctors to assess more exactly the depth and size of cancers before surgery.

■ A vaccine against malignant melanoma is in the developmental stages, and is close to being ready for testing.

DIETARY MEASURES

■ Be sure to eat at least five servings of fruits and vegetables each day, especially those foods rich in the antioxidants beta-carotene, vitamin C, and selenium, such as broccoli, carrots, and citrus fruits. Dr. Harvey Arbesman, Professor of Dermatology at the New York State University at Buffalo School of Medicine and Biomedical Sciences in Buffalo, New York, makes this recommendation based on more than fifty studies of basal cell and squamous cell cancer of the skin and nutrition. His recommendations are supported by research done by Dr. Ken Nelder, professor of dermatology at Texas Tech University. Independent studies have found that people with skin cancer have lower than normal tissue levels of vitamin A, beta-carotene, and selenium. Further, it has been found that increasing the intake of vitamins A, C and E, beta-carotene, and selenium helps to protect against the development of skin cancer.

■ Include in your diet plenty of whole grains, sea vegetables, beans and soybeans, hot peppers, cabbage, tomatoes, onions, rosemary, garlic, grapes, citrus fruits, licorice root, green tea, flaxseed and olive oils, white fish, and maitake, reishi, and shiitake mushrooms. These foods are thought to have antioxidant, anticancer, and immune-boosting properties.

■ A diet high in omega-3 essential fatty acids and low in omega-6 essential fatty acids is important in helping to prevent melanoma. Therefore, you should consume fish oil and olive oil, and *avoid* corn oil, safflower oil, and sunflower oil. Even butter, with its higher ratio of omega-3 to omega-6 oils, is considered safer than eating corn oil insofar as the development of skin cancer is concerned. With a higher omega-6 to omega-3 fat ratio, the production of certain prostaglandins increases dramatically, which in turn increases the genesis and growth of skin tumors. One recent study found that a group of people with melanoma ate about twice as much omega-6 type oils as a similar group of cancer-free individuals. In mice, safflower and sunflower oils have also been shown to spur the growth of melanoma. Thus, eating fish at least twice a week and cooking with olive oil is recommended.

■ Avoid red meat, processed foods, red and yellow dyes, monosodium gluta-mate, nitrites (found in cured meats), saccharin, sugar, dairy products, alco-hol, caffeine-containing drinks, aspartame (NutraSweet), and hydrogenated vegetable oils.

■ Drink at least eight glasses of filtered water daily to keep the body's waste materials flowing out.

NUTRITIONAL SUPPLEMENTS

■ The following nutrients are recommended for people with skin cancer, as well as for cancer prevention:
  • A high-potency multivitamin and mineral supplement. Take this daily.
  • Beta-carotene. Take 10,000 to 25,000 international units daily.
  • Vitamin-B complex. Take a product containing 100 milligrams of most of the major B vitamins daily.
  • Vitamin C. When vitamin C was added to the drinking water of mice with melanoma, their tumors grew more slowly and their survival time increased. Take 1,000 milligrams of vitamin C with bioflavonoids three times a day.
  • Vitamin E. A University of Arizona study reported that the adminis-tration of high doses of supplemental vitamin E prevented ultraviolet-light-induced skin cancers in animals. Take 400 international units of vitamin E daily.
  • Selenium. In laboratory studies on animals exposed to ultraviolet rays, those that were given selenium, either orally or topically, had signifi-cantly less free-radical and pigmentary changes and a lower incidence of skin cancer. Take 100 micrograms of selenium daily.
  • Zinc. Take 50 milligrams daily.
  • Calcium and magnesium. Take 1,500 milligrams of calcium and 750 milligrams of magnesium a day.
  • Folic acid. Take 400 to 800 micrograms daily.
  • Fish oil, flaxseed oil, or olive oil. Take 2 teaspoons daily.

■ If chemotherapy or radiation therapy becomes necessary to treat advanced malignant melanoma, a different regimen of nutritional supplementation is recommended. This is because chemotherapy and radiation therapy expose healthy cells to free-radical damage, depleting antioxidant enzymes, nutrients, and mechanisms. Nutritional support must provide additional antioxidants and nutrients to protect against these damaging effects. The following supplements are recommended:

- A high-potency multivitamin and mineral supplement daily.
- Beta-carotene. Take 100,000 international units daily.
- Vitamin B_{12}. Take 1,000 micrograms daily.
- Vitamin C with bioflavonoids. Take 3,000 to 8,000 milligrams daily, divided into three doses.
- Vitamin E. Take 400 to 800 international units daily.
- Selenium. Take 800 micrograms daily.
- Folic acid. Take 400 milligrams daily.
- Flaxseed oil. Take 1 to 2 tablespoons daily.
- Alpha-lipoic acid. This is a very potent lipid- and water-soluble antioxidant that can get to any place in the body, and that also activates other antioxidants. Take 150 milligrams three times a day.
- Coenzyme Q_{10}. This supplement helps to augment the body's energy needs, is an antioxidant, and may have anticancer properties. Take 100 milligrams three times daily.
- N–Acetylcysteine (NAC). NAC increases the liver's detoxification of wastes. Take 500 milligrams twice a day.
- Pine bark or grapeseed extract. These are powerful antioxidants. Take 50 milligrams of either one three times a day.

HERBAL TREATMENT

■ For a general detoxifying and eliminative combination, mix equal parts of powdered extracts of bloodroot, burdock root, chaparral, dandelion, echinacea, frangula, ginger, licorice, red clover, and violet leaves. Put the mixture into capsules and take two capsules four times a day.

■ Cat's-claw extract is an immune-enhancer and may have anticancer properties as well. Take 1,000 milligrams three times a day.

Caution: Do not take cat's claw if you are pregnant or nursing, if you take anticoagulants (blood-thinners), or if you are an organ-transplant recipient.

■ Milk-thistle extract helps to strengthen the liver and detoxify the system. Take 150 milligrams three times a day.

■ Red-clover extract helps to prevent the formation of new blood vessels that are needed to supply the growing tumor. Take 500 milligrams four times a day.

AROMATHERAPY

■ A soothing bath to which several drops of essential oils of chamomile or lavender has been added can help to relax and calm you if you are suffering from a severe form of skin cancer.

■ *Do not* use bergamot oil on your skin or in your bath if you will be out in the sun unprotected, as it increases the skin's sun sensitivity.

HOMEOPATHY

■ Homeopathic remedies used to treat early basal cell carcinomas *only* (not other types of skin cancer) include *Arsenicum acidum* (for tumors that are dry, red, and hot in an irritable person with nervous headaches), *Conium maculatum, Gallium aparine* (for cancerous lesions associated with chronic urinary problems and/or swelling of the ankles), *Hydrastis* (to dry up ulcerated lesions), *Kali sulfuricum,* and *Lycopodium*. However, no treatment regimens are included here, as it is recommended that you seek the advice of a professional homeopath if you want to treat early basal cell carcinoma homeopathically. If the problem does not resolve quickly with homeopathy, you should use another form of treatment.

OTHER THERAPIES

■ Electrotherapy holds promise as a treatment to inhibit tumor growth. It may be used either on its own or to increase the effectiveness of anticancer drugs. There are studies reporting success in animals, as well as clinical reports of success in treating squamous cell carcinomas in humans. This approach may be very useful in the future for the treatment of primary skin cancers as well as metastases of tumors from other parts of the body to the skin.

■ Photodynamic (light) therapy is used to treat mycosis fungoides, and is being tested for the treatment of basal cell and squamous cell carcinomas. In the 1940s, Mayo Clinic researchers found that cancer cells selectively absorb porphyrins, or light-activated dyes. The cancer cells fluoresce a brilliant red when activated by red light. The porphyrins inside them undergo a chemical change and selectively destroy the cancer cells in the presence of higher doses of the red light. Generally there is a one- to three-day waiting period between cancer diagnosis and treatment, as the only FDA-approved photosensitive chemical, porfimer (Photofrin), also collects in normal kidney, liver, spleen, and pancreas tissue. Thus, time must be allowed for the Photofrin to clear from those organs before treatment is instituted. An argon-pumped laser is used to deliver red light directly to the treatment sites via hair-thin fiberoptic tubes. Within hours of the first treatment, the cancer cells begin to die, and most normal tissues are left unharmed. The main limitation to using this kind of therapy for cancer is that the physician has to be able physically to reach the tumors via fiberoptic tubes to treat them. Because porfimer collects in the skin, and because the skin, obviously, is easily accessible, photodynamic therapy is well suited for treatment of skin cancers, especially mycosis fungoides. It is a very successful, precise, simple, painless, and relatively safe form of light therapy that should enjoy increasing application in the future. However, because porfimer temporarily collects in the skin, there is increased photosensitivity and skin irritation for up to a month after treatment.

■ A diagnosis of, and treatment for, any kind of cancer, including skin cancer, is a source of stress. To reduce the effects of stress on the body, do some type of aerobic exercise and stretching five times a week. This increases the body's circulation and improves one's pyschological outlook as well.

■ Relaxation techniques, yoga, and meditation are helpful to the body, mind, and spirit. See Part Three for examples of easy techniques you can start with.

■ Consider joining a support group or seeking other sources of psychological support. A study by Dr. F.I. Fawzy and colleagues at the UCLA School of Medicine in 1993 demonstrated that melanoma patients had a statistically significant greater rate of survival and freedom from recurrences if they participated in an intensive six-week therapy group shortly after their diagnosis and initial surgery. This study of sixty-eight patients was randomized and controlled, and although it is a small sample, it suggests that mental interventions play an important role in recurrence and survival among people with malignant melanoma. Many people with melanoma also have a psychological need to feel that they are doing all they can to extend and improve the quality of their lives, lessen the feelings of helplessness, and strengthen their sense of hope. This is particularly true for people with late-stage disease, but it also applies to those with relatively good prognoses, who are recommended only to have regular checkups after surgery and who consequently feel as if they are "sitting on a time bomb."

▓ Positive guided imagery, meditation, and/or prayer can be helpful not only mentally and psychologically, but also physicially, and should be practiced daily.

GENERAL RECOMMENDATIONS

▓ The best approach to skin cancer is prevention. Take the following measures to help prevent skin cancer:

- Limit your time in the sun and seek the shade, not a tan.
- Use a sunscreen with a sun protection factor (SPF) rating of at least 15 to guard against the sun's damaging effects. Choose a product that protects against both UVA and UVB rays. Reapply sunscreen to all exposed areas of skin every two hours while you are outside. Remember that clouds and haze do not block harmful UV radiation, so you still need to cover up and apply sunscreen to all exposed skin when it is overcast.
- Wear sunglasses, a broad-brimmed hat, and protective clothing whenever you are outside.
- Stay away from tanning parlors and artificial tanning devices.
- After sun exposure, apply a 5-percent vitamin-E cream. In animal studies, applying vitamin E oil or cream to the skin up to eight hours after sun exposure prevented UV-light-induced skin damage, tumor formation, and immune suppression.

▓ Do not use sunscreen on babies under six months old. Instead, keep them out of the sun entirely.

▓ Do a skin self-examination every three months. (See Part Three for a discussion and illustration of this procedure.) If you find any suspicious spots in your self-exam, don't panic, but do consult a dermatologist as soon as possible. Remember, all skin cancers are curable if discovered early.

Skin Ulcers

If the skin breaks down, with a loss of the top layer of skin and a variable loss of the deeper layers, ulcers form. Skin ulcers, which are most common in older adults, can be a result of diabetes, skin cancer, eczema, infection, trauma, arteriosclerosis, venous stasis, neurologic disease, connective-tissue disease, blood disorders, malnutrition, high blood pressure, or pressure over the bony areas, such as occurs with prolonged bed rest or inactivity. This section focuses particular attention on the most common types, venous stasis leg ulcers due to poor return of blood through the leg veins to the heart.

Venous stasis ulcers account for 80 to 90 percent of leg ulcers in the older population. They affect women more frequently than they do men. These ulcers are generally located near the bottom of the leg, most often behind the inner ankle. They are rapid-forming and irregular, with surrounding swelling, itchy red rashes, and/or darkened pigmentation. Pulses are normal in the ankles and feet.

Ulcers are notoriously difficult to heal, so alternative techniques are a very important addition to medical treatment. Many of the integrative treatment approaches described below can be used successfully for many types of ulcers in addition to venous to stasis ulcers of the leg.

CONVENTIONAL TREATMENT

■ Wear support stockings when up and walking, to prevent new ulcers from forming.

■ Wet dressings and twenty-minute soaks with potassium permanganate, silver nitrate, acetic acid, hydrogen peroxide, Betadine or saline solution three times a day aid in healing and soothing ulcers, and in fighting infection. Whirlpool baths can be used as an alternative to soaks.

■ Your doctor may mechanically debride (remove dead skin) affected areas with forceps and scissors after soaking or whirlpooling. Removing the dead tissue allows fresh, new tissue to grow.

■ Twenty-percent benzoyl peroxide gel, fibrinolysin (Elase), trypsin (Granulex), papain (Panafil), collagenase (Santyl), or other proteolytic enzymes may be used to chemically debride the ulcer. Care should be taken never to apply these products to normal surrounding skin.

■ Medium-strength topical steroids can be applied to any inflamed skin surrounding the ulcer. Care must be taken not to apply the steroid directly to the ulcer, as this will markedly slow healing.

■ A layer of product such as dextranomer (Debrisan) beads, which are tiny, porous spheres, or DuoDERM granules can be applied to wet, soupy ulcers to absorb serum, bacteria, and cellular debris. If the absorbent material is replaced with a new layer before it becomes saturated, it provides continuous deep cleansing, which aids in healing.

■ One of many available synthetic dressings is applied over the clean, debrided ulcer and changed every few days. Opaque hydrocolloid membranes such as DuoDERM; semitransparent, nonadherent membranes such as Second Skin or Vigilon; and translucent, self-adherent polyurethane membranes such as OpSite or Tegaderm are commonly used.

■ In lieu of a synthetic dressing, mupirocin (Bactroban) antibacterial ointment can be applied to the ulcer, covered with a nonstick gauze, and changed every day.

■ An Unna boot compression dressing, made of zinc-oxide-impregnated gauze, can be used if you are mobile and the ulcer is not infected. It is changed on a weekly basis.

■ A more recent development in wound care is bioengineered, cultured living skin substitute. Graftskin (Apligraf) has been found to be up to three times more effective in closing uninfected skin ulcers that have been present for longer than one year than Unna boot compression therapy alone. It is thought to promote healing through tissue regeneration, stimulation of the underlying wound bed, and contraction of the wound edges. It is put on once and left on the ulcer, unless signs of infection develop.

■ Hyperbaric oxygen therapy (HBOT), in which 100-percent pure oxygen is delivered under greater than atmospheric pressure, has become a more widespread treatment for leg ulcers and other wounds. In this treatment, the patient lies comfortably in a chamber while the therapy helps the body to heal its own tissues by enriching the bloodstream with additional oxygen.

■ For chronic, difficult cases, skin grafts are a last resort.

■ All underlying systemic and local diseases that may be contributing to the formation of skin ulcers need to be evaluated and treated.

■ Oral pentoxifylline (Trental) may be prescribed to address the problem of insufficient microcirculation in the legs, if that is believed to be contributing to leg ulcers.

■ Nystatin/triamcinolone (Mycolog), neomycin (Myciguent), parabens preservatives, and lanolin should be avoided. These substances can cause an allergic contact dermatitis, and they also slow healing.

DIETARY MEASURES

■ To aid wound healing, eat a well-balanced diet with plenty of whole grains, lean protein, and green, orange, and yellow vegetables.
■ Drink eight glasses of pure filtered water a day.
■ Avoid junk food, sugar, artificial ingredients, and animal fats.

NUTRITIONAL SUPPLEMENTS

■ Incorporate the following nutrients, which speed healing, into your daily regimen:
  • A high-potency multivitamin and mineral supplement. Take this daily.
  • Beta-carotene. Take 15,000 international units a day.
  • Vitamin B complex. Take a supplement containing 100 milligrams of most major B vitamins twice a day.
  • Vitamin C with bioflavonoids. Take 1,000 milligrams three times a day.
  • Vitamin D. Take 400 to 1,000 international units a day.
  • Vitamin E. Take 400 international units a day. Vitamin E oil can also be applied topically to ulcers that are mostly healed to help to accelerate healing and reduce scarring.
  • Flaxseed oil. Take 1 tablespoon twice a day.
  • Zinc. Take 25 milligrams twice a day, with meals and with 1 milligram of copper.
  • Free-form amino-acid complex. Take this supplement as directed by the manufacturer.

■ Any additional nutritional deficiencies should be determined and additional supplements added as appropriate.

HERBAL TREATMENT

■ Astralagus helps the immune system and healing after surgery.

■ The combination of echinacea and goldenseal helps to support the immune system and prevent infection. Echinacea powder can also be mixed with olive oil to make a paste and applied to the ulcer three times a day. Or you can combine 1 teaspoon of goldenseal powder with the oil from one 800-international-unit vitamin-E capsule and a few drops of olive oil and apply that to the ulcer three times a day for its antiseptic, healing, and soothing qualities.

■ Aloe-vera juice, applied topically, makes a helpful compress for dry ulcers.

■ Calendula ointment is soothing to dry ulcers.

■ Comfrey ointment, applied topically, is helpful if the ulcer is dry.

■ A charcoal pack made with eucalyptus oil can be used if the ulcer is old and contains foul debris.

■ Raw honey, applied locally three times a day, can speed healing.

AROMATHERAPY

■ Tea tree oil, applied to the ulcer every two to three hours, helps to prevent infection. If it is too strong, you can dilute it in an equal amount of olive oil.

HOMEOPATHY

■ *Arnica tincture,* applied externally to the ulcer, is helpful in the first stage of skin breakdown.

■ *Calcarea sulfurica* 9c is best for ulcers that are inflamed, with a thick, yellow, pus-filled discharge. Take one dose three times a day.

■ *Graphites* 12x or 6c is helpful for oozing, burning, stinging ulcers with surrounding skin that looks cracked. Take it three times a day for three days.

■ *Hepar sulphuris* 9c is best for the stage when the ulcer is red and inflamed but does not have much of a discharge. Take a dose three times a day.

■ *Petroleum* 12x or 6c is good for itching, burning ulcers on dry, cracked skin. Take it three times a day for three days.

ACUPRESSURE

See Acupressure Points in Part Three for the locations of these points on the body.

■ Pressing Gallbladder 34, Large Intestine 4, Liver 3, Stomach 36, and the back Bladder points improves circulation. This helps to bring necessary nutrients and take away toxins from the ulcer. Three times a day, gently apply pressure for three minutes to any of these pairs of points that can be reached easily.

OTHER THERAPIES

■ Electrotherapy shows promise as a treatment to promote the healing of skin ulcers. There have been many studies over the last fifty years showing that the application of low-amperage direct current promotes healing of ulcers, among other things. Results of studies done on ischemic, leprous, and decubitus ulcers can readily be extrapolated to apply to the treatment of other ulcers, including the common venous stasis leg ulcer. Electrotherapy can also increase blood flow in the capillaries in the skin, which is important because insufficient blood flow is a major factor in leg ulcers. In the accelerated ulcer and wound healing found with electrotherapy, no adverse effects have been reported. In fact, after electrotherapy, highly contaminated wounds have been found to be less contaminated with bacteria. Thus, electrical stimulation for ulcers is an excellent noninvasive therapy of great efficiency and low social costs which needs to be much more widely studied and applied.
■ Ultraviolet-light therapy with a heat lamp can be used to dry ulcers if they are soupy and wet.
■ Massaging the area around the ulcer daily helps to increase local blood flow and aid in healing.

GENERAL RECOMMENDATIONS

■ Elevate your feet by nine inches in bed for one hour at midday and one hour at night.

■ Avoid all trauma to the skin to prevent further skin breakdown and the onset of new ulcers.

■ Use only a mild soap, such as Purpose, and warm water for washing the surrounding normal skin. Dry the skin gently and use a mild moisturizer to prevent drying and cracking of the skin, which can increase the risk of new ulcer formation.

Sunburn

The sun's ultraviolet rays are very strong, and being out unprotected for just a few hours at midday can cause a bad sunburn. There are two types of ultraviolet (UV) rays, designated ultraviolet-A UVA and ultraviolet-B UVB. Both are harmful. If the sun is reflected off water, metal, snow, or sand, its effects intensify. Higher altitude also increases the intensity of the sun's burning rays.

Sunburns, like other burns, are classified as first-degree, second-degree, third-degree, and fourth-degree, depending on how many layers of skin and underlying structures they involve. Most sunburns are first-degree burns. First-degree sunburns involve only the epidermis and are characterized by pain, heat, and redness of the top layer of the skin. Symptoms appear from one hour to one day after exposure, and peak about one day later. Second-degree sunburns go through part of the skin layers under the epidermis, in the dermis, and damage the small blood vessels and elastic fibers in the skin. Immediately, there is painful redness due to swollen capillaries, and much later there is wrinkling and sagging of the skin. This type of sunburn is extremely painful, with swelling, blistering, and seeping of fluids. Rarely, a sunburn is severe enough to be classified as a third- or fourth-degree burn.

If a second-degree sunburn is larger than the size of a quarter, you should seek professional medical advice. Sunburns of the face, palms, soles, and joints can cause serious problems, no matter how small their size or how severe they are. Burns in these areas should always be checked out by a physician and watched carefully. If the area of sunburned skin is large enough, you may develop chills, fever, and weakness. All sunburns should also be watched for signs of infection, especially after the skin has peeled.

Perhaps the worst aspect of sunburn is that the incidence of malignant melanoma, a form of skin cancer that can be life-threatening if not treated early and successfully, increases dramatically in those who have experienced severe sunburns as a child or young adult. Other type of skin cancer, such as squamous cell carcinoma and basal cell carcinoma, also have been found to be closely related to a history of sunburn.

■ The best approach to sunburn is to prevent it in the first place. Take the following measures to protect yourself:

- Apply a sunscreen with a sun protection factor (SPF) of 15 or higher to all exposed areas of skin whenever you go outside or ride in a car. Get a product that protects against *both* UVA and UVB rays. Apply it to all exposed areas thirty minutes before you expect to go out, and reapply it if you are out in the direct sun for over an hour.
- Wear a hat, sunglasses, and loose, long-sleeved, light-colored clothing. There is a line of clothing called Solumbra, made by Sun Precautions of Everett, Washington, that has an SPF rating of 30.
- Try not to go outdoors between 10:00 AM and 2:00 PM, when the ultraviolet light is most intense.
- Be just as cautious on cloudy or foggy days as you are on sunny days, as 80 percent of the sun's rays get through the clouds.

■ To soothe a sunburn, bathe or soak the involved area for thirty minutes in lukewarm water to which oatmeal or baking soda has been added. Use 1 cup of oatmeal or baking soda per bathtubful of water.

■ While cooling the burn, remove any watches, rings, belts, bracelets, or anything else potentially constricting from the affected area before the burned skin swells around these items.

■ Benzocaine- and lidocaine-containing sprays such as Americaine and Solarcaine are available over the counter for pain relief.

■ An over-the-counter painkiller such as acetaminophen (in Tylenol and many other products), aspirin (Bayer and others), or ibuprofen (Advil, Nuprin, and others) can be taken for pain.

■ An oral antihistamine such as diphenhydramine (Benadryl, Diphenhist, and others), chlorpheniramine (Chlor-Trimeton, Teldrin, and others), hydroxyzine (Atarax, Hyzine-50, Vistaril), or cetirizine (Zyrtec) can be helpful for itching that develops as the sunburn heals.

■ Using an antibacterial soap helps prevent secondary infection.

■ If the sunburn is deeper than the very superficial layers of your skin, your physician may prescribe a topical cortisone cream that is soothing and speeds healing.

■ Do not burst any blisters over the burns. They form a natural bandage that helps the skin to heal.

■ For severe burns, your physician may recommend a short course of oral prednisone to aid in healing.

■ *Never* apply butter, petroleum jelly, or any other greasy substance to a sunburn. This will only trap the heat and can cause a burn to deepen.

DIETARY MEASURES

■ With any kind of burn, there is a greatly increased need for protein and energy, as the injured tissues' requirements skyrocket and your metabolism speeds up. Therefore, eat lots of lean, high-quality protein foods.

■ Eat plenty of green and yellow vegetables. These help to provide beta-carotene and vitamin C, both of which are important in the healing process.

■ Include pumpkin seeds and oysters in your diet. These foods help to supply much-needed zinc.

■ Make sure to drink plenty of filtered water to replace fluids lost through the burn.

NUTRITIONAL SUPPLEMENTS

■ Beta-carotene aids in healing. Take 25,000 international units twice a day for three days, then 10,000 international units twice a day for two weeks.

■ Vitamins A and E and selenium are important antioxidants and free-radical scavengers. Sunburn increases the number of free radicals attacking skin cells. Take 25,000 international units of vitamin A, 400 international units of vitamin E, and 200 micrograms of selenium a day for two weeks. You can also combine vitamin A, vitamin E, flaxseed oil, zinc oxide paste, and aloe vera gel and apply the mixture to the burn twice a day to soothe and speed healing. Once the burn is mostly healed, you can apply vitamin-E cream or oil twice a day to the areas of the burn to prevent scarring.

■ Vitamin C and bioflavonoids are necessary for the production of new collagen, a major protein component of skin. Take 1,000 milligrams three times a day for two weeks. You can also mix 2 tablespoons of powdered vitamin C into ½ cup of aloe-vera gel and spray this on the affected area twice a day until the burn heals.

■ Flaxseed oil supplies essential fatty acids that are vital for healthy skin and skin repair. Take 2 tablespoons daily for two weeks.

▓ Zinc aids in healing and strengthens the immune system. Take 30 milligrams twice a day for two weeks.

HERBAL TREATMENT

▓ Aloe vera gel is the most important herbal therapy for mild sunburns. Applying the gel directly from the fresh plant to the burn eases the pain and keeps the burn from turning white and from blistering. Break open the stem of a live plant and apply the gel to your sunburn several times a day. Some people prefer commercial aloe preparations, which smell better and go on more easily. The gel works on several enzyme systems to decrease pain, reduce inflammation, speed wound healing, and stimulate new skin-cell growth. Aloe also has antibacterial and antifungal properties, and it increases the amount of blood bringing healing resources to the areas of sunburned tissue.

▓ Calendula cream can be applied directly to the sunburn for soothing relief of pain. It also has antiseptic properties and helps to prevent scarring.

▓ Comfrey cream can be used to help increase tissue regrowth and promote healing. Or soak a clean cloth in comfrey root tea and apply it as a compress to the sunburned areas for fifteen minutes twice a day.

▓ Echinacea stimulates the immune system to prevent and fight infection, important after a second-degree sunburn. Drink 1 to 2 teaspoons of tincture of echinacea immediately after a burn, and apply a few drops directly to the burn to benefit from echinacea's mild antiseptic properties.

▓ Gotu kola, taken orally with vitamin-C supplements, helps to speed healing of skin tissue by stimulating collagen synthesis. It also fights infection. Take 200 milligrams of gotu kola extract or a cup of gotu kola tea twice a day to get its benefits.

▓ Nettle lotion or ointment, applied directly to the burn, is soothing.

▓ Plantain is one of the most popular American folk medicines for burns. Juice from the fresh leaves of the plantain is very soothing when applied directly to mild sunburn.

▓ St. John's wort is also frequently helpful to reduce the pain, inflammation, healing time, and scarring of a first-degree burn. Apply a few drops of the tincture directly to the burn. Or, if you have the dried herb readily available, make a preparation by steeping 1 to 2 teaspoons of the dried herb in a few ounces of vegetable oil and apply that to the burn.

■ Green tea or black tea extracts, applied topically, may help to prevent sunburn and thus skin cancer. This was reported at the 1998 meeting of the American Association for Cancer Research. Ordinary tea bags that have been steeped in boiling water and then cooled are particularly recommended for sunburned eyelids. You can also add four tea bags to a quart of water, boil, then cool to lukewarm. Soak a towel in the tea and place the towel over the sunburned skin. Keep reapplying tea-soaked towels for about thirty minutes or until the pain resolves.

AROMATHERAPY

■ Lavender oil can be dripped directly on the sunburn. It is said to have remarkable pain-relieving and burn-healing powers. Remember never to ingest essential oils, though, as even a small amount can be toxic.

■ Combine lavender essential oil and aloe vera to get the benefits of both. Add ⅛ teaspoon of lavender oil to 4 ounces of aloe vera juice and spray it on sunburned skin as often as needed. For an added cooling effect, keep it in the refrigerator. Shake the bottle before each use.

■ A bath made by adding 20 drops each of lavender and chamomile oils to a tubful of cool water is very soothing. Soak for at least ten minutes to get some relief from the pain of the sunburn.

■ Tea tree oil, applied directly to the burn, soothes sunburn and helps to prevent infection. If it is too irritating when applied directly, dilute it in a bit of water first.

HOMEOPATHY

■ *Apis mellifica* 12c or 30x is good for a sunburn that is very swollen and feels a lot better with applications of cold. Take one dose every two to three hours.

■ *Calendula* 6c or 12x is helpful if the pain from the burn is relatively mild. Take one dose every two to three hours.

■ *Urtica urens* 6c or 12x is good if the sunburned skin is very itchy and stinging badly, or if there are severe shooting pains. Take a dose every two to three hours.

■ The following homeopathic tinctures are very helpful when applied directly to the sunburn:

- *Hypericum.* Add 20 drops to 4 ounces of cool water to make a soak for painful burns where nerves have been damaged.
- Rescue Remedy. This useful remedy is derived from a combination of flowers.
- *Urtica urens.* Add 20 drops of the tincture to 4 ounces of tepid water to make a soak to relieve the itch and sting of sunburned skin, especially if severe shooting pains are also present.

ACUPRESSURE

See Acupressure Points in Part Three for the locations of these points on the body.

■ Press the Golden Points near the sunburned area at least three times a day to increase local blood flow which will remove toxins and bring needed nutrients.

■ To relieve the pain of the sunburn and speed healing, press the Bladder 65 acupoint on each foot for three minutes, three times a day. The Bladder 65 points are on the outside edges of the feet, in the depressions under the bone just beyond the joint joining the fifth toe to the foot. With your thumb on top of the foot and your fingers under the sole of the foot, use your index finger to press the acupoint. Your finger should be pointed toward the fifth toe, with your nail edge pointing up underneath the bone.

GENERAL RECOMMENDATIONS

■ Dipping gauze in ordinary whole milk and applying it to the sunburn for fifteen minutes is very soothing. Be sure to wash the milk off thoroughly afterward. Repeat this every two to four hours. The fat content of whole milk makes it very calming to burned skin.

Surgery

Sometimes, surgical removal of a mole, benign tumor, skin cancer, or malignant melanoma lesion is required. Occasionally, these are large excisions involving flaps or grafts of skin. In this section, we will look at some conventional and alternative techniques that can be used to help to reduce fear prior to surgery, speed recovery after surgery, and aid in the healing of the surgical wound.

CONVENTIONAL TREATMENT

- Rest after surgery, following your doctor's directions.
- Protect the wound from sun exposure.
- An ice pack can be applied to the areas over the arteries that supply the wound, to temporarily slow the local blood flow and, thus, surgery-related bleeding.
- Lidocaine with procaine (EMLA) cream or topical lidocaine (ELA-Max, Xylocaine) can be spread on the skin before the shot of lidocaine to further reduce any pain you may feel when a "numbing medicine" injection is given.
- A neomycin/polymyxin B/bacitracin combination (Neosporin, Polysporin) ointment or silver sulfadiazine (Silvadene, SSD, Thermazene) cream applied to the wound twice a day speeds wound healing by almost 30 percent.
- An over-the-counter medication such as acetaminophen (in Tylenol and many other products), aspirin (Bayer and others), or ibuprofen (Advil, Nuprin, and others) can be used for pain relief. If such medications are not sufficient, your doctor may prescribe a stronger medicine.
- Watch for signs of infection, such as redness, extreme pain, local swelling, and pus-filled discharge. If any such sign develops, consult your physician.

DIETARY MEASURES

- Eat a healthy, whole-foods-based diet with plenty of whole grains, fruits, vegetables, and lean protein.
- Juices high in beta-carotene, such as carrot, beet, celery, and garlic juice, speed healing.

■ Keep well hydrated by drinking at least six glasses of pure water daily.
■ Avoid high-fat foods, sugars, caffeine, alcohol, and refined foods with lots of preservatives and artificial ingredients.

NUTRITIONAL SUPPLEMENTS

■ The following nutritional supplements are suggested to speed healing. They should be started two weeks prior to surgery and continued for one month afterward:
  • A high-potency multivitamin. Take this daily.
  • Beta-carotene. Take 25,000 international units daily.
  • Vitamin-B complex. Take a product containing 100 milligrams of most of the major B vitamins daily. Also take an additional 500 milligrams of pantothenic acid twice a day.
  • Vitamin C with bioflavonoids. Take 1,000 milligrams three times a day.
  • Vitamin D. Take 400 international units daily.
  • Vitamin E. Take 400 international units daily.
  • Free-form amino acids, especially arginine and glycine. Take these as recommended by the manufacturer twice a day.
  • Flaxseed oil. Take 1 teaspoon twice a day.
  • Zinc. Take 25 milligrams twice a day, with meals and with 1 milligram of copper.

■ Soon after surgery, a combination of equal parts of vitamin-E oil, vitamin-A oil, flaxseed oil, and zinc-oxide cream can be applied directly to the area twice a day to speed healing.
■ When the wound is mostly healed, applying vitamin-E oil topically twice a day helps to reduce scarring.

HERBAL TREATMENT

■ Astragalus extract helps immune function and healing after surgery. Take it as directed by the manufacturer.
■ A combination of echinacea and goldenseal extracts helps to support the immune system and prevent infection. Take it as directed by the manufac-

turer. Echinacea is also available in ointment form, and can be applied twice a day to the wound to speed healing. Or combine 1 teaspoon of powdered goldenseal extract with the oil from one 800-international-unit vitamin-E capsule and a few drops of olive oil to make a paste, and apply it to the wound three times a day for its antiseptic, healing, and soothing qualities.

■ Aloe-vera gel, applied topically, is helpful for wounds which are already partially healed. Apply it as directed by the manufacturer.

■ Calendula ointment is soothing. Apply it as directed by the manufacturer.

■ Comfrey ointment is helpful if the wound is dry. Apply it as directed by the manufacturer.

■ Raw honey, applied locally three times a day, can speed healing.

■ Distilled witch hazel, applied locally twice a day, can speed healing and stop bleeding.

AROMATHERAPY

■ Tea tree oil, applied to the wound every two to three hours, helps to prevent infection. If it is too irritating in its pure form, it can be diluted in a bit of olive oil.

HOMEOPATHY

■ Taking a dose of *Arnica* 30c three times a day for two days before surgery and one dose of *Arnica* 200c as soon as possible after surgery helps to reduce the swelling and soreness and speed healing. As an alternative to the single dose of *Arnica* 200c, you can continue taking a dose of *Arnica* 30c three to four times a day for two days after the procedure.

■ Take a dose of *Ledum* 6c three to four times a day, starting on day three after the last dose of *Arnica*.

■ *Silica* is best for wounds that become infected easily, heal slowly, and are inflamed, painful, and pus-filled.

■ There have been many studies in the medical literature showing that electrotherapy increases blood flow to healing tissues, reduces local swelling, speeds scar formation, and improves flap and graft survival after surgical incision. Several groups of scientists have shown in the laboratory that electric currents induce human fibroblasts (cells that produce connective tissue) to significantly increase their rate of DNA and collagen synthesis, as well as their migration to sites where they are needed. Many controlled studies support the use of electrotherapy to aid in wound healing after surgery, and this is a modality whose usefulness has not been fully utilized.

■ Relaxation techniques should be practiced prior to surgery to calm the body and emotions. This practice has been shown to improve the surgical outcome.

■ Guided imagery and visualization exercises can improve your frame of mind prior to and after surgery, speed healing, and reduce pain after surgery. The night before, repeatedly visualize, to the smallest detail, the surgery going easily and without complications. After surgery, try to picture your pain, giving it size, shape, and color, and then visualize yourself throwing it out of the room into space.

Varicose Veins
and Spider Veins

As 75 percent of people over the age of sixty-five know, veins that have become swollen, raised, and snakelike are called varicose veins. If one or more of the one-way valves in superficial veins no longer functions normally, the blood headed back to the heart can pool or even flow backward. This stretches the vein and makes it impossible for other nearby valves to close properly as well. The vein becomes swollen and kinked, and blood stagnates in the vein. The veins turn purple, dark blue, or cranberry in color.

Varicose veins are most common on the thighs, the backs of the calves, the insides of the legs, and the ankles. In addition to being cosmetically displeasing, varicose veins often feel heavy, burn, itch, or throb, and the feet and ankles can swell. The legs may feel hot and heavy and become sensitive to pressure. Symptoms generally worsen during the day, especially with prolonged standing. The severity of the appearance of the varicose veins does not necessarily correspond to the severity of the associated pain and soreness. People with only a few visible varicosities can suffer from severe pain from them.

Varicose veins run in families, and affect women more frequently because of premenstrual or menopausal hormones, birth control pills, and pregnancy. In fact, they occur in 40 percent of pregnant women. Other factors that contribute to varicose veins include advancing age, muscular atrophy in the legs, poor circulation, smoking, prolonged bed rest, overweight, lack of exercise, prolonged standing or sitting, tight clothing, high heels, excessive heavy lifting, and chronic constipation.

In addition to being painful and tiring, varicose veins can cause other problems. These include blood clots and inflammation in the veins, and bleeding (either under the skin or on the surface) if the distended vein is accidentally cut or bumped. The presence of many varicosities prevents the delivery of enough nutrients and oxygen to the tissues of the legs and delays removal of wastes from leg tissues. Then the skin around the varicosities may become very thin, discolored, hardened, and prone to ulcers.

Very tiny dilated capillaries, usually on the face, legs, and thighs, are called spider veins. They are typically a red or bluish color and can be short unconnected lines or come together in a "sunburst" pattern or a spiderweb-like pattern just under the surface of the skin. They are not an early sign of varicose veins and are not a dangerous problem. Spider veins often run in families, and tend to be more common in women, especially with the hormonal changes of puberty and pregnancy. Injury to a part of the body or wearing tight hosiery may bring out unwanted spider veins in the involved area. Spider veins also occur on the face in those with fair skin, rosacea, and chronic, unprotected sun exposure.

CONVENTIONAL TREATMENT

■ Sclerotherapy, in which a concentrated salt solution is injected directly into a blood vessel, may be recommended for varicose veins or spider veins. The injection causes the sides of the blood vessel to stick together. The vessel then turns into an almost invisible scar over a period of several weeks. Surrounding veins take over for the ones that have been sclerosed, and return the blood to the heart. There are some risks with this procedure, however, including pain, a burning sensation, muscle cramps, brownish discoloration, and recurrence of spider veins and small varicosities.

■ Lasers such as the tunable dye laser are particularly good for treating spider veins and varicose veins of the face and legs.

■ If you have severe varicose veins in your legs, your doctor may recommend surgery to remove all or part of the involved veins. A vascular surgeon may ligate, or tie off, a blood vessel. Or he or she may "strip" the vein by making two small incisions, in the upper thigh and the lower leg, and threading the cut vein out through the lower incision with the aid of a guide wire.

■ Cover-up cosmetics such as Covermark or Dermablend can be used to disguise noticeable spider veins on the face or legs.

■ Electrotherapy to spider veins of the face helps to minimize their prominence. In this procedure, a tiny needle is inserted in the capillary, an electric current is run through it, and the capillary is destroyed.

■ To prevent or avoid aggravating spider veins on the face, apply a sunscreen with a sun protection factor (SPF) of 15 or higher to your face thirty minutes before going outside. Do this on a daily basis.

■ Drink at least eight glasses of filtered water daily.

■ Eat a well-balanced high-fiber diet with lots of whole grains, fish, steamed vegetables, and fruits, especially citrus rinds, berries, and cherries.

■ Carrot, celery, parsley, cucumber, spinach, turnip, beet, and watercress juices are recommended.

■ Include in your diet foods that are high in rutin, a bioflavonoid that maintains the strength and integrity of capillary walls. Buckwheat pancakes and kasha, made from buckwheat, are tasty sources of rutin.

■ Lemon peel helps to relieve varicosities as well, as it contains flavonoids that reduce the leakiness of capillaries and veins. Try adding lemon peel to all your fruit juices.

■ Onion skin is one of the best sources of quercetin, another bioflavonoid that decreases capillary fragility. Cook with whole, unpeeled onions whenever possible, throwing away the skin before eating.

■ Spanish peanuts' reddish, papery skins contain compounds that decrease capillary fragility and leakiness. Have a few handfuls of Spanish peanuts a day if you enjoy them.

■ Avoid fried foods, fatty foods, sugar, salt, alcohol, processed foods, fatty meats, and whole milk cheeses and dairy products.

NUTRITIONAL SUPPLEMENTS

■ Vitamin C, bioflavonoids, and vitamin E help to improve circulation and reduce pain from varicosities. Bioflavonoids also strengthen venous walls and connective tissue that supports blood vessels, and vitamin E also acts as a blood thinner to improve circulation. Take 1,000 milligrams of vitamin C and 300 milligrams of a bioflavonoid complex three times daily, and 200 international units of vitamin E twice daily. Take an additional 1,000 milligrams of rutin daily.

■ Essential fatty acids also help to decrease pain from varicose veins. Take 500 to 1,000 milligrams of black currant seed, borage, or evening primrose oil a day to reduce pain.

■ Take 25,000 international units of beta-carotene daily.

■ Take a vitamin-B complex plus an additional 60 milligrams of vitamin B_6 daily for several months.

▓ Horse-chestnut seed offers perhaps the best herbal relief for the swelling, pain, itching, fatigue, and tenseness associated with varicose and spider veins. Clinical studies show that horse chestnut improves circulation in the legs, decreases inflammation, and strengthens the capillaries and veins. Combine ten parts distilled witch hazel with one part tincture of horse chestnut and apply this mixture externally to the affected areas as needed to help ease discomfort. Look for an extract of horse chestnut that provides a daily dosage of 50 milligrams of aescin, one of the key compounds that strengthens capillary cells and reduces fluid leakage. You can also take 500 milligrams of oral horse chestnut three times a day. It usually takes about 3 months to see benefits, so be patient.

Caution: Do not exceed the recommended oral dosage of horse chestnut extract, because larger doses can be toxic.

▓ Bilberry extract stimulates new capillary formation, strengthens capillary walls, and enhances the effect of vitamin C in reducing blood-vessel fragility. Take 20 to 40 milligrams three times a day.

▓ Butcher's broom extract improves varicosities by constricting and strengthening veins. Take 300 milligrams three times a day.

▓ Gingko biloba extract enhances tissue oxygenation and circulation. Take 40 milligrams three times a day.

▓ Grapeseed extract also improves circulation. Take 50 milligrams three times a day.

▓ Gotu kola extract is helpful for venous insufficiency, water retention in the ankles, foot swelling, and varicose veins. Take 200 milligrams three times a day.

▓ Hawthorn extract contains vitamin C, bioflavonoids, zinc, and sulfur, all of which are helpful for varicose veins. Take 200 milligrams three times a day.

▓ Distilled witch hazel is soothingly astringent when applied to areas with varicosities by means of a cotton ball dipped in the extract. Several studies in animals have shown that witch hazel helps to strengthen blood vessels as well.

AROMATHERAPY

■ Aromatherapy can lessen the pain and improve the appearance of varicose and spider veins. The essential oils of cypress, geranium, ginger, juniper, lavender, lemon, neroli, peppermint, and rosemary help to improve local circulation in the areas of varicosities. Use up to 10 drops of any of these oils, or a combination, in a quart of water to soak clean cloths to make compresses. Use warm compresses for fifteen minutes, then cool compresses for an equal amount of time. Repeat this for as long as you like to "exercise" the veins (the cold makes the blood vessels smaller, while the heat makes the veins bigger). After using the compresses, massage your legs with a massage oil to which a few drops of essential oil have been added, always stroking upward toward your heart. Regular leg massage is very helpful for varicosities of all sizes. You can also use the essential oils listed above to make a soothing warm bath.

HOMEOPATHY

■ *Carbo vegetabilis* 30x or 15c is best if your skin looks mottled, with white-colored legs and blue, distended veins. Take one dose three times a day.
■ *Ferrum metallicum* is best for visibly swollen veins. Take it as directed by the manufacturer.
■ *Hamamelis virginiana* 12x or 6c is best for swollen leg veins that are painful to the touch and feel bruised. Take one dose three times a day for up to five days. *Hamamelis,* or homeopathic witch hazel, can also be used topically. Apply the lotion to especially painful varicose veins and wrap the legs in lotion-soaked bandages. Leave the bandages in place for as long as possible, then use again only as needed for pain relief.
■ *Pulsatilla* 6c is best if there is stinging pain accompanying spider or varicose veins. Take a dose every three to four hours.

ACUPUNCTURE

■ Hong Jin, a licensed acupuncturist practing in Hacienda Heights, California, reports having good results with acupuncture treatments for varicose and spider veins. She places needles along the meridians and the coordinating internal organs of the affected blood vessels. With regular treatments, she says, patients experience a gradual improvement in their varicosities and related symptoms. Consult a qualified acupuncturist if you are interested in trying this type of treatment.

ACUPRESSURE

See Acupressure Points in Part Three for the locations of these points on the body.

■ Pressure to the Spleen 9 points for three minutes three times a day helps to relieve water retention and varicose veins. The Spleen 9 points are located on the insides of the legs, below the knees and under the large bulge of the bone.

■ Other acupoints that help to relieve water retention include Conception Vessel 6, Spleen 6, Kidney 2, and Kidney 6. Again, pressure should be applied to all points bilaterally for three minutes three times a day for maximum results. Conception Vessel 6 is located two finger-widths directly below the belly button. The Spleen 6 points are found four finger-widths above the inner ankle bone on the inner calf. The Kidney 6 points are one thumb-width below the insides of the ankle bones. The Kidney 2 points are located in the middle of the inside arches of the feet.

■ Points that improve circulation include Bladder 23, 25, and 27; Gallbladder 30 and 34; and Liver 3.

OTHER THERAPIES

■ Reflexology to the areas of the feet corresponding to the colon, liver, and adrenal glands has been found to be helpful for varicose veins.

GENERAL RECOMMENDATIONS

■ If you are pregnant or otherwise predisposed to varicose veins, wear support hose from morning until bedtime. Support stockings help the veins to push the blood upward from the legs to the heart.

■ Rest and elevate your legs and feet often, preferably above the level of your heart. Avoid standing or sitting in one position for a long time. If you have to stand a lot, try to contract and relax your calf muscles to promote good circulation. Do not sit on your legs or with your knees crossed.

■ Walking is one of the best preventive and therapeutic measures for varicose veins. It tones and enlarges muscles, which in turn press on the veins to push the blood back toward the heart. Leg exercises also help lymphatic drainage in the legs, lessening fluid retention and varicosities.

■ Avoid tight, constricting clothing such as girdles, tight knee socks, and hose with elastic leg bands. Wear comfortable, loose-fitting clothes. Wear flat or low-heeled shoes.

■ Maintain a normal weight. Excessive weight puts a lot of pressure on the fragile capillaries and veins in your legs.

■ Avoid becoming constipated, as straining with bowel movements puts added pressure on the veins.

Vitiligo

Vitiligo appears as sharply defined chalk-white spots, streaks, and patches of skin and hair where normal pigmentation has been lost due to destruction of the melanocytes, or pigment cells. Once the melanocytes are destroyed, no more melanin, or pigment, is made in these sites. The white patches usually appear symmetrically on both sides of the body. Vitiligo affects approximately 1 percent of the population. The condition is more common in dark-skinned people and, while noticeable in people with light-colored skin, it can be extremely distressing to people with darker complexions. It most often develops between the ages of ten and thirty. Common sites of pigment loss include exposed areas of the skin, such as the central face, fingers, hands, wrists, body folds, sites of injury, and the hair. The mucous membranes and areas around moles are other commonly affected sites.

Vitiligo is thought to be an autoimmune problem in which the body attacks its own pigment cells and kills them. There is often a precipitating factor such as stress or illness in a predisposed person. Thirty percent of people with this disorder have a family history of vitiligo, so there is obviously a genetic component. In addition, there is often a family or personal history of other connective-tissue or endocrine disease also related to an immune problem. These include alopecia areata, thyroid disease, diabetes, Addison's disease (a disorder of the adrenal glands), and pernicious anemia.

Vitiligo is a chronic disease, and its course is variable. Most commonly, it comes on rapidly, followed by a period of stability or slow progression of the problem. In about 30 percent of cases, the affected skin may begin to repigment naturally in sun-exposed areas as melanocytes migrate in from surrounding normal skin or from deep in the hair follicles. Skin that recovers in this way or with treatment usually shows small dots of repigmentation around involved hair follicles.

CONVENTIONAL TREATMENT

■ Smaller depigmented areas can be stained with a product such as Vitadye or Dy-O-Derm, which dyes the skin and makes the vitiligo less noticeable. Self-tanning agents can also be used.

■ Psoralens plus ultraviolet light (PUVA) therapy, a combination of concentrated UVA light therapy and an oral medication, psoralen, that intensifies the effects of the light, is the mainstay of conventional treatment for vitiligo. The oral medication is taken several hours before the light therapy, which is administered in a special light box at the dermatologist's office and takes several minutes. Or, a topical psoralen solution, 8-methoxypsoralen, may be painted on the depigmented spots thirty minutes before UVA-light therapy, and washed off afterward. Care must be taken for the next three days to protect areas of skin that have been painted or, if an oral psoralen drug is used, the entire body and the eyes. An eye exam must be done before starting therapy and routinely thereafter. It generally takes at least six months, with treatments three times a week, to see good results from PUVA treatment. However, PUVA is up to 85 percent effective in over 70 percent of patients, as long as the hands and feet are not affected (the skin of the hands and feet does not usually respond to this therapy). Possible risks of PUVA therapy include nausea, sunburn, and severe dryness of the skin in the short term, and an increased risk of photoaging, skin cancers, and cataracts over the long term.

■ A trial of a strong corticosteroid cream or oral prednisone for one or two weeks is often useful. Topical steroids are frequently effective for vitiligo in children. If there is no repigmentation after a month, the topical or oral steroids should be stopped.

■ Minigrafting is a procedure that involves removing vitiliginous skin and transplanting small sections of normally pigmented skin into the areas of depigmentation. The melanocytes from the transplanted skin slowly spread out to repigment the entire involved area. However, one big risk with this treatment is that vitiligo will develop at the donor sites of normal skin as well.

■ There is the hope that in the future, new sheets of the individual's own normal skin can be grown and transplanted to areas of pigment loss after removal of the vitiliginous skin. A small number of the person's normally pigmented skin cells can be removed and grown in a culture medium until new sheets of normal skin are formed. This procedure can now be used for burn patients, and the hope is that this technology can soon be used for people with vitiligo as well.

■ If the vitiligo is very extensive, permanent depigmentation of the remaining pigmented area with 20 percent monobenzylether of hydroquinone cream is an option. The cream is applied twice a day, and treatment may take up to a year to complete. Skin irritation is a common side effect. However, the success rate is over 90 percent, and most people are happy with the permanent results.

NUTRITIONAL SUPPLEMENTS

■ A small study at the Department of Dermatology of the University of Alabama Birmingham Medical Center found that supplementation with folic acid, vitamin B_{12}, and vitamin C resulted in noticeable repigmentation of the subjects' skin. I therefore suggest taking a vitamin-B complex containing 100 milligrams of each of the major B vitamins and at least 400 micrograms of folic acid daily; 1,000 micrograms of vitamin B_{12} daily, and 2,000 milligrams of vitamin C twice daily.

HOMEOPATHY

■ Homeopathic remedies that may be recommended for vitiligo include *Alum, Natrum carbonicum, Phosphorus, Sepia, Silica*, and *Sulfur*. The exact remedy is best chosen by a qualified homeopath.

GENERAL RECOMMENDATIONS

■ Opaque cosmetic cover-ups such as Dermablend and Covermark can be exactly matched to your normal skin tone. Such products are commonly used for small areas of pigment loss, especially on the face and hands. However, they do rub off and have to be reapplied during the day.
■ Apply a sunscreen with a sun protection factor (SPF) of 30 or higher on a daily basis to all depigmented spots to protect the affected skin from sunburn and photoaging. A sunblock containing zinc oxide and titanium dioxide is preferable. Do this even if you do not anticipate being outdoors, as your skin is exposed to sunlight through windows in your home and car. Areas of vitiligo no longer have any protective pigment, burn easily, and are more susceptible to developing skin cancer. A product called Total

Block combines an SPF of 60 with antioxidants and cover-up protective liquid makeup to cover and protect areas of vitiligo in a cosmetically pleasing way.

■ Avoid skin trauma as much as possible, as cuts and abrasions frequently are followed by vitiligo in the affected areas.

Warts

Warts are caused by a viral infection of the cells in the outermost layer of skin or mucous membranes. They are very common, and more than sixty types of human papillomaviruses, which cause different types of warts, are known. Warts occur most frequently in older children when the virus enters the skin through a cut. The wart then appears one to eight months later, and is easily spread by scratching or rubbing. Unfortunately, warts often spread from one location of the body to another and recur after treatment or with time. However, with the exception of genital warts, which are usually sexually transmitted, most warts do not spread from one person to another. Again except for genital warts, which have been linked with cervical cancer, most warts are harmless. They can be annoying and cosmetically displeasing, however. Untreated, most warts last between six months and two years, unless the person's immune system is severely compromised, in which case they last longer. People who are immunosuppressed also are much more susceptible to getting warts, and in much greater numbers.

Warts vary in size from about two to ten millimeters (approximately one-sixteenth to three-eighths inch), usually have clear borders, and are generally firm and flesh-colored. Contrary to popular belief, they do not have "roots" or "seeds." However, capillaries (tiny blood vessels) can appear as tiny black dots within the wart. Warts can be flat, cauliflower-like, or needle-shaped. They most frequently appear as hard, flesh-colored, round *common warts* on the fingers, hands, and knees. A variant that occurs on the soles of the feet are called *plantar warts.* These are usually painful. *Flat warts,* flesh-colored and flat-topped, most frequently appear on the face, wrists, and backs of the hands. *Filiform warts* are long and slender and develop on the eyelids, armpits, and necks of overweight, middle-aged people. *Digitate warts* have fingerlike projections and are dark-colored. *Genital warts* are pink and cauliflower-shaped.

There are almost as many traditional and alternative treatments for warts as there are types of viruses causing the warts. Alternative treatment methods are directed not only against the virus, but also toward strengthening the immune system through proper diet and supplements. Warts can be very resistant to treatment, however, and take one to two months of conscientious therapy to resolve. Genital warts require immediate treatment, as they can be a precursor to cervical cancer.

CONVENTIONAL TREATMENT

■ Topical solutions such as Duofilm or Occlusal, made from salicylic and/or lactic acids, can be applied to the wart one to three times a day. First soak the wart in water for ten minutes to soften it, and follow by paring the wart down so that the medicine will be better absorbed. Apply the acid with care, protecting the normal surrounding skin, which can easily become irritated. Acid-containing plasters such as TransPlantar or Trans-Ver-Sal may be easier to use, as you apply them nightly and leave them on for twenty-four hours.

■ Oral cimetidine (Tagamet), a drug originally used to treat stomach ulcers, has been found to fight viruses that cause warts and to boost the immune system. Oral cimetidine has been helpful in over two-thirds of cases, eliminating warts within three months. It is usually most helpful in children. The cost can be prohibitively high, though.

■ Liquid nitrogen, applied to the wart for three to ten seconds in the dermatologist's office, is often curative, as it destroys the cells of the wart. However, the treated area burns and throbs for a few minutes while and after the liquid nitrogen is sprayed on. As with most other wart treatments, more than one application may be necessary to completely get rid of warts.

■ Curettage, or cutting off, of the wart is another option. It can be done alone or combined with other therapies.

■ Carbon dioxide laser treatments to remove warts are one of the newer therapies.

■ Dinitrochlorobenzene (DNCB) is a chemical that can be painted on warts. It works by causing a local autoimmune reaction.

■ Large, resistant warts can be injected with the anticancer drug bleomycin (Blenoxane). This can be painful, but is also usually very effective.

■ The power of suggestion has been used by dermatologists for many years to treat warts, especially in children. The warts are usually painted with a colored solution or one that glows in the dark. Then the child is told that over the next several days the warts will magically disappear. It is thought that the power of suggestion boosts the child's immune system to get rid of the warts.

■ Tretinoin (Retin-A) gel, applied topically, is often used for flat warts of the face. Another topical medication, fluorouracil (Efudex, Fluoroplex) cream, may also be used for flat facial warts.

■ Imiquimod (Aldara) cream is an immune-response modifier that is very helpful for external genital warts. It is put on the warts at bedtime three times a week, and washed off six to ten hours later, on arising. It can be used for up to sixteen weeks, with results seen as early as four weeks. As with topical antiviral therapies, possible side effects include local redness, flaking, swelling, itching, and burning.

■ A podophyllum solution (Podocon-25, Podofin) may be applied to genital warts by a dermatologist. It is then washed off at home by the patient six to twelve hours later. It is a powerful irritant, however, and it must be washed off immediately if the area treated becomes painful, inflamed, or very itchy.

■ Podofilox (Condylox) is a newer drug, similar to but not as strong as podophyllum. It can be applied at home for genital warts. Caution still has to be used not to apply the medication to normal skin or to leave on for too long. Skin erosion, pain, and inflammation are unwanted possibilities if instructions for the use of this drug are not strictly followed.

■ Trichloroacetic acid (TCA) is often used in the treatment of genital warts.

DIETARY MEASURES

■ A diet rich in whole grains, fresh vegetables, garlic, and alfalfa sprouts is suggested.

■ Foods high in vitamin A, such as dark-green and yellow vegetables, eggs, and cold-water fish, should be emphasized.

■ Avoid refined grains, sugar, caffeine, excess fat, and processed foods.

NUTRITIONAL SUPPLEMENTS

■ The following supplements should be taken for one month for first-time episodes of warts, and for up to four months if the warts tend to recur. These nutrients increase immunity and speed healing:

• Vitamin A. Take 25,000 international units a day.

• Beta-carotene. Take 50,000 international units a day.

- Vitamin B$_1$ (thiamine). Take 1.5 milligrams a day.
- Vitamin B$_6$ (pyridoxine). Take 10 milligrams a day.
- Vitamin C with bioflavonoids. Take 500 milligrams a day.
- Vitamin E. Take 400 international units a day.
- Shiitake mushroom extract. Take 300 to 500 milligrams twice a day.
- Zinc. Take 50 milligrams a day.

■ The following topical regimen using vitamin A can be used until the wart dissolves: In the morning, crush a vitamin-A capsule in enough water to make a paste and apply the paste to each wart. Cover with a bandage. In the afternoon, put a drop of castor oil on each wart, and in the evening apply a drop of lemon juice to each wart. Repeat this daily. This is especially helpful for plantar warts.

■ Vitamin E, used topically, is a slower treatment, often taking several months. You can apply the oil from a 400-international-unit capsule to the warts three times a day and cover with an adhesive bandage. Better yet, combine the vitamin-E oil with the vitamin-A paste described above.

HERBAL TREATMENT

■ Alfalfa tea can be helpful. Steep 1 tablespoon of the seed or 2 ounces of the dried leaf in 1 quart of boiling water. Drink a cup three times a day.

■ Thuja, also known as arbor vitae, can be made into a lotion or ointment and applied directly to the wart on a daily basis.

■ The inner side of a fresh banana skin can be placed against the wart and held in place with a tight dressing. Replace with a new piece of banana skin every day until the wart dissolves.

■ Basil contains many antiviral compounds. Apply some fresh crushed basil leaves to the wart, and cover with a bandage. Repeat this daily for one week.

■ Bloodroot ointment, which contains skin-irritating compounds and protein-dissolving enzymes, may be applied to the wart several times a day.

■ The juice of buttercup flowers and leaves can be applied directly to the warts several times a day.

■ Celandine is thought to contain a chemical that inhibits the replication of the wart virus, as well as skin irritants and enzymes that destroy the wart proteins. Squeeze the latex from the fresh stems of celandine plants and apply the gel directly to the wart once or twice a day until the wart has resolved. Or, if the fresh plant is not available, you can apply a strong tea made from the herb to the wart twice a day.

■ The sap from the stem or root of the dandelion is corrosive, and can be used to destroy the wart if it is applied locally every day.

■ Garlic oil, fresh grated garlic, and crushed garlic are very toxic to warts. Apply any of these forms of garlic directly to the warts and cover with a tight dressing, taking care not to get any of the garlic on the surrounding normal skin. Do this twice a day until the warts have disappeared.

■ Pineapple is rich in proteolytic enzymes that can destroy warts. Cut a square of pineapple peel and tape the inner side to plantar warts overnight. Remove the peel and soak your foot in hot water in the morning. File down any peeling skin. Repeat this treatment nightly as necessary.

■ If you live near a willow tree, tape a piece of the moistened inner bark from the willow tree to the wart. Change it daily. Willow contains a large amount of salicylic acid, a chemical traditionally used to treat warts.

HOMEOPATHY

■ *Antimonium crudum* 12x or 6c is recommended for dry, itchy warts. Take a dose three times a day for up to three days.

■ *Causticum* 12x or 6c is best for warts near the fingernails that are flat, painful, and bleed easily. Take a dose three times a day for up to three days.

■ *Dulcamara* 6c is good for hard, flat, transparent warts of the hands. Take a dose three times a day for up to three days.

■ *Mercurius cyanatus* 12x or 5c is best for plantar warts. Take a dose twice a day for up to five days.

■ *Nitricum acidum* 6c is best for large, painful, jagged warts. Take a dose three times a day for up to three days.

■ *Thuja occidentalis* 6c is recommended for fleshy, cauliflower-shaped warts and for warts that are bleeding or stinging. Take a dose three times a day for up to ten days. *Thuja* tincture can also be applied directly to the wart twice a day. Discontinue early if there is no effect, however, as internal remedies will be necessary.

ACUPUNCTURE

■ A study by Dr. Xu Yihou of Wuhan Municipal Hospital of Traditional Chinese Medicine in Wuhan, China, found that of twenty-eight people treated with acupuncture for flat facial warts, two-thirds were clinically cured. All of those cured had had their warts for less than a year. In cases that had been present for more than two years, the effect of acupuncture was minimal. Consult a qualified acupuncturist if you are interested in trying this type of treatment.

OTHER THERAPIES

■ Warts can be treated very successfully with hypnotherapy. An article published in 1959 in the British medical journal *The Lancet* showed that when a suggestion was made that the warts on only one side of the patient's body would disappear, this was followed by one-sided cure in nine out of ten patients!

■ The use of guided imagery in the treatment of warts serves as a great example of belief activating our own ability to heal via our central nervous, circulatory, and immune systems. To treat warts, spend three minutes a day imagining them dissolving away. Do this every day for a period of at least three weeks.

GENERAL RECOMMENDATIONS

■ Do not pick or scratch at a wart. This will not get rid of it, but may cause it to spread or become infected.

Wrinkles

As most people know only too well, wrinkles on the face are lines that develop as one ages. They are usually due a combination of many factors, which can include common facial movements that are repeated for years, dryness, smoking, overuse of astringents, overzealous scrubbing of the face, and, most importantly, unprotected overexposure to the sun. These are the *extrinsic aging factors*—changes we bring on ourselves due to our lifestyle choices. Deep wrinkles are most often caused by excessive chronic sun exposure. Deep wrinkles around the lips also develop with long-term smoking.

Intrinsic aging is a function of genetic inheritance and advancing age. As we get older, our skin loses its small blood vessels, reducing the blood supply that nourishes it. Meanwhile, oil and sweat glands produce less sebum and perspiration. Some hair follicles shrink, leaving us with less hair. With time, skin gets thinner and loses some of the supporting collagen that had made it firm, plump, and able to hold moisture. Oxidative (free radical) damage causes the formation of insoluble collagen, which is inelastic and unable to absorb water well, and does not plump up. With the loss of moisture, lines and wrinkles form. We do not usually find these changes cosmetically pleasing.

Fortunately, there are many conventional and alternative ways to prevent and treat wrinkling of the skin.

CONVENTIONAL TREATMENT

■ Alpha-hydroxy and beta-hydroxy acids encourage old skin layers to peel off and regenerate younger-looking skin after several weeks and months of their use. These compounds are found in many cosmetic and skin-care products. Gluconolactone, a polyhydroxy-acid derivative of a naturally occurring sugar acid found in the skin, has antioxidant functions, normalizes cell renewal and exfoliation, and strengthens skin barrier functions, all helping to reduce fine wrinkling. It is more hydrating and gentler than alpha-hydroxyacids, and therefore can be used on all skin types, including sensitive skin. Gluconolactone is the active ingredient in a line of products marketed under the brand name Exuviance.

■ Vitamin-A derivatives are very popular and helpful for the topical treatment of wrinkles. Tretinoin emollient cream (Renova) is the only prescription retinoid just for wrinkles. Retinol (RoC) cream, available over the counter, is another vitamin-A product. It is less potent than tretinoin.

■ Chemical peels performed every three months at a dermatologist's or plastic surgeon's office have become increasingly popular as a way to deal with wrinkles. There are now a great variety of superficial, medium, and deep peels that are available for treating wrinkles of different depths. Superficial "lunchtime peels," improve wrinkles, while the deeper peels actually remove them.

■ Wrinkles can be replaced with collagen or other materials injected directly into the wrinkles by a dermatologist or plastic surgeon. This procedure needs to be repeated approximately every six months to maintain the effect.

■ Local injections of diluted botulinum toxin (Botox) have become very popular. The toxin is injected into the muscle between the eyebrows, where it paralyzes the muscle, eliminating wrinkles for about three to six months.

■ Laser resurfacing, with the advent of less painful lasers and techniques, has become an increasingly popular way to treat wrinkles. The erbium:YAG laser gives a more superficial laser dermabrasion, but has a shorter recuperative period than the superpulsed carbon dioxide laser, which is used to remove deep wrinkles.

■ Microdermabrasion, also known as the "power peel," has gained in popularity in recent years. In this technique, four to six half-hour superficial dermabrasions are done at one- to two-week intervals to reduce the signs of aging. Deeper dermabrasions have been used for years for deep wrinkling and scarring.

■ A face lift can be done to tighten the skin and remove the appearance of unwanted wrinkles. Increasingly, people are resorting to this procedure when they are in their forties, instead of waiting until later.

DIETARY MEASURES

■ Good nutrition benefits your skin, as the skin offers a visible reflection of what is going on inside you. Eat a healthy, well-balanced, nutritious diet high in vegetables, complex carbohydrates, and lean protein foods.

■ Drink plenty of pure water to keep your skin well hydrated.

■ Avoid alcohol, which contributes to premature aging of the skin.

NUTRITIONAL SUPPLEMENTS

■ The following oral supplements are recommended to protect against harmful oxidation and to slow the wrinkling process:
  - A high-potency multivitamin and mineral complex. Take this daily.
  - Beta-carotene complex. Take 50,000 international units a day.
  - Vitamin C with bioflavonoids. Take 500 to 1,000 milligrams three times a day.
  - Vitamin E. Take 400 to 800 international units a day.
  - Selenium. Take 100 to 200 micrograms a day.

■ Consuming foods and supplements rich in vitamins A, C, and E is important, but topical application of creams containing forms of these vitamins, plus the natural hormone dehydroepiandrosterone (DHEA) can be much more effective. For example, using a 10-percent topical vitamin-C product allows you to get approximately thirty times the level of vitamin C to the top layer of wrinkled skin as compared with ingesting megadoses of vitamin C. The following topical antioxidant vitamin and supplement creams are excellent for the treatment and prevention of wrinkles:
  - Ten-percent vitamin-C lotion. Apply this daily. Be careful, as not all preparations of topical vitamin C are effective; the vitamin C must be converted to the L-ascorbic acid form of the vitamin. Cellex-C and C Scape Serum are two products that have been shown to produce a marked decrease in the appearance of wrinkles with regular use.
  - Five-percent vitamin-E cream. Apply this daily.
  - Coenzyme Q_{10} (ubiquinone) cream. Apply this daily. Studies have shown that this antioxidant can decrease the depth of facial wrinkles noticeably after just one month of daily use.

■ DHEA cream. Apply this daily.

HERBAL TREATMENT

Most natural antiwrinkle creams work either as antioxidants that mop up damaging free radicals or as emollients that moisturize and soften the skin and reduce the appearance of fine wrinkles.

■ Topical preparations made from fruit acids, or alpha-hydroxy acids, have been successfully used to fight fine wrinkling. Glycolic acid is one commonly used fruit acid. You can also go directly to the source, using the inside of a lemon, lime, papaya peel, or pineapple peel to gently smooth over your skin in the evening before going to bed. These fruits naturally contain alpha-hydroxy acids that slough off dead skin cells, revealing fresh new skin cells underneath.

■ Herbs such as calendula, fennel, horsetail, and licorice are added to skin-care preparations, as they stimulate the skin cells and make the skin appear younger.

■ Carrot, horse chestnut, and rosemary are antioxidants that can be added to topical preparations to help reverse fine wrinkling.

■ Cocoa butter is a major emollient used in antiwrinkle skin lotions and cosmetics, especially for dry, wrinkled skin around the eyes, the corners of the mouth, and the neck.

■ Coconut, almond, avocado, and olive oil are other emollients that can help reduce the appearance of fine wrinkles.

■ Many cosmetics contain combinations of vitamins and herbal products. Provitamin B_5, vitamin C, vitamin E, vitamin A, glycolic acid, alpha-hydroxy acid, beta-hydroxy acid, and papaya are now being included in all kinds of cleansers, toners, moisturizers, sunscreens, and cosmetics produced by many different manufacturers.

AROMATHERAPY

■ Combine 1 drop of rose oil and 2 drops of everlasting oil with 1 ounce of rose hip seed oil. Apply the mixture each morning to wrinkled areas after cleansing. Store it in a dark glass bottle.

ACUPUNCTURE

■ Acupuncture has been used for centuries in traditional Chinese medicine as a beauty treatment. It activates local blood circulation, reduces wrinkling, and diminishes pigmentation of the facial skin. In 1991, Drs. L. Schnitzler and A. Adrien reviewed a large number of cases over several years in France. Electroacupuncture was used to treat slack skin and wrinkles of the face and neck, and significant improvements were noted in 70 percent of the patients after ten to fifteen sessions. Periodic maintenance treatments were needed to preserve the results. No harmful side effects were noted. Consult a qualified acupuncturist if you are interested in trying this type of treatment.

ACUPRESSURE

See Acupressure Points in Part Three for the locations of these points on the body.

■ Press the bottom of each cheekbone below each pupil for three minutes three times a day to help tone facial muscles and reduce wrinkling.

■ A commercial electroacupressure device was recently developed by a chiropractor for facial toning and to preserve a youthful appearance. It is marketed under the brand name Rejuvenique. You wear a contoured mask for fifteen to thirty minutes four times a week for sixty to ninety days. You may then go to a maintenance schedule of once a week if you desire, or continue the four-times-a-week regimen if you find the electrical micropulsations relaxing yet invigorating. The inner lining of the mask has contacts at key acupressure points. A module containing a 9-volt battery connects to the mask and delivers microimpulses to the facial contact cushions. This device is said to tighten and tone the muscles of the face, which in turn tightens and tones the overlying skin, reducing the appearance of lines and wrinkles. It is also said to increase the skin's microcirculation, increasing the delivery of nutrients to the skin cells and the removal of excess wastes and toxins, as well as stimulating local lymphatic drainage, decreasing facial puffiness, and allowing the pores to close naturally.

OTHER THERAPIES

■ Massage relaxes and nourishes facial tissues, minimizing wrinkling. Pat your cheeks and the sides of your face for twenty seconds each morning. Also, massage each side of your face with your fingertips from top to bottom for sixty seconds each evening.

GENERAL RECOMMENDATIONS

■ Every morning, apply a sunscreen with a sun protection factor (SPF) of 15 or higher to all sun-exposed areas. Reapply the sunscreen every few hours if you are outdoors.

■ Wear a hat and UV-filtering sunglasses outside.

■ Do not use tanning beds. If you do use an artificial tanning product, remember to use sunscreen as well—the tan does not protect you against sun damage.

■ Use a moisturizing cleanser or soap to wash your skin.

■ After cleansing your face, apply a moisturizer. Reapply it several times during the day in dry weather or when spending time in a dry environment, such as an airplane cabin or a centrally heated building in winter.

■ Limit your use of astringents, which are drying.

■ If you smoke, quit. In addition to causing heart and lung problems, smoking turns your skin yellow, leathery, and wrinkled. This is a result of both nicotine, which reduces microcirculation in the skin, and the repeated facial posture associated with smoking.

■ Avoid cycles of gaining and losing weight. This leaves the skin sagging and wrinkled.

PART THREE

Skin-Care Treatments and Techniques

Introduction

In Part One, we looked at conventional dermatology and a variety of alternative approaches to skin problems, including nutritional therapies, herbal remedies, aromatherapy, homeopathy, acupuncture, stress reduction techniques, electrotherapy, light therapy, and mind-body medicine. Part Two offered an integrative medical approach to dealing with some thirty common and/or challenging skin conditions to enable you to combine conventional medical treatments with alternative therapies to come up with an approach that is right for you and your skin problem.

In Part Three, you will find detailed instructions that will help you to care for your skin, hair and nails all the time, regardless of their state of health. Various diagnostic procedures and treatments are also described. This section will show you how to perform a skin self-exam, which is something everyone should do at least once a month. The preparation of herbal poultices, tinctures, oils, teas, and baths will be simply explained. Various stress-reduction techniques will also be described in easy-to-follow terms.

Being comfortable with the details of both basic skin care and natural treatment techniques will allow you to feel confident while choosing skin treatments that integrate the best of what both traditional dermatology and alternative dermatology have to offer.

Acupressure Points

According to traditional Chinese medicine, the body is criss-crossed by twelve meridians, or channels through which the body's vital energy flows. An acupressure point (or acupoint) is a point located along one of the twelve meridians that has increased sensitivity and that can exert a powerful effect on specific organs or body systems when pressed repeatedly. The figures that follow will help you to find the exact locations of many acupoints commonly used to help restore balance and health to the skin.

Most acupoints are found in small hollows between bones, muscles, and tendons. Use your most sensitive index finger, middle finger, or thumb to find the site and apply pressure. There is usually a slight sensitivity or tenderness at the point itself. Pressure should be applied gently at first and then increased slightly until a mild sensation is felt.

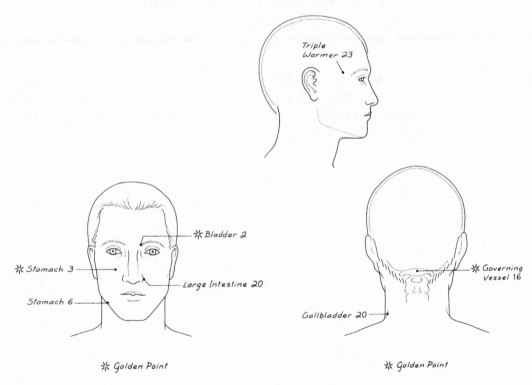

Triple Warmer 23

✳ Bladder 2

✳ Stomach 3

Large Intestine 20

Stomach 6

✳ Governing Vessel 16

Gallbladder 20

✳ Golden Point

✳ Golden Point

Acupressure Points

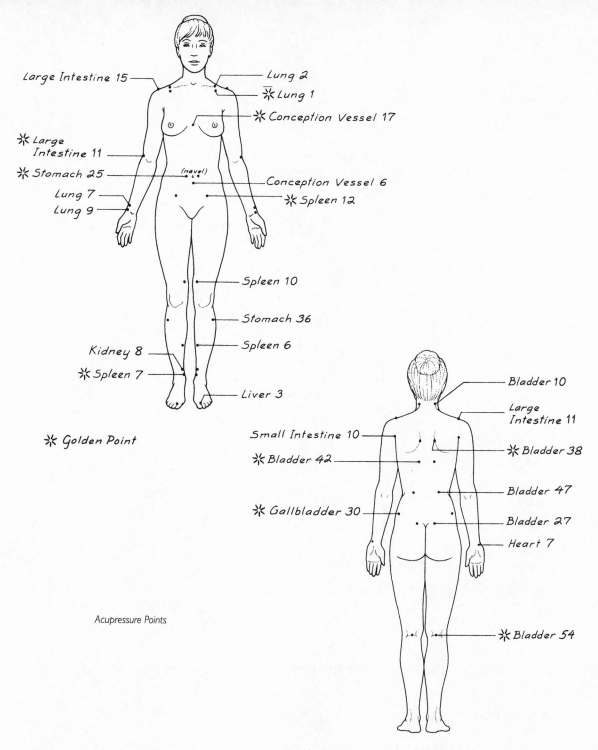

Large Intestine 15

Lung 2
Lung 1
Conception Vessel 17

Large
Intestine 11

Stomach 25

(navel)

Conception Vessel 6
Spleen 12

Lung 7
Lung 9

Spleen 10

Stomach 36

Kidney 8
Spleen 6

Spleen 7

Liver 3

✳ Golden Point

Acupressure Points

Bladder 10

Large
Intestine 11

Small Intestine 10

Bladder 38

Bladder 42

Bladder 47

Gallbladder 30

Bladder 27

Heart 7

Bladder 54

✳ Golden Point

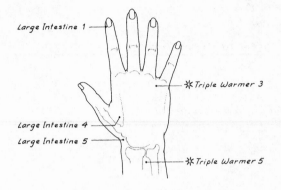

Large Intestine 1

※ Triple Warmer 3

Large Intestine 4

Large Intestine 5

※ Triple Warmer 5

※ Golden Point

Acupressure Points

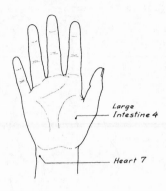

Large Intestine 4

Heart 7

Acupressure Points

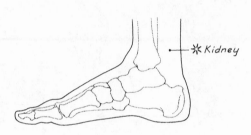

※ Kidney

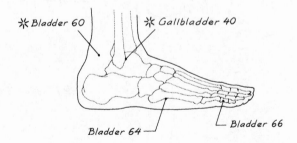

※ Bladder 60

※ Gallbladder 40

Bladder 64

Bladder 66

※ Golden Point

Acupressure Points

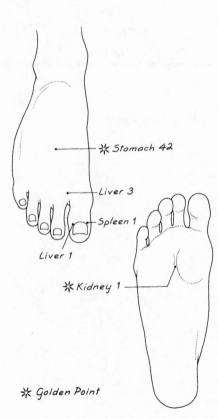

※ Stomach 42

Liver 3

Spleen 1

Liver 1

※ Kidney 1

※ Golden Point

Acupressure Points

Bodywork

Bodywork is the term used to refer to massage and more than eighty other therapies involving touching or moving the body. The most widely used types of bodywork in the United States are massage, deep tissue techniques, pressure-point techniques, and movement integration. Bodywork methods have gained general acceptance as complementary medical therapies that reduce stress and improve a person's general physical and mental well-being. They are also very useful for the treatment of specific medical problems including those of the skin.

MASSAGE

Everyone needs the human touch to thrive, and it can greatly aid in the healing process. Massage helps psychologically to reduce anxiety and pain through its calming effect on the nervous system and its relaxation of the voluntary muscles. Massage also speeds healing by increasing the local blood flow. This brings an increased blood supply, with oxygen, nutrients, and disease-fighting components, to the affected area. In a small study of healthy women at the Center for Research in Complementary and Alternative Medicine in West Orange, New Jersey, researchers found that more than half of the subjects had substantially more and better functioning immune-system cells after just one hour of full-body massage. Massage also helps in the elimination of toxins from the body by increasing the working of the intestines.

Swedish, or European, massage is the best known type of massage. This technique uses long gliding strokes, kneading, and friction. Another type of massage is lymphatic massage, which is directed at encouraging the movement of lymph through the lymphatic vessels. Lymphatic massage can promote quick recovery from an illness or disease by opening up blocked lymphatic vessels and moving metabolic waste products rapidly through the body so they can be eliminated. Also, lymphatic massage changes the levels of neurohormones excreted in the urine, and this affects the levels of neurohormones acting on the brain and nervous system. Thus, by removing neurotoxins and changing the levels of neurohormones, lymphatic massage directly affects and improves a person's emotional and nervous state.

There are professional massage therapists practicing all over the country. To locate one in your area, you can contact the American Massage Therapy Association or the American Physical Therapy Association (see Resource Organizations in the Appendix).

DEEP TISSUE TECHNIQUES/ROLFING

Rolfing is the most famous of the deep tissue techniques. In a series of ten hour-long, deep, often painful treatments, the fascia surrounding the muscles are physically separated from one another. These fascia fibers, which form tough sheaths that cover all the muscles in the body, are thought to get stuck together and hold the body out of alignment. Rolfing is done to bring the body into better alignment, and has been shown to reduce anxiety and the tension held in the body. The Rolf Institute of Structural Integration can assist you in finding a trained practitioner in your area (see Resource Organizations in the Appendix).

PRESSURE-POINT TECHNIQUES

Pressure-point techniques are aimed at effecting change throughout the body by means of manipulating or applying pressure to certain key points. These therapies include reflexology, color zone therapy, and reiki. Acupressure also is a pressure-point technique.

Reflexology

Reflexology is performed by about 25,000 practitioners worldwide. It is helpful in relieving stress, improving the blood supply, and speeding nerve impulses. Specific parts of the hands and feet are thought to correspond to and affect every organ and gland in the body through the medium of the spinal cord and brain. In reflexology, precise pressure is applied to reflex areas of nerve endings in the hands and feet. The local pressure produced by reflexology is thought to release blockages of energy flow that have caused pain and disease throughout the body.

In her book *Feet First* (Fireside Books, 1988), Laura Norman notes that after reflexology treatments, her clients' skin seems to glow. Reflexology treatments reduced the puffiness and dark circles under their eyes and diminished their skin-tension lines and skin tightness. This is because the treatments increased circulation and elimination of toxins, and also relaxed the muscles and thought processes. For skin problems in general, she recommends massaging the reflex areas of the feet corresponding to the thyroid, lymphatics, pituitary, liver, kidneys, adrenal gland, and solar plexus. In cases of eczema and psoriasis, Ms. Norman advises also massaging the spleen, pancreas, intestines, and spine reflex areas of the feet.

Color Zone Therapy

A new technique, color zone therapy, combines color therapy and zone therapy with the addition of positive meditations. Zone therapy is similar to reflexology, but key points on the hands and face, in addition to the feet, are stimulated to treat the whole body via the glands and internal organs. Color and verbal meditations are used to assess and treat health problems, eliminating contributing negative attitudes and replacing them with positive beliefs, thoughts, and images. For example, in the case of hair loss, it is recommended that one visualize the color yellow along with zone therapy of the areas of the hands, feet, and face associated with the pituitary, thyroid, nervous system, thymus, adrenal glands, liver, and kidneys. For the treatment of genital herpes, massage of these same areas of the feet is recommended, in addition to massage of areas corresponding to the ovaries or prostate and the spleen. The color indigo is to be visualized. In the treatment of shingles, the color green is imagined, and reflex areas of the nervous system in addition to the glands, liver, and spleen are stimulated. For types of skin cancer, green or indigo are suggested visualization colors. For most other skin problems, the color yellow is visualized. Improvements in skin conditions are thought to be mediated through increased blood flow, relaxation of the muscles and mind, and positive mind-body interactions.

Reiki

Reiki is similar to acupressure. It is specifically concerned with moving energy through the body in order to balance it. Reiki is thought to affect the energy field and the endocrine system. Thus, healing occurs in the body as a whole, and is not specific to a particular disease. Followers of reiki believe that because our skin comes into direct contact with the world, it is a symbol for making contact with others, as well as drawing boundaries between ourselves and others. Reiki therapy is aimed at helping those with skin problems to break through the boundaries they have made between themselves and the world, as symbolized by rashes from within or injuries from outside the boundaries of their skin. This is done in part through the medium of touch, which crosses our boundaries both literally and figuratively, by reaching into our feelings.

I have heard anecdotal reports from a dermatologist who uses reiki on many of her patients, along with conventional medical therapies. Patients previously resistant to treatment have responded, often much faster and with fewer side effects than normally encountered. She claims to have had success using reiki on patients with atopic dermatitis, severe eczema, psoriasis, vitiligo, severe acne, lupus, lichen planus, pemphigus, Hansen's disease (leprosy), exfoliative dermatitis, and postherpetic neuralgia. She recommends the treatment mostly to patients who are open to alternative forms of therapy so that they can learn to use the technique on themselves. In this way they become responsible in part for their own healing. It is a simple technique to learn, but you need a strong commitment to practice it regularly.

MOVEMENT INTEGRATION

Movement-integration techniques teach better ways to move one's body so as to improve health. These therapies are helpful for decreasing stress and improving overall well-being. Two of the most popular movement-integration techniques are the Alexander and Feldenkrais techniques.

Alexander Technique

The Alexander Technique focuses on teaching you to change unhealthy habits of posture and movement with the goal of increasing total coordination. The teacher guides you through a series of simple movements that help you to achieve greater control in your activities and to develop better, less stressful responses to any stimuli. The American Society for the Alexander Technique can help you to locate a teacher of the technique in your area (see Resource Organizations in the Appendix).

Feldenkrais Technique

The Feldenkrais technique consists of two components. The first, known as awareness through movement, involves directed exercise sessions with specific sequences of movement designed to address problems in the body and increase bodily awareness. The second component, functional integration, involves passive exercise, in which a practitioner manipulates and moves various parts of the body in specific ways. The Feldenkrais Guild of North America can assist you in finding a practitioner in your area (see Resource Organizations in the Appendix).

Therapeutic Touch

Therapeutic touch involves the transfer of energy from one person to another to enhance the healing process. It has been called "healing meditation." Developed in 1972 by a nurse, Delores Krieger, and Dora Kunz, a healer, this technique is rapidly gaining acceptance. It is currently practiced in over eighty hospitals in the United States.

In a meditative state, a therapeutic touch practitioner holds his or her hands a short distance away from the person being treated to sense and "smooth out" the person's aura, or energy field. The client, who begins the twenty- to thirty-minute session in a relaxed state, can experience different feelings, ranging from the release of previously suppressed emotions to a quiet, calm sense of well-being.

In clinical studies, therapeutic touch has been shown to relieve pain, decrease stress and anxiety, and improve autonomic nervous system functioning. It has also been seen to change the activity of enzymes in the body, raise hemoglobin levels, reduce inflammation, and speed wound healing. A 1981 study found that therapeutic touch was better at reducing anxiety in hospitalized patients than either casual touch or talking. This finding was confirmed in two independent studies in 1984 and 1990, respectfully.

Some practitioners believe in and teach slightly different forms of healing using the human energy field. One of the best known is Barbara Brennan, a former NASA research scientist who has researched the human energy field for over twenty years. She has written books and developed lectures and courses to teach her form of energy healing.

Relatively speaking, the usefulness of therapeutic touch and its variants has only just begun to be explored scientifically, but these techniques can certainly be applied to the treatment of skin problems.

Guided Imagery Techniques

Guided imagery uses the power of the imagination to create a positive physical response. It can reduce stress, slow the heart rate, stimulate the immune system, accelerate healing, and reduce pain. Guided imagery is a flow of thoughts in which specific images, sounds, smells, tastes, and tactile sensations are suggested or imagined. These images can be devised by a therapist as a way of suggesting healing, or you yourself can create healing images as a way of understanding the meaning of your symptoms and of accessing your inner healing resources. Imagery is a rich, symbolic, and highly personal language that represents internal reality, which may or may not correspond to external reality. If you are particularly good at worrying yourself sick, you will probably also be very good at learning how to improve your health with positive imagery, as the internal processes are very similar.

Imagery is the form in which the nervous system stores, accesses, and processes information. It is thus a key interface between the mind and the body. Guided imagery is thought to work by sending messages from the more highly evolved centers of the brain, in the cerebral cortex, to the lower centers of the brain, which regulate such basic functions as breathing, heart rate, blood flow, blood pressure, immunity, temperature, waking rhythms, hunger, thirst, and digestion. When people imagine hearing things, the auditory cortex is activated, creating imaginary realities and sending impulses to the lower centers of the nervous system to which they respond in the same ways they would to external realities. Likewise, the sensory cortex shows activity when you imagine feeling things, and the visual cortex is active when you imagine seeing things.

Imagery is very useful in medicine because it directly affects your physiology. It also helps you to develop insight and perspective on your illness. This in turn can help you to cope with your condition. Just as important, imagery is closely linked with your emotions. Emotions are often at the root of many common health conditions, but are locked within the unconscious. Imagery can help in clarifying attitudes, emotions, behaviors, and lifestyles that may be, at least in part, causing or worsening the illness. Imagery can help you to understand the needs an illness may represent and fulfill in your life. Then you can develop other healthier ways to better meet those needs.

Imagery is often used successfully in conjunction with hypnosis, neurolinguistic programming (NLP), relaxation, meditation, biofeedback, and counseling. After receiving proper instruction by a guided-imagery specialist, you can also find guided imagery to be a highly effective form of self-care done at home. Skin conditions that may respond particularly well to the use of guided imagery include psoriasis, acne, cancer, eczema, genital herpes, pain, and warts. It is a highly cost-effective complementary technique that can be used to increase your sense of empowerment and self-control, and thus help to improve your health and quality of life. It should certainly be tried in cases of intractable, chronic, or difficult skin problems. For a detailed explanation and instruction in guided imagery, including descriptions of specific visualizations for certain disorders, I recommend consulting Gerald Epstein's book *Healing Visualizations: Creating Health Through Imagery* (Bantam New Age Books, 1989).

Hair Care

When your hair looks its best, you feel more healthy and attractive. Conversely, if you are having a "bad hair day," it is harder to feel as good about your appearance. No matter what length, color, or type your hair is, you can develop healthy habits to keep it looking its best.

Always remember that, in general, "less is best" when it comes to the care of your hair. That means using fewer hair products, doing less blow-drying and brushing, minimizing the use of dyes, curling irons, and rollers, and, as much as possible, avoiding permanents, tight hairstyles, and sun exposure. The following are some tips for achieving and maintaining a healthy, attractive head of hair:

- Use shampoos, hair sprays, creams, gels, mousses, and conditioners specifically formulated for your type of hair, whether it is dry, oily, fine, coarse, and/or chemically treated. Shampoos can be cleansing, moisturizing, volumizing, or low in alkaline for chemically treated hair. Conditioners can be oil-free, protein-rich, and body-building, or they can be moisturizing for dry or chemically treated hair. Conditioners can also be for daily use or deep, leave-in conditioners for coarse, dry hair.
- Use warm but not hot water to wash your hair. Hot water will dry your scalp, making dandruff more likely.
- Do not overwash your hair. One soaping per shower or bath is all that is needed.
- As you get older, shampoos that add moisture, thickness, and volume to the hair are helpful. Weekly leave-in conditioners as well as natural conditioners become more important with age as well.
- Use a wide-toothed comb to get the tangles out of your hair after washing.
- If you use a blow-dryer, do not use the hottest setting. Using a diffuser on your blow-dryer is best for permed hair to better distribute the heat.
- Use the lower speeds of the blow-dryer to style your hair.
- Gently brush out your hair, and do not overbrush.
- Use your own brushes and combs. Keep them clean by removing hair and soaking them in warm water each week.
- Minimize your use of curling irons and rollers, which are hard on the hair.

■ Minimize your use of harsh chemical treatments, dyes, and perms, especially if you are pregnant or nursing. Shampoos and dyes made from natural products are less damaging to your hair.

■ Do not tightly braid your hair or pull it back in tight ponytails. This pulls on the roots of your hair and leads to hair loss.

■ Do not use plain rubber bands, which tear and pull at your hair.

■ Regular trims to cut off split and broken ends become more important as your hair becomes older.

■ Shield your hair and scalp from the damaging effects of sunlight with bathing caps and broad-brimmed hats.

Herbal Treatments

Herbs and herbal products come in many forms and can be used in an even greater number of ways to promote the health of your skin. You may choose to buy your herbs in the form of commercial teas, tinctures, oils, creams, powders, capsules, or tablets. Or you may want to make your own herbal preparations from the leaves, flowers, roots, or bark of various herbs.

In this section you will find easy-to-follow directions for how to make your own herbal treatments if you are interested in getting fresher, more potent herbal formulations, saving money, or just having some fun as you maintain and improve the health of your skin with herbs.

INFUSIONS (TEAS)

You make an herbal infusion just like you would any other tea—by steeping the parts of the plant in hot water, and then drinking it. To make herbal tea from pre-bagged tea, simply follow the manufacturer's directions. If you are using the whole herb, unless the label specifies otherwise, use 2 heaping tablespoons of the herb and 8 ounces of water for every cup of tea.

To make a tea from the leaf or flower of the herb, place the herb in a cup or teapot, boil the water, and pour the water over the herb. Use only a china or glass teapot or cup, not metal or plastic. Cover the container and allow the herbal tea to steep for five to ten minutes.

If you are making a tea from the root or bark of the herb, place the herb in the water and bring to a boil. Reduce the heat and simmer for ten minutes, then steep for another five minutes.

When the tea is done steeping, strain out the herb, allow the tea to cool to a comfortable drinking temperature, and serve. To treat skin problems topically, you can also use a strong herbal tea to make a compress. Simply soak a clean cloth in the tea and apply it to the affected area.

TINCTURES

Tinctures use alcohol to draw out, concentrate, and preserve the active properties of an herb. A few drops of this concentrated form of the herb can be added to a cup of tea or a glass of spring water, used to make a compress, or added to oil and used for a body massage.

Many herbal tinctures are readily available in natural foods stores, drugstores, and other outlets. If you would like to make your own, however, you can. Loosely fill a glass bottle or jar with the herb of your choice (crumble or cut up the pieces first). Add pure alcohol, such as vodka, to cover the herbs. Seal the bottle or jar tightly and shake it. Store it for two weeks in a place where the temperature stays between 70°F and 80°F. Shake the bottle or jar daily. When the two weeks are up, strain out the herbs and collect the residue. The tincture is now ready to use. If you are concerned about the alcohol component of the tincture, add the prescribed number of drops to ¼ cup of boiling water or very hot tea and wait for five minutes or so to allow the alcohol to boil off.

OILS

An herbal oil is a good way to get the beneficial properties of an herb directly to an area of the body that is injured or affected by illness. To make an herbal oil, wash fresh herbs and let them dry overnight. Crumble or dry the herbs and place them in a glass bottle or jar. Add almond oil or light virgin olive oil until the oil covers the herb parts by about an inch. Seal the container tightly.

Let the jar stand in a very warm place, such as out in the sun during the day and near a heat source such as a radiator, for two weeks. When the two weeks are up, strain the herbal parts out of the oil Your herbal oil is now ready to use. If you will not use all of the oil in a matter of days, store it in the refrigerator to keep it from turning rancid.

POULTICES

Poultices are another good way to get the benefits of a medicinal herb directly to the skin. They are best for areas that need wet compresses.

There are two basic ways of making a poultice. The first works best with plant parts that contain a significant amount of moisture, and you need the fresh herb—the fresher the better. On a flat surface, place fresh herb parts on a piece of clean, loosely woven cloth such as lightweight cotton, cheesecloth, gauze, linen, or muslin. Fold the cloth over several times to cover and contain the herb, then run a rolling pin over the cloth until the herb is completely crushed and herbal juices have been released into (and contained by) the poultice. Unwrap the cloth a layer at a time until you come to a completely wetted area. Apply the wet area of the cloth to the affected area of the skin, then wrap the poultice in a dry towel to hold it in place for at least twenty minutes. You can leave the poultice in place overnight, if necessary.

Another way of making a poultice adds soothing warmth to the treatment, and can utilize either fresh or dried herb. Put a strainer, steamer, or sieve over a pot of rapidly boiling water. Place either chopped fresh herbs or dried herbs in the strainer. Reduce the heat, cover the pot and sieve, and simmer for about five minutes. Remove the sieve from the heat and remove the softened and warmed herbs from the sieve. Spread the herbs on a piece of clean, loosely woven cloth such as lightweight cotton, cheesecloth, gauze, linen, or muslin and, when the poultice has cooled sufficiently, apply the resulting poultice to the affected area of skin. Be careful to test the temperature before applying it to avoid burning yourself. To hold the poultice in place and preserve the heat, wrap it with a clean dry towel or cloth. The poultice should be left in place at least twenty minutes, and may be left on overnight.

BATHS

There are a number of ways to prepare herbal baths that can help with a variety of skin conditions. A very simple, soothing herbal bath can be made by dissolving aloe vera gel or several drops of herbal tincture in a tubful of hot bath water. You can also use whole or dried herbs to make a bath. The easiest technique is to take a square of cheesecloth, place herbs in the center, draw the sides together, and tie them together to form a pouch. Let the pouch sit under the faucet as hot water fills the tub—much as you would pour hot water over a teabag . Once you are in the bath, you can squeeze the pouch to release herb-treated water over affected skin or, as long as you are using only leaves and other soft herbal parts, you can gently massage the affected skin with the pouch of herbs.

Light Therapy

Full-spectrum, colored, ultraviolet, and laser light are useful therapies for chronic pain, cancer, and immune disorders. Natural sunlight can help to reestablish the body's natural rhythm, which is important to maintain or reestablish good health. Controlled sun exposure can also be helpful for certain disorders, such as eczema and psoriasis. Colored-light therapy has been used successfully to enhance relaxation and pain relief and to speed wound healing.

When we see natural, full-spectrum sunlight, the energy of the sunlight is converted into electrical impulses by photoreceptors in our eyes. These electrical sparks travel through the optic nerve to the hypothalamus, a structure located deep in the brain. The hypothalamus then sends chemical messengers called neurotransmitters to different organs throughout the body to control the autonomic (involuntary or automatic) functions and maintain good health. It has recently been theorized that light is also important in stimulating other areas of the brain, including the cerebral cortex, the motor cortex, the limbic system, and the brain stem. Thus, motivation, thinking, creativity, memory, body movements, emotions, coordination, and balance, as well as the body's optimal absorption of nutrients, are thought to be influenced by the amount of natural sunlight we expose ourselves to. "Malillumination" or "photocurrent deficit" from inadequate full-spectrum light exposure adversely affects one's health in many ways. Therefore, a good supply of natural light is essential for balanced health.

Colored-light therapy is beginning to be used to treat a wide range of health problems, including stress, anxiety, chronic pain, allergies, and wound healing. Hopefully, it will have a bigger place in the future in the treatment of dermatologic problems that are made worse by stress or anxiety or are characterized by pain. It will also become increasingly important in the treatment of allergic reactions of the skin and poorly healing wounds.

As early as 1942, scientists showed that red light stimulates the sympathetic nervous system, while white and blue light act on the parasympathetic nervous system. They also discovered that some colors stimulate hormone production, while others diminish it. Earlier, it had been found that certain colors can affect certain diseases. For example, symptoms of smallpox and measles were reduced when patients were put in rooms with red windows. Dr. Norman Shealy, the founder of the American Holistic Medical Academy, uses flashing opaque white or violet lights to effect relaxation, and to decrease stress and chronic pain. Dr. Shealy believes that the brain responds uniquely to specific colors and, therefore, responds uniquely to different frequencies of flashing light. He also thinks that the way in which each light frequency specifically alters the production of neuro-chemicals in the brain accounts for the different positive treatment results. Other physicians use red-light therapy to treat allergies, wounds, localized pain, and stress.

Certainly, the future of light therapy is bright. Light treatments are inexpensive and in many cases can be used at home, in conjunction with other therapies, to help to clear a large variety of skin problems.

Meditation Techniques

There are many approaches to meditation, but, in general, one tries to achieve a calm, focused, nonthinking awareness in the present moment. Thus, one is neither preoccupied with past memories nor planning future events. In *concentrative meditation,* you narrow your focus, paying close attention to your breath, an image, or a sound to calm the mind and permit a greater awareness to come to the surface. In *mindful meditation,* you pay nonjudgmental attention to your changing thoughts, emotions, and perceptions, but in the present only, with the goal of gaining a broad, sweeping awareness of everything you perceive.

Practitioners of *transcendental meditation* (TM) focus on a single object, word, or phrase. Numerous studies have shown that TM causes a generalized decrease in heart rate, respiratory rate, and blood levels of stress hormones, and helps the body to enter a healthy, relaxed state. With TM, there is increased activity of alpha waves in the brain. This type of brain wave is associated with both relaxation and increased alertness. According to Dr. Joan Borysenko, a pioneer in the field of mind-body medicine and former codirector of Harvard University's Mind-Body Clinic, one becomes "more in touch with the inner physician, allowing the body's own inner wisdom to be heard." Some teachers of TM claim that this approach can be used to treat eczema and psoriasis and the stressors that cause flare-ups of these diseases. This self-care technique can easily be practiced at home, and shows a great deal of promise in the management of acute and chronic dermatologic problems, as well as for overall good health. However, meditation is not recommended for individuals who are predisposed to mental illness, in whom it may worsen stress and psychiatric symptoms.

Nail Care

As with your skin and hair, when your nails look their best, you feel more healthy and attractive. And as is true with both hair and skin care, "less is best" when it comes to the care of your nails. That is, avoid over-manicuring, overpolishing, or working with your nails. Moisturize and protect them, just as you do your skin and hair, to keep them at their best.

The following are some tips for achieving and maintaining healthy, attractive fingernails and toenails:

- Keep your nails and hands well moisturized. Moisturizers containing collagen and vitamin E are especially good for the nails. They are most effective if put on after soaking your nails in warm water and patting dry.
- File your nails in one direction only, not back and forth.
- Keep toenails clipped straight across, not curved or pointed, to avoid ingrown toenails. Also, do not clip toenails too short or clip them in at the sides.
- Use a fine-textured emery board, not a metal nail file. Metal files are hard on the nails.
- Moisturize and gently push back your cuticles. Do not cut them.
- Do not manicure your nails too frequently or apply nail products too often.
- If you have sensitive skin and nails, look for fragrance-free and formaldehyde-free polishes and non-acetone polish removers.
- If you wear polish, let your nails go "bare" for a few days each month to let the air get to them.
- Use protective cotton-lined vinyl gloves to wash dishes, work with cleansers, or work in the garden.
- Never bite your nails. Do not use them as prying tools.

Relaxation Techniques

We have seen that many skin problems are triggered by or flare up in response to stress and anxiety, and can therefore be improved with mind and body relaxation techniques. The body responds to anxiety-provoking thoughts and events with muscle tension. Increased muscle tension in turn increases the feeling of anxiety. Thus, we can experience an increasing cycle of tension or relaxation mentally, emotionally, and physically. Deep muscle relaxation reduces muscle tension and thus reduces the feeling of anxiety. Progressive relaxation is a technique you can use to consciously aid muscle relaxation.

After getting into a comfortable position, you progressively tighten and then loosen the muscles of your body in an ordered, systematic way. Start with your right and then your left hand and arm, move up to the muscles of your face, and then proceed downward, tensing and relaxing the muscles of your abdomen and then your lower body—again, first the right side and then the left. With each muscle group tightening and then relaxing, focus on how different these feelings are and how good the relaxation feels, physically and mentally. Breathe deeply, inhaling with the tensing of each set of muscles and exhaling with each muscle relaxation to maximize the effect of this exercise. To promote relaxation, practice the following for fifteen minutes twice a day:

- Get into a comfortable position, lying down or in a chair with your head supported.
- Clench your right hand tightly into a fist, noticing the tension in your hand and forearm. Relax your hand. Contrast the feeling of looseness and relaxation in your right hand with the feeling of tension you just experienced.
- Repeat with the left hand. Finally, clench both hands at the same time.
- Bend your elbows and tense your biceps and notice the feeling of tautness. Relax, straightening out your arms and concentrating on how different the feeling of relaxation is from the feeling of tension. Repeat.
- Repeat all of the following once, concentrating each time on first the feeling of tension and then the feeling of relaxation:
  - Wrinkle your forehead tightly, then relax and smooth it out.
  - Frown deeply, noticing the tension develop in your forehead, then relax and notice how your brow becomes smooth again.

- Close your eyes and squint them together tightly, then relax them.
- Clench your jaw, biting hard, then relax your jaw, parting your lips slightly.
- Press your tongue against the roof of your mouth, then relax.
- Purse your lips into a tight "O," then relax them. Your forehead, scalp, eyes, jaw, tongue, and eyes should now all feel relaxed.

■ Press your head all the way back, then roll it all the way to the right. Then roll it all the way to the left. Finally, bring your head forward, pressing your chin as up close to your chest as you can. Feel the tension in your throat and the back of your neck before you return your head to a comfortable position and relax deeply.

■ Shrug your shoulders up tightly next to your head, then relax and drop them back down. Your neck, throat, and shoulders should now feel deeply relaxed.

■ Breathe in deeply, holding your breath and noticing the tension. Exhale and notice how you relax as you do so. Repeat this several times.

■ Tighten your stomach, hold, then relax.

■ Arch your lower back, then relax.

■ Tighten your buttocks and thighs, pressing your heels down as hard as you can to tense your thighs. Relax.

■ Tense your calves by curling your toes downward, then relax.

■ Tense your shins by bending your toes toward your face, then relax.

■ Concentrate on the feeling of heaviness throughout your body from your feet up to your face as you allow the relaxation to spread upward and deepen, letting go more and more.

If you practice this routine faithfully every day, you should become proficient at it after a week or two.

Skin Care

When your skin looks and feels its best, you are healthier and feel more attractive. How you treat your body as a whole has a big effect on the way your skin looks, feels, and functions. For your skin to look its best, you should not smoke (and should avoid secondhand smoke) or use recreational drugs. You should also eat plenty of fresh fruits and vegetables; get adequate amounts of vitamins, minerals, amino acids, and essential fatty acids; and drink plenty of pure water.

Through experience, you know if your skin tends to hold moisture normally, to be dry or oily, or to be made up of a combination of dry and oily areas. You should use a basic skin-care regimen appropriate for your skin type to help keep your skin looking, feeling, and functioning at its best. No matter what you skin type is, though, keep in mind that "less is best" is a good general philosophy, and be sure to apply a good broad-spectrum sunscreen each day. The following are lifestyle tips that apply to all skin types:

- Do not smoke. Smoking decreases the flow of blood to the skin and also promotes wrinkling.
- Take vitamin C, a B-vitamin complex, vitamin E, bioflavonoids, L-proline, L-lysine, and grapeseed extract supplements daily. These are antioxidants that help to prevent free-radical damage to the skin. Proline and lysine are necessary amino acid building blocks of normal skin that help to maintain its tone and flexibility.
- Avoid "yo-yo" dieting—cycles of significant weight loss followed by weight gain. This stretches the skin out when you gain weight, and causes it to sag when you lose weight.
- Drink at least eight 8-ounce glasses of filtered water a day. This keeps the skin hydrated, which keeps it younger-looking and helps to prevent dry skin.
- Eat at least five servings of fruit and vegetables a day. They contain valuable antioxidants that prevent free-radical damage to the body and skin. Blueberries, blackberries, garlic, kale, strawberries, and spinach are particularly high in valuable antioxidants.

DAILY REGIMEN FOR NORMAL SKIN

- Use a low-alkaline soap or cleanser to wash your face every day.
- Put on a light moisturizer.
- Apply a broad-spectrum sunscreen with a sun protection factor (SPF) of at least 15. Reapply it frequently if you are spending time outdoors or in your car.

DAILY REGIMEN FOR DRY SKIN

- Cleanse your skin with a creamy cleanser or superfatted soap.
- Moisturize your face and body every day. Natural moisturizers include aloe, apricot, avocado, coconut, jojoba, olive, and sesame oils, as well as cocoa butter. Reapply moisturizer as needed during the day.
- If your skin is very dry, apply a heavier moisturizing cream before going to bed.
- After cleansing and moisturizing, apply a sunscreen with a sun protection factor (SPR) of 15 before going out in the morning. Reapply it frequently if you are spending time outdoors or in your car.

DAILY REGIMEN FOR OILY SKIN

- Use a cleanser that also contains a toner to help reduce oiliness. However, make sure that the cleanser is not too drying, as your skin may react by producing more oil.
- If you do not currently have an active flare-up of acne, you can make a facial steam bath to cleanse your pores by adding a few drops of peppermint oil to a pot of hot water. Place your face over the pot and cover your head with a towel to hold in the steam.
- After washing your face, put on a small amount of a noncomedogenic, oil-free moisturizer.
- Use a separate toner once or twice a week to remove extra oil from your face. One good natural toner is diluted witch hazel. Sage is also a good natural astringent that tightens your skin and is very helpful for toning.
- An exfoliating scrub can be made from ground cornmeal, oatmeal, apricot seeds, and/or almonds combined with a small amount of water or plain

yogurt. Do not overscrub active acne flare-ups, however, as this will make the problem worse.

■ Always remember to put on a noncomedogenic broad-spectrum sunscreen with a sun protection factor (SPF) of 15 or higher before going out.

■ Use only noncomedogenic, oil-free cosmetics.

DAILY REGIMEN FOR COMBINATION SKIN

■ Wash your face every day with a gentle cleanser.

■ Put a light moisturizer on the dry part or parts of your face, usually the cheeks.

■ Apply a gentle, alcohol-free toner once or twice a week to the oily parts of your face, usually the nose, chin, and forehead. Toners containing sage or diluted witch hazel make good natural astringents.

■ Don't forget to apply a noncomedogenic, oil-free sunscreen with a sun protection factor (SPF) of 15 or higher before you finish your regimen.

■ Use only noncomedogenic, oil-free cosmetics.

Skin Self-Examination

Everyone should give him- or herself a full-body skin self-examination once a month to check for any suspicious spots or changes in moles that may signify a developing problem, especially skin cancer. A good time to do this is after a bath or shower, in a location with excellent lighting. To perform a skin self-exam, you will need both a full-length mirror and a hand mirror.

The following are instructions for examining your skin:

- When you first start doing skin self-exams, take some time to learn where existing moles and blemishes are, and how they usually look and feel.
- First, examine the front of your body from head to toe in a full-length mirror.
- Next examine the back of your body from head to toe in the mirror.
- Raise your arms and look at your right and left sides from head to toe in the full-length mirror.
- Next, carefully check your upper arms, forearms, palms, and fingernails. Look at one side of your body at a time.
- Examine the front, back, and sides of each leg.
- Check the spaces between the toes and the soles of each foot.
- Using the hand mirror, carefully look at the back of your neck and your scalp, parting your hair to do so.
- Also using the hand mirror, examine your back and buttocks for skin changes.

It may feel awkward at first, but with practice it will become second nature. If you notice any new spots; any change in the size, shape, or color of an existing mole; or a skin lesion that does not heal, don't panic, but do call your dermatologist promptly. Remember, all types of skin cancer are curable if caught early enough. By doing this self-exam once a month, you can help to ensure that if you do develop a problem, your chances of a complete cure will be excellent.

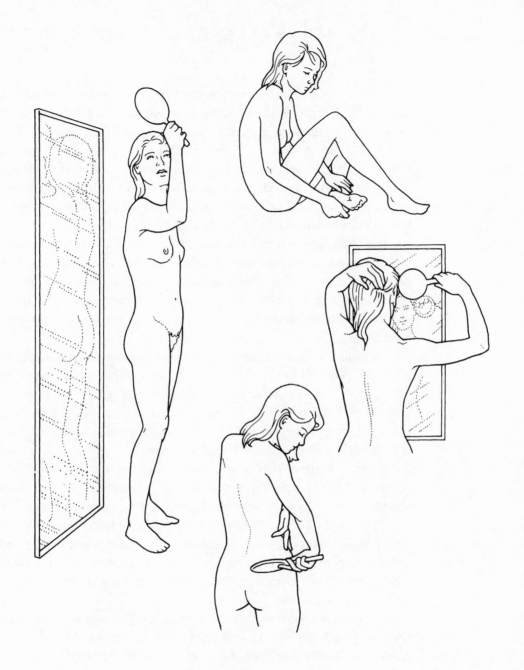

Skin Self-Examination

Sound and Music Therapy

For thousands of years it has been recognized that sound and music have the ability to enhance healing. In recent years, sound therapists have found that certain sounds create a feeling of well-being or calm. These sounds also act to slow a person's respiration and heart rate, produce changes in skin temperature, decrease muscle tension, lower blood pressure, change brain-wave frequencies, increase blood flow to the brain and body, and increase mental functioning. Even ultrasonic waves, which cannot be heard by the human ear, can affect human health.

Sound therapy's effectiveness may be due to the link between the ear, brain, and autonomic (automatic) nervous system. The autonomic vagus nerve connects to all of the body's internal organs. Our emotional responses are controlled by the limbic system in the brain, to which the ear and the autonomic nervous system—and thus all the body's organs—are linked.

According to Steve Halpern, Ph.D., a composer and musician, the human body responds to sound in two main ways: rhythm entrainment and resonance. In rhythm entrainment, the heartbeat begins to pulse in sync with the external rhythm of the music. In fact, studies suggest that the intrinsic rhythms of the heart, brain, and other organs have a special synchronicity that, when disturbed, results in illness.

When different pitches or frequencies of sound stimulate the body to vibrate in different areas, this is described as *resonance*. Usually, high sound resonates in the higher parts of the body, and lower sounds stimulate the lower parts of the body to vibrate. In fact, some people are trained in "toning," making elongated vowel sounds that resonate throughout the body and specific parts of the brain, depending on the pitch of the tone. Toning is thought to synchronize brain waves, release stress, and greatly improve one's sense of well-being.

The greatest therapeutic effects of music are generally produced when you understand and like the particular musical selection. In Hal Lingerman's book *The Healing Energies of Music* (Quest Books, 1995), the author includes a very informative chapter on music to improve one's health. In it, he details a list of musical pieces specific for different emotional purposes, including releasing anger, calming anger, and relieving fear. Music ideal for imagery, meditation, and prayer, and music to enhance courage, is also listed. Thus, new interest in music as a form of therapy has taken hold and can certainly be applied to a vast array of skin problems.

There is also an increasing interest in the development of sound-based treatment devices, such as the Infratonic QGM and other cymatic instruments. These instruments produce specific sound frequencies to achieve specific therapeutic results such as pain relief or stress reduction. The Infratonic QGM device simulates the infratonic sound which is emitted from the hands of qigong masters when they are practicing their art. Tested on over 1,000 hospitalized patients, the device is said to produce *qi,* or vital energy, that can be very helpful in the production of pain relief, muscular relaxation, increased circulation, and increased alpha waves in the brain. In China, it is medically recognized nationally as an effective instrument for pain reduction. It is currently pending FDA approval in this country.

Cymatic devices, which have been used worldwide for about thirty years, use computer-generated, highly specific audible waves applied directly to the skin to reestablish the body's healthy equilibrium. This therapy stimulates the natural regulatory and immunologic systems of the body via direct contact or by way of acupuncture meridians. The sound waves pass through healthy tissues but reestablish healthy resonance in sick tissues, thus producing an optimum metabolic state for a particular cell or organ. In this way, the body is helped to heal itself.

The TENS unit, which generally produces electric frequencies, can also generate vibratory frequencies that greatly reduce generalized itching. It can thus produce biologically active resonance, with subharmonics of musical notes having the greatest biologic effect.

Music has been used since the 1950s to facilitate psychotherapy, as it can evoke a wide range of emotions, depending on the musical composition. It can also be combined with guided imagery and breathing to bring about a very powerful emotional release or to tap into the unconscious mind. Music therapy is also currently very important in modern hospital settings to elevate mood, reduce the perception of physical discomfort, aid in relaxation, and reduce anesthesia requirements.

Sound and music therapy should grow in importance in the healing of the future. They are certainly low-cost complementary treatments with no side effects. Perhaps various forms of sound and music therapy can be used for the diagnosis as well as the treatment of diverse health problems in the future. The benefits of relaxation and pain reduction through sound therapy can certainly be used to help treat difficult dermatologic conditions such as psoriasis, eczema, and melanoma today.

Yoga

Yoga is a key component of Ayurvedic medicine, which started in India in the second century BC, and is the one of the oldest medical approaches known. The Ayurvedic meaning of *yoga* is "union," referring to the integration of physical, mental, and spiritual energies, which together improve a person's well-being. Ultimately, the aim of yoga is to help one achieve increased vitality and spiritual awareness. Yogic postures, breathing exercises, and forms of meditation are excellent forms of preventive medicine, having been shown in numerous studies to reduce stress, anxiety, and allergies. Yoga also lowers blood pressure, heart rate, pain perception, and tendency toward addictions. Various forms of yoga have also been shown to improve sleep, memory, intelligence, motor skills, metabolic and respiratory functions, the tone of the nervous systems endocrine system, and visual and auditory perceptions.

Breathing exercises are done to help remove energy blockages and increase the steady flow of the life force, or *prana,* throughout the body. A person who suppresses unpleasant feelings may also unwittingly restrict his or her breathing. Conversely, proper breathing can help to bring about a needed emotional release. If the mind is calm and focused, the breathing will be even and calm, and vice versa. Therefore, breathing exercises are frequently done before the actual yoga exercise is started. According to yoga masters, spiritual awareness can be achieved through yoga after dedicated practice for many years.

The best-known type of yoga is hatha yoga. This is further divided into meditative and therapeutic forms. Meditative poses help to align the spine and head, increasing relaxation and calmness of the mind. Therapeutic poses are suggested to reduce back, neck, and joint pain, and to improve one's overall health while maintaining the mind in a relaxed openness.

Alternative-health expert and author Dr. Deepak Chopra and others have become very popular in applying Ayurvedic techniques, including yoga, to the prevention and treatment of Western medical problems. In fact, some insurance companies are now covering the expenses of yoga training, a sign of the cost-effectiveness of yoga in health care. Thus, yoga can certainly be used to improve skin problems and should be used as a complementary skin therapy to an even greater degree in the future. Yoga can be practiced at home, but it should first be learned from a professional teacher. There are professional practitioners of yoga and yoga classes throughout the country.

Appendix

Glossary

acne. A skin condition most common in adolescence, with plugging and inflammation of the pores of the face, neck, back, shoulders, and chest. The hair follicles become clogged with sebum (oil), keratin, bacteria, and/or yeast. Types of acne lesions include blackheads, whiteheads, papules, pustules, and cysts. Also known as acne vulgaris ("common acne").

actinic keratosis. A small red or brown rough, scaly precancerous growth on chronically sun-exposed skin. Actinic keratoses should be treated so that they do not progress to become cancerous.

acupoints. Points on the surface of the skin that correspond to specific internal organs and systems. They are located along the channels in the body through which *chi*, or the vital life force, runs. Acupuncture and acupressure utilize these points to restore balance in the body.

acute disease. An illness or symptom that comes on quickly and, generally, has a limited duration.

adaptogen. A substance, usually a type of herb, that increases the body's resilience to stress. Adaptogens work by supporting the adrenal glands to help the body to adapt to problems and avoid collapsing.

age spots. *See* Solar lentigines.

alpha-hydroxy acids (AHAs). Acid extracts derived from fruits or milk that act as mild exfoliants and are used in many moisturizers and anti-aging creams.

androgenic alopecia. The most common form of hair loss. Caused by an excess of androgens, or male hormones, hair loss generally becomes noticeable in middle-aged men and older women. Also known as male pattern baldness.

androgens. Hormones that are important in the development of acne in teenagers and hair loss (androgenic alopecia) in middle-aged men and older women. Commonly referred to as male hormones, they are in fact present in people of both sexes.

antimicrobial. Germ-fighting.

antioxidant. Any of a group of substances, including vitamins, minerals, and enzymes, that prevent or reduce the cellular destruction caused by free radicals.

astringent. A substance that cleanses oily residue from the skin with a cooling, tingling, or tightening function.

athlete's foot. A fungal infection of the feet, with red sores or flaking between the toes and/or red scaling and blistering on the sole of the foot.

atopic dermatitis. A chronic, red, itchy skin condition in people with an inherited tendency toward allergies. Also known as atopic eczema.

basal cell carcinoma. The most common form of skin cancer, accounting for about 90 percent of skin cancer cases in the United States. It usually lookes like a skin-colored or pink bump or nodule, usually with a "pearly," smooth surface. It is generally slow-growing and occurs on sun-exposed areas, especially the head, ears, and neck.

benign. Not malignant (cancerous).

benzoyl peroxide. A first-line treatment for acne that acts as a drying agent and a mild antibiotic.

beta-hydroxy acids. Any of a class of acids, usually derived from fruits, that are used as exfoliants. Salicylic acid is a beta-hydroxy acid.

biopsy. A diagnostic procedure in which a sample of tissue is removed and examined under a microscope for signs of cancer cells and other identifying cells.

blackhead. An open, clogged comedone found in acne that is dark in color because of the pigment melanin.

blister. A small swellings of the skin filled with watery material.

boil. *See* Furuncle.

botulinum toxin (Botox). A purified version of the toxin that causes botulism, given in a local injection to prevent and minimize wrinkles by temporarily paralyzing muscles that cause frown lines between the eyebrows and across the forehead. The treatment lasts for three to six months.

bovine collagen. Collagen derived from cows. A purified form of bovine collagen may be injected locally into the skin to temporarily fill wrinkles and make them seem to disappear.

broad-spectrum sunscreen. A sunscreen that filters out both ultraviolet-A (UVA) and ultraviolet-B (UVB) rays from the sun.

cancer. Any of a group of diseases in which cells become abnormal and divide too often, out of control, and not in order.

cellulite. A type of fatty tissue containing bands of collagen fibers. The skin looks dimpled because the collagen fibers inhibit the cellulite's ability to stretch.

chemical peel. A procedure used to reduce wrinkling, actinic keratoses, and age spots. In this technique, a liquid acid solution is painted on the skin to encourage top layers of the skin to peel off. The amount of skin removed depends on the type and strength of the solution used, and on how long it is left on.

chronic disease. An illness that has a long duration, frequent recurrences, and/or a progressive course. There is no natural tendency to recover, although many chronic diseases can be managed successfully.

cold sores. Tiny single or clustered clear fluid-filled blisters caused by the herpes simplex virus. The blisters usually form around the lips.

collagen. A protein in the dermis of the skin that gives the skin its strength and thickness and is important in scar formation.

comedone. An acne lesion that may be open (a blackhead) or closed (a whitehead). A comedone forms when a hair follicle or pore becomes plugged with excess sebum (oil), dead skin cells, and bacteria.

congenital nevi. Moles that are present at birth or that appear during a baby's first year. They are benign, but large ones have an increased chance of becoming cancerous.

contact dermatitis. An irritant or allergic reaction to a substance that touches one's skin. It is usually characterized by a red, itchy rash developing in the areas touched.

corticosteroid. Any of a group of anti-inflammatory drugs used topically and orally to treat many skin conditions, such as eczema and psoriasis.

cryosurgery. A procedure in which liquid nitrogen is used to freeze and then blister off a skin lesion.

curettage. The use of a curette (a sharp, spoon-shaped instrument) to scrape away skin cells. It is most often used to treat basal cell carcinomas.

cutaneous. Related to the skin.

cyst. A small closed sac containing keratin, cellular debris, sebum, and micro-organisms.

dandruff. The shedding of light-colored dead skin cells from the scalp.

dermabrasion. The use of a rapidly rotating wheel or circular brush to sand off the top layer of the skin and reduce scars and wrinkles.

dermatitis. A general term for inflammation of the skin, with redness, pain, and/or itching.

dermis. The innermost layer of the skin, located beneath the epidermis.

double-blind study. An optimum model for medical studies. In double-blind studies, neither the person conducting the experiment nor the subjects being tested know which subjects are receiving the drug being tested and which are being given placebo.

dysplastic (atypical) nevi. Irregularly shaped, large, and/or colored moles that are benign but that have a slightly higher chance than other moles of becoming cancerous.

eczema. A form of dermatitis that is not caused by germs and is not contagious. Also known as atopic dermatitis.

elastin. Elastic fibers in the dermis that allow the skin to stretch and contract repeatedly as it moves.

electrodesiccation. The direct use of electric current to destroy growths, stop bleeding, and treat facial spider veins, among other things.

epidermis. The outer layer of the skin, lying above the dermis.

exfoliant. A substance that sloughs off the outer, older layer of skin cells. Exfoliating scrubs may be used for acne or to make the skin look younger.

fat-soluble vitamin. Any of a group of vitamins that are stored in fat, such as vitamins A, D, E, and K. Fat-soluble vitamins stay in the body much longer than water-soluble vitamins do.

fever blisters. *See* Cold sores.

folliculitis. Infection of one or more hair follicles or pores, caused by bacteria or, less often, by fungi.

free radicals. High-energy, unstable molecules or fragments of molecules that damage parts of cells and play a role in the aging process.

furuncle. A tender, red, inflamed lesion. Also known as a boil.

herpes zoster. A condition characterized by a painful cluster of blisters on a reddish base, caused by a reactivation of the chickenpox virus many years after the original outbreak of chickenpox. Also called shingles.

homeopathic remedy. In homeopathy, a medicine given according to the Law of Similars, which holds that like shall be cured by like.

hyperpigmentation. The darkening of certain skin areas, due to pregnancy, wound healing, or other factors.

hypoallergenic. A term applied to products or substances that are considered less likely to cause allergic reactions. There are currently no legal guidelines declaring which ingredients can and cannot be used in products labeled as hypoallergenic, however.

hypopigmentation. The lightening of patches of skin that occurs with aging or wound healing, as a side effect of some skin treatments, or due to other factors.

impetigo. A contagious bacterial skin infection that can be spread by physical contact. It is more common in children than in adults.

keloid. A hard, fleshy scar caused by overgrown scar tissue.

keratin. The strong, protective protein that makes the cells of the skin's topmost, horny layer, and of the hair, fingernails, and toenails very tough.

keratolytic. The property of tending to loosen and remove cells in the skin's outermost horny layer.

laser. Any of many different types of machines that produce a concentrated light beam. The word *laser* is an acronym for *l*ight *a*mplification by *s*timulated *e*mission of *r*adiation.

laser resurfacing. A technique in which a laser is used to remove superficial layers of skin to reduce wrinkling and photoaging.

lesion. An injury, wound, infected patch, or other abnormal area of skin.

macule. A flat spot on the skin that may be any color from red to black, and that is characteristic of many types of skin problems or lesions.

male pattern baldness. *See* Androgenic alopecia.

malignant. Cancerous.

melanin. The pigment produced by specialized cells called melanocytes that gives skin its color and protects against ultraviolet radiation.

melanoma. The most dangerous type of skin cancer. It looks like a multicolored or dark, irregularly shaped mole or patch, and needs to be treated immediately, before it metastasizes (spreads). If untreated, melanoma can be life-threatening.

meridian. One of the fourteen or more channels in the body through which, in Chinese medical philosophy, the vital energy (called *qi,* or *chi*), runs.

metastasize. To spread, as cancer, to other parts of the body from the earliest, primary spot.

Moh's surgery. An excision technique in which a microscope is used to map each microscopic piece of tissue to be removed and examine it for cancerous cells before deciding whether the next microscopic layer of tissue also should be cut away. Moh's surgery is used in hard-to-treat or recurrent nonmelanoma skin cancers.

mole. A dark growth on the skin composed of noncancerous clusters of melanocytes (pigment-producing cells).

mycosis fungoides. A cancer of the lymphatic system that usually first appears on the skin. Also known as T-cell lymphoma.

nervine. A type of herb that helps the nervous system by acting as a tonic, relaxant, or stimulant.

nevus. Medical term for a mole (the plural is *nevi*).

PABA. *See* Para-aminobenzoic acid.

papule. A small bump that may be red, white, or flesh-colored.

Para-aminobenzoic acid (PABA). A common ingredient in sunscreens. People with sensitive or allergy-prone skin should use PABA-free products.

photoaging. Damage to the skin caused by exposure to sunlight over time. This includes much of the wrinkling, lines, and brown spots that develop after years of being exposed to the sun.

pores. Tiny openings in the skin through which perspiration and sebum (oil) empty onto the skin's surface. Also known as hair follicles.

pruritus. Medical term for itching.

psoriasis. A noncontagious skin condition in which skin cells turn over at a very fast rate, producing red, thickened areas of skin covered with silvery scales.

pustule. A pus-filled bump.

qi. The vital life energy that, in Chinese medical philosophy, runs throughout the body along lines known as meridians. When the vital force is in balance, there is health. When it is out of balance, there is disease. Also spelled *chi*.

radiation therapy. A treatment in which high-energy rays are used to kill cancer cells. It is sometimes used to treat nonmelanoma skin cancers, especially in older adults or the infirm.

ringworm. A fungal skin infection that causes ring-shaped patches of reddened and/or scaly skin.

rosacea. A skin condition characterized by facial redness, thin red facial lines, swelling, and papules. It is most common in middle-aged adults. Also known as acne rosacea.

sclerotherapy. A treatment for spider veins in which an irritating solution is injected into a cosmetically displeasing vein. This causes the opposing linings of the vessel to swell and stick together, and the vein closes down and fades.

sebaceous glands. Glands in the skin that produce sebum, the moisturizing lubricant for the skin.

seborrheic dermatitis. An inflammatory rash in areas with large numbers of sebaceous (oil) glands, such as the eyebrows, scalp, behind the ears, and at the corners of the nose. The rash is reddish with yellowish, greasy scales, and is thought to be caused by the yeast *Pityrosporum ovale*. Also known as seborrhea.

sebum. A waxy, oily substance that surfaces through hair follicles to moisturize the skin.

shingles. *See* Herpes zoster.

solar lentigines. Medical term for age or liver spots caused by cumulative sun exposure. They are flat, brown macules that usually develop on the face, hands, and back.

spider veins. Patches of dilated or broken tiny red or purple blood vessels that look like spider webs, sunbursts, branching trees, or short broken lines. They usually form on the legs of middle-aged women. Also known as telangiectasia.

squamous cell carcinoma. The second most common type of skin cancer, which originates in the squamous cells of the epidermis. It is usually found on the ears, face, and hands, and manifests itself as a red nodule or a pink, scaly patch that can ulcerate and crust. It needs to be treated aggressively, as it will metastasize (spread) if left untreated.

stratum corneum. The top layer, or surface horny layer, of the epidermis.

subcutaneous layer. The large network of fat cells and connective tissue beneath the dermis that stabilizes the skin above it and insulates the organs beneath it.

sun protection factor (SPF). A measurement used in grading the effectiveness of sunscreens in protecting the skin from the ultraviolet-B (UVB) rays of the sun. It describes the relative length of time you can stay exposed to the sun before you sunburn, as compared to not using any sunscreen. Dermatologists recommend using a broad spectrum sunscreen with an SPF of 15 or higher, which allows you to stay out in the sun fifteen times longer without burning than if you had no sunscreen on at all.

sunblock. A cream containing titanium dioxide and/or zinc oxide that protects the skin from the harmful rays of the sun by reflecting ultraviolet (UV) rays. Some sunblocks also contain compounds that absorb the UV radiation.

sunscreen. A substance that protects the skin from the harmful rays of the sun by absorbing the ultraviolet rays.

suntan lotion. A lotion that offers little or no sun protection, but is used to moisturize the skin and enhance tanning.

surgical excision. Cutting into the skin around a growth using surgical instruments to remove a lesion and closing the wound with stitches. The lesion is usually sent to a pathologist for examination under a microscope.

telangiectasia. *See* Spider veins.

tonic. A type of herb used to nurture and enliven the body as a means of enhancing health and preventing illness.

tumor. An abnormal overgrowth of tissue that may be either benign or malignant.

ultraviolet-A (UVA) radiation. Long wavelengths of light given off by the sun. UVA radiation has been associated with skin damage that may lead to melanoma, photoaging, and nonmelanoma skin cancer.

utraviolet-B (UVB) radiation. Short wavelengths of light given off by the sun. UVB radiation causes sunburns and skin cancer.

vesicle. A small blister that contains clear, watery liquid.

water-soluble vitamin. Any of a group of vitamins that are soluble in water. As a result, they are constantly being eliminated through the sweat, urine, and other body fluids. B-complex vitamins and vitamin C are examples of water-soluble vitamins.

whitehead. A closed comedone, or clogged pore, that shows up as a tiny white or flesh-colored bump, usually on the face, typical of acne.

xerosis. Medical term for dry skin.

References

PART ONE: THE ELEMENTS OF HEALTH CARE FOR YOUR SKIN

Understanding Your Skin, Hair, and Nails

Graham-Brown and Bourke, *Mosby's Color Atlas and Text of Dermatology* (London: Mosby International Limited, 1998).

Moschella, Sam, and Harry Hurley, *Dermatology* (Philadelphia, PA: W.B. Saunders Company, 1985).

Conventional Approaches to Skin Care

Becker, R.O. *Cross Currents: The Promise of Electromedicine, The Perils of Electropollution* (Los Angeles, CA: Jeremy P. Tarcher, 1990).

Eisenberg, D., "Alternative Therapies for Cutaneous Disorders," *Archives of Dermatology* 133 (March 1997): 379–380.

Ely, Haines, "Shocking Therapy: Uses of Transcutaneous Electric Nerve Stimulation in Dermatology," *Dermatologic Clinics* 9(1) (January 1991): 189–197.

Fawzy, F.I., N.W. Fawzy, C.S. Hyun, R. Elashoff, D. Guthrie, J.L. Fahey, and D.L. Morton, "Malignant Melanoma: Effects of an Early Structured Psychiatric Intervention, Coping, and Affective State on Recurrence and Survival 6 Years Later," *Archives of General Psychiatry* 50 (1993): 681–689.

Fleischer, A.B., Jr., S.R. Felman, S.R. Rapp, D.M. Reboussin, M.L. Exum, and A.R. Clark, "Alternative Therapies Commonly Used Within a Population of Patients with Psoriasis," *Cutis* 58(3) (September 1996): 216–220.

Foulds, I.S., and A.T. Barker, "Human Skin Battery Potentials and Their Possible Role in Wound Healing," *British Journal of Dermatology* 109(5) (November 1983): 515–522.

Graham-Brown, Robin, and John Bourke, *Mosby's Color Atlas and Text of Dermatology* (London: Mosby International Limited, 1998).

Green, Lawrence J., *The Dermatologist's Guide to Looking Younger* (Freedom, CA: The Crossing Press, 1999).

ItchStopper.com. World Wide Web address, http://www.ItchStopper.com, accessed 1 November 1997.

Moschella, Sam, and Harry Hurley, *Dermatology* (Philadelphia, PA: W.B. Saunders Company, 1985).

Reich, J.D., and P.P. Tarjan, "Electrical Stimulation of Skin," *International Journal of Dermatology* 29(6) (July–August 1990): 395–400.

Sampere, C.T., J.A. Guasch, C.M. Paladino, M. Sanchez Casalongue, and B. Elencwajg. "Spinal Cord Stimulation for Severely Ischemic Limbs," *Pacing and Clinical Electrophysiology* 12(2) (February 1989): 273–279.

Scheman, Andrew J., and David Severson, *Pocket Guide to Medications Used in Dermatology* (Baltimore, MD: Williams & Wilkins, 1997).

Diet and Nutrition

Balch, James, and Phyllis Balch, *Prescription for Nutritional Healing.* 2nd Ed. (Garden City Park, NY: Avery Publishing Group, 1990).

Carper, Jean, *Food—Your Miracle Medicine* (New York, NY: HarperCollins, 1993).

Editors of *Prevention* Magazine, *Healing with Vitamins* (Emmaus, PA: Rodale Press, 1996).

Editors of *Prevention* Magazine, *Prevention's Food and Nutrition.* (New York, NY: Berkley Books, 1996).

Fugh-Berman, Adriane, *Alternative Medicine: What Works* (Baltimore, MD: Williams and Wilkins, 1997).

Garrison, Robert, Jr., and Elizabeth Somer, *The Nutrition Desk Reference* (New Canaan, CT: Keats Publishing, 1995).

Murray, Michael, *Encyclopedia of Nutritional Supplements* (Rocklin, CA: Prima Publishing, 1996).

Somer, Elizabeth, *The Essential Guide to Vitamins and Minerals* (New York, NY: HarperCollins, Inc., 1995).

Herbal Medicine

Alive Research Group, *Encyclopedia of Natural Healing* (Blain, WA: Natural Life Publishing, 1997).

Alternative-Medicines.com. World Wide Web address: http://www.alternative-medicines.com/herbdesc.htm, accessed 2 December 1997.

Bertram, P.D., "Melanosis Coli: A Consequence of 'Alternative Therapy' for Psoriasis," *American Journal of Gastroenterology* 88(6) (June 1993): 971.

Bossuyt L., and A. Dooms-Goossens, "Contact Sensitivity to Nettles and Chamomile in 'Alternative' Remedies," *Contact Dermatitis* 31(2) (1994): 131.

Caceres, A., L. Giron, S. Alvarado, and M. Torres, "Screening of Antimicrobial Activity of Plants Popularly Used in Guatemala for the Treatment of Dermatomucosal Diseases," *Journal of Ethnopharmacology* 20(3) (August 1987): 223–237.

Crissey, J.T., and L.C. Parish, "Plant Dermatitis: A Brief Retrospect," *Clinics in Dermatology* 4 (2) (April–June 1986): 1–4.

Duke, James A., "Herbal Alternatives for 50 Common Ailments," *New Age Journal's Annual Guide to Holistic Living* (1998): 59–60.

Editors of *Prevention* Magazine, *New Choices in Natural Healing* (Emmaus, PA: Rodale Press, 1995).

Editors of *Prevention* Magazine, *The Doctor's Book of Home Remedies* (Emmaus, PA: Rodale Press, 1990).

Ferguson, J.E., R.J. Chalmers, and D.J. Rowlands, "Reversible Dilated Cardiomyopathy Following Treatment of Atopic Eczema with Chinese Herbal Medicine," *British Journal of Dermatology* 136(4) (April 1997): 592–593.

Goff, S., and I. Levenstein, "Measuring the Tropical Preparations Upon the Healing of Skin Wounds," *Journal of the Society of Cosmetic Chemists* 15 (1964): 509–518.

Gundidza, M., and A. Kufa, "Skin Irritant and Tumour Promoting Extract from the Latex of *Euphorbia bougheii*," *Central African Journal of Medicine* 39 (3) (March 1993): 56–60.

Hallowell, Christopher, "The Plant Hunter," *Time* Vol. 150, No.19 (Fall 1997), pp. 17–22.

Heggers, J.P., Pelley, R.P., and M.C. Robson, "Beneficial Effects of Aloe in Wound Healing," *Phytotherapy Research* 7 (1993): S48–52.

Hoffman, David, *The Complete Illustrated Holistic Herbal* (Rockport, MA: Element Books, 1996).

Hoffman, Ronald L., "Detox Your Body," *New Age Journal's Annual Guide to Holistic Living* (1998): 62–63.

Keville, Kathi, *Herbs for Health and Healing* (Emmaus, PA: Rodale Press, 1996).

Klein, Alan D., "Aloe Vera," *Journal of the American Academy of Dermatology* 18 (1988): 714–720.

Knight, T.E., and B.M. Hausen, "Melaleuca Oil (Tea Tree Oil) Dermatitis," *Journal of the American Academy of Dermatology* 30(3) (March 1994): 423–427.

Lorenzetti, L. J., R. Salisbury, J. Beal, and J. Baldwin, "Bacteriostatic Property of Aloe Vera," *Journal of Pharmaceutical Science* 53 (1964): 12.

Ludeman, Kate, L. Henderson, and H. Basayne, *Do-It-Yourself Allergy Analysis Handbook* (New Canaan, CT: Keats, 1979).

Lushbaugh, C.C., and D.S. Hale, "Experimental Radiodermatitis Following Beta Irradiation," *Cancer 6* (1953): 690–697.

Markowitz, S.B., C.M. Nunez, S. Klitzman, A.A. Munshi, W.S. Kim, J. Eisinger, and P.J. Landrigan, "Lead Poisoning Due to Hai Ge Fen. The Porphyrin Content of Individual Erythrocytes," *Journal of the American Medical Association* 271(12) (March 23–30 1994): 932–934.

Medline. World Wide Web address: *http://www.medline.com/alternative health/ message board*, accessed 30 November 1997.

Ody, Penelope, *Home Herbal* (New York, NY: Dorling Kindersley, 1995).

Ody, Penelope, *The Complete Medicinal Herbal* (New York, NY: Dorling Kindersley, 1993).

Pazzaglia, M., N. Venturo, G. Borda, and A. Tosti, "Contact Dermatitis Due to a Massage Liniment Containing *Inula helenium* Extract," *Contact Dermatitis* 33(4) (October 1995): 267.

Plotkin, M., and R. Schultes, "Virola: A Promising Genus for Ethnopharmacological Investigation," *Journal of Psychoactive Drugs* 22(3) (July-September 1990): 357–361.

Rodriguez, P., J. Blanco, S. Juste, M. Garces, R. Perez, L. Alonso, and M. Marcos, "Allergic Contact Dermatitis Due to Burdock (*Arctium lappa*)," *Contact Dermatitis* 33(2) (August 1995): 134–135.

Sasseville, D., and K.H. Nguyen, "Allergic Contact Dermatitis from *Rhus toxicodendron* in a Phytotherapeutic Preparation," *Contact Dermatitis* 32(3) (March 1995): 182–183.

Selvaag, E., B. Eriksen, and P. Thune, "Contact Allergy Due to Tea Tree Oil and Cross Sensitization of Colophony," *Contact Dermatitis* 31(2) (1994): 124.

Sheehan, M., and D.J. Atherton, "One-Year Follow-Up of Children Treated with Chinese Medicinal Herbs for Atopic Eczema," *British Journal of Dermatology* 130 (1994): 488–493.

Siegers, C.P., E. von Hertzberg-Lottin, M. Otte, and B. Schneider, "Anthranoid Laxative Abuse—A Risk for Colon Cancer?" *Gut* 34(8) (August 1993): 1099–1101.

Stansbury, Jill, "Power Plants for Dermatitis," *Let's Live* (March 1999): 68–73.

Strickland, F., R. Pelley, and M. Kripke, "Prevention of Ultraviolet Radiation-Induced Suppression of Contact and Delayed Hypersensitivity by *Aloe barbadensis* Gel Extract," *Journal of Investigative Dermatology* 102(2) (1994): 197–204.

The Burton Goldberg Group, *Alternative Medicine: The Definitive Guide* (Fife, WA: Future Medicine Publishing, 1995).

Vukovic, Laurel, "The Best Herbs for Every Stage of Your Life," *Natural Health* (September-October 1998): 121–149.

Aromatherapy

Schiller, David, and Carol Schiller, *Aromatherapy for Mind and Body* (New York, NY: Sterling Publishing, 1996).

The Burton Goldberg Group, *Alternative Medicine: the Definitive Guide* (Fife, WA: Future Medicine Publishing, 1995).

Wilson, Roberta, *Aromatherapy for Vibrant Health and Beauty* (Garden City Park, NY: Avery Publishing Group, 1995).

Hay, Isabelle, M. Jamieson, and A. Ormerod, "Randomized Trial of Aromatherapy," *Archives of Dermatology* 134(11) (November 1998): 1349–1352.

Homeopathy

Callinam, Paul, *Family Homeopathy* (New Canaan, CT: Keats Publishing, 1995).

Castro, Miranda, *The Complete Homeopathy Handbook* (New York, NY: St. Martin's Press, 1990).

Horvilleur, Alain, *The Family Guide to Homeopathy* (Alexandria, VA: Health & Homeopathy Publishing, 1986).

Lockie, Andrew, and N. Giddes, *The Complete Guide to Homeopathy* (New York: DK Publishing, 1995).

Monte, Tom, with editors of *Natural Health,* "Homeopathy," *New Age Journal's Annual Guide to Holistic Living* (1998): 58, 121–124.

Ross, Barry, *The Family Health Guide to Homeopathy* (Berkeley, CA: Celestial Arts, 1992).

The Burton Goldberg Group, *Alternative Medicine: The Definitive Guide* (Fife, WA: Future Medicine Publishing, 1995).

Ullman, Dana, *The Consumer's Guide to Homeopathy* (New York, NY: Tarcher/Putnam, 1995).

Weiner, Michael, and K. Goss, *The Complete Book of Homeopathy* (Garden City Park, NY: Avery Publishing Group, 1989).

Acupuncture and Acupressure

Acupuncture.com. World Wide Web address http://www.acupuncture.com/ Experiences.

Bauer, Cathryn, *Acupressure for Everybody* (New York, NY: Henry Holt and Company, 1991).

Cao, LQ, and T. Wang, "The Change of the Concentration of Substance P in the Rats 'Channel Point' Skin and Plasma in the Acupuncture Analgesia," *Chen Tzu Yen Chiu (Acupuncture Research)* 14(4) (1989): 452–462.

Gach, Michael, *Acupressure's Potent Points* (New York, NY: Bantam Books, 1990).

Hu, X., B. Wu, J. Xu, X. Huang, and J. Hau, "Studies on the Low Skin Impedance Points and the Feature of its Distribution Along the Channels by Microcomputer," *Chen Tzu Yen Chiu (Acupuncture Research)* 18(2) (1993): 163–167.

Jacobs, Jennifer, MD, consultant editor, *Encyclopedia of Alternative Medicine* (Boston, MA: Journey Editions, 1996).

Kimura, M., F. Mastrogiovanni, S. Toda, K. Kuroiwa, K. Tohya, R. Sugata, and M. Ohnishi, "An Electron Microscopic Study of the Acupuncture or Moxibustion Stimulated Regional Skin and Lymph Node in Experimental Animals," *American Journal of Chinese Medicine* 16(3-4) (1988): 159–167.

Lee, J.S., S.K. Ahn, and S.H. Lee, "Factitial Panniculitis Induced by Cupping and Acupuncture," *Cutis* 55(4) (April 1995): 217–218.

Markowitz, S.B., C.M. Nunez, S. Klitzman, A.A. Munshi, W.S. Kim, J. Eisinger, and P.J. Landrigan, "Lead Poisoning Due to Hai Ge Fen. The Porphyrin Content of Individual Erythrocytes," *Journal of the American Medical Association* 271(12) (March 23–30, 1994): 932–934.

Rosenfeld, Isadore, *Dr. Rosenfeld's Guide to Alternative Medicine* (New York, NY: Fawcett Columbine, 1996).

Rosted, P. "A Protocol for Successful Treatment of Chronic Skin Diseases with Acupuncture," *American Journal of Acupuncture* 20(4) (1992): 321–326.

Shoukang, L., "Acupuncture and Moxibustion in the Treatment of Dermatoses," *Journal of Traditional Chinese Medicine* 13(1) (1993): 69–75.

The Burton Goldberg Group, *Alternative Medicine: The Definitive Guide* (Fife, WA: Future Medicine Publishing, 1995).

Woodham, Anne, and D. Peters, *Encyclopedia of Healing Therapies* (New York, NY: Dorling Kindersley Publishing, 1997).

Yihou, X., "Treatment of Facial Skin Diseases with Acupuncture. A Report of 129 Cases" *Journal of Traditional Chinese Medicine* 10(1) (1990): 22–25.

Other Skin Therapies

Benoit, L.J., and E.H. Harrell, "Biofeedback and Control of Skin Cell Proliferation in Psoriasis," *Psychological Reports* 46(3 part 1) (June 1980): 831–839.

Bilkis, Michael, and K. Mark, " Mind-Body-Medicine....Practical Applications in Dermatology," *Archives of Dermatology* 134 (November 1998): 1437–1441.

Domar, A.D., J.M. Noe, and H. Benson, "The Preoperative Use of the Relaxation Response with Ambulatory Surgery Patients," *Journal of Human Stress* 13 (B) (Fall 1987): 101–107.

Fawzy, F.I., N.W. Fawzy, CS Hyun, R. Elashoff, D. Guthrie, J.L. Fahey, and D.L. Morton, "Malignant Melanoma: Effects of an Early Structured Psychiatric Intervention, Coping, and Affective State on Recurrence and Survival 6 Years Yater," *Archives of General Psychiatry* 50 (1993): 681–689.

Fugh-Berman, Adriane, *Alternative Medicine: What Works* (Baltimore, MD: Williams and Wilkins, 1997).

Goodman, M., "An Hypothesis Explaining the Successful Treatment of Psoriasis with Thermal Biofeedback: A Case Report," *Biofeedback and Self Regulation* 19(4) (December 1994): 347–352.

Grossbart, Ted, and Carl Sherman, *Skin Deep* (Santa Fe, NM: Health Press, 1992).

Healthy.Net. World Wide Web address http://www.healthy.net/library/articles/RBUllman/sayingsk.htm, accessed 24 January 1998.

Hughes, H.H., R. England, and D.A. Goldsmith, "Biofeedback and Psychotherapeutic Treatment of Psoriasis: A Brief Report," *Psychological Reports* 48(1) (February 1981): 99–102.

Kidd, C.B., "Congenital Ichthyosiform Erythroderma Treated by Hypnosis," *British Journal of Dermatology* 78(2) (February 1966):101–105.

Mason, A.A., "A Case of Ichthyosiform Erythroderma of Brocq Treated by Hypnosis," *British Medical Journal* 2(1952): 422–423.

Mine, H., "Itch and the Heat Tolerance Scale: Effects of Thermographic Biofeedback," *Shinrigaku Kenkyu (Japanese Journal of Psychology)* 62(6): 335–341.

O'Sullivan, Richard, G. Lipper, and E. Lerner, "The Neuro-Immuno-Cutaneous-Endocrine Network: Relationship of Mind and Skin," *Archives of Dermatology* 134 (November 1998): 1431–1435.

Putt, S.C., L. Weinstein, and M.T. Dzindolet, "A Case Study: Massage, Relaxation, and Reward for Treatment of Alopecia Areata," *Psychological Reports* 74(3, part 2) (1994): 1315–1318.

Rice, B.I.; and J.V. Schindler, "Effect of Thermal Biofeedback-Assisted Relaxation Training on Blood Circulation in the Lower Extremities of a Population with Diabetes," *Diabetes Care* 15(7) (July 1992): 853–858.

Schneck, J.M., "Hypnotherapy for Ichthyosis," *Psychosomatics* 7(4) (July-August 1966):233–235.

Seville, R.H., "Psoriasis and Stress," *British Journal of Dermatology* 97(3) (September 1977): 297–302.

Shapiro, Debbie, *Your Body Speaks Your Mind: How Your Thoughts and Emotions Affect Your Health* (Freedom, CA: The Crossing Press, 1997).

Susskind, W., and R.J. McGuire, "The Emotional Factor in Psoriasis," *Scottish Medical Journal* 4(1959): 503–507.

The Burton Goldberg Group, *Alternative Medicine: The Definitive Guide* (Fife, WA: Future Medicine Publishing, 1995).

Thomsen, Robert, "Spirituality in Medical Practice," *Archives of Dermatology* 134 (November 1998): 1443–1446.

Tsushima, William, "Current Psychological Treatments for Stress-Related Skin Disorders," *Cutis* 42 (November 1988): 402–404.

Vedic-Health.Com. World Wide Web address http://www.vedic-health.com/intro.html, accessed 21 September 1997.

PART TWO: COMMON SKIN PROBLEMS

Acne

Jin, L, "Treatment of Adolescent Acne with Acupuncture," *Journal of Traditional Chinese Medicine* 13(3) (1993): 187–188.

Athlete's Foot

Caceres, A., B. Lopez, X. Juarez, J. del Aguila, and S. Garcia, "Plants Used in Guatemala for the Treatment of Dermatophytic Infections. 2. Evaluation of Antifungal Activity of Seven American Plants," *Journal of Ethnopharmacology* 40(3) (December 1993): 207–213.

Bedsores

Anthony, D. "The Treatment of Decubitus Ulcers: A Century of Misinformation in the Textbooks," *Journal of Advanced Nursing* 24 (1996): 309–316.

Comorosan, S., R. Vasilco, M. Arghiropol, L. Paslaru, V. Jieanu, and S. Stealea, "The Effect of Diapulse Therapy on the Healing of Decubitus Ulcer," *Romanian Journal of Physiology* 30 (1–2) (January-June 1993): 41–45.

Griffin, J.W., R.E. Tooms, R.A. Mendius, J.K. Clifft, R. Vander Zwaag, and F. el-Zeky, "Efficacy of High Voltage Pulsed Current for Healing of Pressure Ulcers in Patients with Spinal Cord Injury," *Physical Therapy* 71(6) (June 1991): 433–442, 442–444.

Itoh, M., J.S. Montemayor, Jr., E. Matsumoto, A. Eason, M.H. Lee, and F.S. Folk, "Accelerated Wound Healing of Pressure Ulcers by Pulsed High Peak Power Electromagnetic Energy (Diapulse)," *Decubitus* 4(1) (February 1991):24–25, 29–34.

Kloth, L.C., and J.A. Feedar, "Acceleration of Wound Healing with High Voltage, Monophasic, Pulsed Current," *Physical Therapy* 68(4) (April 1988): 503–508.

Mawson, A.R., F.H. Siddiqui, J.J. Biundo, Jr., "Enhancing Host Resistance to Pressure Ulcers: A New Approach to Prevention," *Preventive Medicine* 22(3) (May 1993): 433–450.

Salzberg, C.A., S.A. Cooper-Vastola, F. Perez, M.G. Viehbeck, and D.W. Byrne, "The Effects of Non-Thermal Pulsed Electromagnetic Energy on Wound Healing of Pressure Ulcers in Spinal-Cord-Injured Patients: A Randomized, Double-Blind Study," *Ostomy Wound Management* 41(3) (April 1995): 42–44, 46, 48.

Stefanovska, A., L. Vodovnik, H. Benko, and R. Turk, "Treatment of Chronic Wounds by Means of Electric and Electromagnetic Fields. Part 2. Value of FES Parameters for Pressure Sore Treatment," *Medical and Biological Engineering and Computing* 31(3) (May 1993): 213–220.

Vodovnik, L., and R. Karba, "Treatment of Chronic Wounds by Means of Electric and Electromagnetic Fields. Part 1. Literature Review," *Medical and Biological Engineering and Computing* 30(3) (May 1992): 257–266.

Wood, J.M., P.E. Evans 3d, K.U. Schallreuter, W.E. Jacobson, R. Sufit, J. Newman, C. White, and M. Jacobson, "A Multicenter Study on the Use of Pulsed Low-Intensity Direct Current for Healing Chronic Stage II and Stage III Decubitus Ulcers," *Archives of Dermatology* 129(8) (August 1993): 999–1009.

Bites and Stings, Insect and Spider

Hill, N., C. Stam, S. Tuinder, and R.A. van Haselen, "A Placebo Controlled Clinical Trial Investigating the Efficacy of a Homeopathic After-Bite Gel in Reducing Mosquito Bite Induced Erythema," *European Journal of Clinical Pharmacology* 49(1-2) (1995): 103–108.

Osborne, S.E., "Summer First Aid: Natural Ways to Tell Bugs to Bug Off, Flies to be Gone and Bees to Flit Away," *Vegetarian Times* 238 (June 1997): 78–83.

Bruises

Pinnel, S.R., S. Murad; and D. Darr, "Induction of Collagen Synthesis by Ascorbic Acid. A Possible Mechanism," *Archives of Dermatology* 123(12) (December 1987): 1684–1686.

Burns

Castillo, E., H. Sumano, T.I. Fortoul, and A. Zepeda, "The Influence of Pulsed Electrical Stimulation on the Wound Healing of Burned Rat Skin," *Archives of Medical Research* 26(2) (Summer 1995): 185–189.

Cold Sores

Kurokawa, M., H. Ochiai, K. Nagasaka, M. Neki, H. Xu, S. Kadota, S. Sutardjo. "Antiviral Traditional Medicines Against Herpes Simplex Virus, Poliovirus, and Measles Virus in Vitro and Their Therapeutic Efficacies for HSV-1 Infection in Mice," *Antiviral Research* 22(2–3) (October 1993): 175–188.

Liao, S.J., and T.A. Liao, "Acupuncture Treatment for Herpes Simplex Infections. A Clinical Case Report," *Acupuncture and Electro-Therapeutics Research* 16(3–4) (1991): 135–142.

Dermatitis (Rashes)

Qinglin, Yang, "Acupuncture Treatment of 139 Cases of Neurodermatitis," *Journal of Traditional Chinese Medicine* 13(2) (1993): 3–4.

Eczema

Bjorna, H., and B. Kaada, "Successful Treatment of Itching and Atopic Eczema by Transcutaneous Nerve Stimulation," *Acupuncture and Electro-Therapeutics Research* 12(2) (1987): 101–112.

Department of Psychiatry, University of Oxford, "Treatment of Atopic Dermatitis: A Comparison of Psychological and Dermatological Approaches to Relapse Prevention," *Journal of Consulting and Clinical Psychology* 63(4) (August 1995): 624–635.

Grossbart, T., and C. Sherman, *Skin Deep. A Mind/Body Program for Healthy Skin* (Santa Fe, NM: Health Press, 1992).

Hoffman, David, *The Complete Illustrated Holistic Herbal* (Rockport, MA: Element Books, 1996).

http:www.medline.com/alternative health/message board; accessed 20 January 1997 through 25 October 1997.

http:www.members.aol.com/evenstar8/role.html/Healthimed; accessed 20 January 1997 through 25 October 1997, 3 December 1997.

Keville, Kathi, *Herbs for Health and Healing* (Emmaus, PA: Rodale Press, 1996).

Latchman, Y., G.A. Bungy, D.J. Atherton, M.H. Rustin, and J. Brostoff, "Efficacy of Traditional Chinese Herbal Therapy in Vitro. A Model System for Atopic Eczema: Inhibition of CD23 Expression on Blood Monocytes," *British Journal of Dermatology* 132 (1995): 592–598.

Lockie, Andrew, *The Family Guide to Homeopathy* (New York, NY: Fireside Books, 1989).

Meredith, Sheena, *The Natural Way With Eczema. A Comprehensive Guide to Effective Treatment* (Rockport, MA: Element Books, 1994).

Ody, Penelope. *Home Herbal* (New York, NY: Dorling Kindersley, 1995).

Ody, Penelope, *The Complete Medicinal Herbal* (New York, NY: Dorling Kindersley, 1993).

Sheehan, M., and D.J. Atherton, "One-Year Follow-Up of Children Treated with Chinese Medicinal Herbs for Atopic Eczema," *British Journal of Dermatology* 130 (1994): 488–493.

Sheehan, M., and D.J. Atherton, "A Controlled Trial of Traditional Chinese Medicinal Plants in Widespread Non-Exudative Atopic Eczema," *British Journal of Dermatology* 126 (1992): 179–184.

Sheehan, M., H. Stevens, L.S. Ostlere, D.J. Atherton, J. Brostoff, and M.H. Rustin, "Follow-Up of Adult Patients with Atopic Eczema Treated with Chinese Herbal Therapy for 1 Year," *Clinical and Experimental Dermatology* 20 (1995): 136–140.

Sheehan, M., M.H. Rustin, D.J. Atherton, C. Buckley, D.J. Harris, J. Brostoff, L. Ostlere, and A. Dawson. " Efficacy of Traditional Chinese Herbal Therapy in Adult Atopic Dermatitis," *Lancet* 340 (4 July 1992): 13–17.

Spence, D.S., "Homeopathic Treatment of Eczema," *British Homeopathic Journal* 80(2) (April 1991): 74–81.

The Burton Goldberg Group, *Alternative Medicine: The Definitive Guide* (Fife, WA: Future Medicine Publishing, 1995).

Traub, M., *Dermatological Diagnosis and Natural Therapeutics* (Kailua Kona, HI: 1995).

Ullman, Dana, *The Consumer's Guide to Homeopathy* (New York, NY: Tarcher/Putnam, 1995).

Xu, X.J., P. Banerjee, M.H. Rustin, and L.W. Poulter, "Modulation by Chinese Herbal Therapy of Immune Mechanisms in the Skin of Patients with Atopic Eczema," *British Jounal of Dermatology* 136 (1997): 54–59.

Hives

Chen, Chung-Jen, and H.S. Yu, "Acupuncture Treatment of Urticaria," *Archives of Dermatology* 134 (November 1998): 1397–1399.

Horvilleur, Alain, *The Family Guide to Homeopathy* (Alexandria, VA: Health & Homeopathy Publishing, 1986).

Itching

Lundeberg, T., L. Bondesson, and M. Thomas, "Effect of Acupuncture on Experimentally Induced Itch," *British Journal of Dermatology* 117(6) (December 1987): 771–777.

Monk, B.E., "Transcutaneous Electronic Nerve Stimulation in the Treatment of Generalized Pruritus," *Clinical and Experimental Dermatology* 18(1) (January 1993): 67–68.

Ward, L., E. Wright, and S.B. McMahon, "A Comparison of the Effects of Noxious and Innocuous Counterstimuli on Experimentally Induced Itch and Pain," *Pain* 64(1) (January 1996): 129–138.

Poison Ivy, Oak, and Sumac

Liao, S.J., "Acupuncture for Poison Ivy Contact Dermatitis. A Clinical Case Report," *Acupuncture and Electro-Therapeutics Research* 13(1) (1988): 31–39.

Psoriasis

Abels, D., R. Theodore, and J. Bearman, "Treatment of Psoriasis at a Dead Sea Dermatology Clinic," *International Journal of Dermatology* 34(2) (February 1995): 134–137.

Callinan, Paul, *Family Homeopathy* (New Canaan, CT: Keats Publishing, 1995).

Editors of Reader's Digest, *Reader's Digest Family Guide to Natural Medicine* (Pleasantville, NY: The R.D. Association, 1993).

Evans, Mark, *The Ultimate Natural Health and Healing Book* (New York, NY: Lorenz Books, 1997).

Fine, R.M., "Psoriasis and Autoimmune Disease," *International Journal of Dermatology* 27(1) (January–February 1988): 17–18.

Fleischer, A.B., Jr., S.R. Felman, S.R. Rapp, D.M. Reboussin, M.L. Exum, and A.R. Clark, "Alternative Therapies Commonly Used Within a Population of Patients with Psoriasis," *Cutis* 58(3) (September 1996): 216–220.

Goodman, M, "An Hypothesis Explaining the Successful Treatment of Psoriasis with Thermal Biofeedback: A Case Report," *Biofeedback and Self-Regulation* 19(4) (1994): 347–351.

Jerner, B., M. Skogh, and A. Vahlquist, " A Controlled Trial of Acupuncture in Psoriasis: No Convincing Effect," *Acta Dermato-Venereologica* 77(2) (March 1997): 154–156.

Liao, S.J., and T.A. Liao, "Acupuncture Treatment for Psoriasis: A Retrospective Case Report." *Acupuncture and Electro-Therapeutics Research* 17(3) (July–September 1992): 195–208.

Monte, Tom, and the editors of *Natural Health* Magazine, *The Complete Guide to Natural Healing* (New York, NY: Berkley, 1997).

Pagano, John, *Healing Psoriasis: The Natural Alternative* (Englewood Cliffs, NJ: The Pagano Organization, 1996).

Price, M.L., I. Mottahedin, and P.R. Mayo, "Can Psychotherapy Help Patients with Psoriasis?" *Clinical and Experimental Dermatology* 16(2) (March 1991): 114–117.

Reeves, W.H., D.E. Fisher; R. Wisniewolski; A.B. Gottlieb, and N. Chiorazzi, "Psoriasis and Raynaud's Phenomenon Associated with Autoantibodies to U1 and U2 Small Nuclear Ribonucleoproteins," *The New England Journal of Medicine* 315(2) (10 July 1986):105–111.

Seville, R.H., "Stress and Psoriasis: The Importance of Insight and Empathy in Prognosis," *Journal of the American Academy of Dermatology* 20(1) (January 1989): 97–100.

Shealy, Norman, *The Complete Family Guide to Alternative Medicine* (Rockport, MA: Element Publishing, 1996).

The Burton Goldberg Group, *Alternative Medicine: The Definitive Guide* (Fife, WA: Future Medicine Publishing, 1995).

Traub, M., *Dermatological Diagnosis and Natural Therapeutics,* 3rd ed. (Kailua Kona, HI: by the author, 1995).

Ubogui, J., F. Stengel, M. Kien, L. Sevinsky, and L. Lupo, "Thermalism in Argentina," *Archives of Dermatology* 134 (November 1998): 1411–1412.

Walsh, D., "Using Aromatherapy in the Management of Psoriasis," *Nursing Standard* 11(13–15) (18 December 1996): 53–56.

Weil, Andrew, "Soothing Psoriasis, Naturally." *Self Healing.* January 1999, 2–3.

Winchell, S., and R. Watts, "Relaxation Therapies in the Treatment of Psoriasis and Possible Pathophysiologic Mechanisms," *Journal of the American Academy of Dermatology* 18(1) (January 1988): 101–104.

Zachariae, R., H. Oster, P. Bjerring, and K. Kragballe, "Effects of Psychologic Intervention on Psoriasis: A Preliminary Report," *Journal of the American Academy of Dermatology* 34(6) (June 1996): 1008–1015.

Rosacea

http://www.acupuncture.com/Experiences

Xu, Yihou, "Treatment of Facial Skin Diseases with Acupuncture—A Report of 129 Cases," *Journal of Traditional Chinese Medicine* 10(1) (March 1990): 22–25.

Scleroderma

Francaviglia, N., C. Silvestro, M. Maiello, R. Bragazzi, and C. Bernucci, "Spinal Cord Stimulation for the Treatment of Progressive Systemic Sclerosis and Raynaud's Syndrome," *British Journal of Neurosurgery* 8(5) (1994): 567–571.

Kruk, M., M. Borkowski, E. Wojtal, and R. Gorewicz, "Rheographic Evaluation of the Changes in Blood Flow after Superficial Electric Stimulation in Patients with Raynaud's Disease or Syndrome," *Polski Tygodnik Lekarski (Polish Medical Weekly)* 44(43–45) (23 October–6 November 1989): 921–923 (Polish).

Maeda, M., H. Kachi, N. Ichihashi, Z. Oyama, and Y. Kitajima, "The Effect of Electrical Acupuncture-Stimulation Therapy Using Thermography and Plasma Endothelin Levels in Patients with Progressive Systemic Sclerosis," *Journal of Dermatology Science* 17(2) (June 1998): 151–152.

Shingles

http://www.acupuncture.com/Experiences

Skin Cancer

Fawzy, F.I., N.W. Fawzy, C.S. Hyun, R. Elashoff, D. Guthrie, J.L. Fahey, and D.L. Morton,. "Malignant Melanoma: Effects of an Early Structured Psychiatric Intervention, Coping, and Affective State on Recurrence and Survival 6 Years Later," *Archives of General Psychiatry* 50 (1993): 681–689.

Schauble, M.K., M.B. Habal, and H.D. Gullick, "Inhibition of Experimental Tumor Growth in Hamsters by Small Direct Currents," *Archives of Pathology and Laboratory Medicine* 101(6) (June 1977): 294–297.

Sollner, W., M. Zingg-Schir, G. Rumpold, and P. Fritsch, "Attitude Toward Alternative Therapy, Compliance with Standard Treatment, and Need for Emotional Support in Patients with Melanoma," *Archives of Dermatology* 133 (1997): 316–321.

Skin Ulcers

Assimacopoulos, D., "Low Intensity Negative Electric Current in the Treatment of Ulcers of the Leg Due to Chronic Venous Insufficiency.

Preliminary Report of Three Cases," *American Surgeon* 115(5) (May 1968): 683–687.

Assimacopoulos, D., "Wound Healing Promotion by the Use of Negative Electric Current," *American Surgeon* 34(6) (June 1968): 423–431.

Bach, S., K. Bilgrav, F. Gottrup, and T.E. Jorgensen, "The Effect of Electrical Current on Healing Skin Incision. An Experimental Study," *European Journal of Surgery* 157(3) (March 1991): 171–174.

Baker, L.L., R.Chambers, S.K. Demuth, and F. Villar, "Effects of Electrical Stimulation on Wound Healing in Patients with Diabetic Ulcers," *Diabetes Care* 20(3) (March 1997): 405–412.

Biedebach, M.C., "Accelerated Healing of Skin Ulcers by Electrical Stimulation and the Intracellular Physiological Mechanisms Involved," *Acupuncture and Electro-Therapeutics Research* 14(1) (1989): 43–60.

Carley, P.J., and S.F. Wainapel, "Electrotherapy for Acceleration of Wound Healing: Low Intensity Direct Current," *Archives of Physical Medicine and Rehabilitation* 66(7) (July 1985): 443–446.

Gault W.R., and P.F. Gatens, Jr., "Use of Low Intensity Direct Current in Management of Ischemic Skin Ulcers," *Physical Therapy* 56(3) (March 1976): 265–269.

Jiang, H., "Acceleration of Epidermis Proliferation by Direct Current Stimulation (An Experimental Study)," *Chung-Hua Cheng Hsing Shao Shang Wai Ko Tsa Chih (Chinese Journal of Plastic Surgery and Burns)* 8 (2) (June 1992): 136–138, 166–167 (Chinese).

Jivegard, L., L.E. Augustinsson, C.A. Carlsson, and J. Holm, "Long-Term Results by Epidural Spinal Electrical Stimulation (ESES) in Patients with Inoperable Severe Lower Limb Ischemia," *European Journal of Vascular Surgery* 1(5) (October 1987): 345–349.

Kaada, B., and M. Emru, " Promoted Healing of Leprous Ulcers by Transcutaneous Nerve Stimulation," *Acupuncture and Electro-Therapeutics Research* 13(4) (1988): 165–176.

Loubser, P.G., D. Cardus, L.R. Pickard, and W.G. McTaggart, "Effects of Unilateral, Low-Freqency, Neuromuscular Stimulation on Superficial Circulation in Lower Extremities of Patients with Peripheral Vascular Disease," *Medical Instrumentation* 22(2) (April 1988): 82–97.

Mulder, G.D., "Treatment of Open-Skin Wounds with Electric Stimulation," *Archives of Physical Medicine and Rehabilitation* 72(6) (May 1991): 375–377.

Page, C.F., and W.R. Gault, "Managing Ischemic Skin Ulcers," *American Family Physician* 11(2) (February 1975): 108–114.

Sampere C.T., J.A. Guasch, C.M. Paladino, M. Sanchez Casalongue, and B. Elencwajg, "Spinal Cord Stimulation for Severely Ischemic Limbs," *Pacing and Clinical Electrophysiology* 12(2) (February 1989): 273–279.

Wolcott, L.E., P.C. Wheeler, H.M. Hardwicke, and B.A. Rowley, "Accelerated Healing of Skin Ulcer by Electrotherapy: Preliminary Clinical Results," *Southern Medical Journal* 62(7) (July 1969): 795–801.

Surgery

Im, M.J., W.P. Lee, and J.E. Hoopes, "Effect of Electrical Stimulation on Survival of Skin Flaps in Pigs," *Physical Therapy* 70(1) (January 1990): 37–40.

Lundeberg, T., J. Kjartansson, and U. Samuelsson, "Effect of Electrical Nerve Stimulation on Healing of Ischemic Skin Flaps," *Lancet* 8613(2) (24 September 1988): 712–714.

Politis, M.J., M.F. Zanakis, and J.E. Miller, " Enhanced Survival of Full-Thickness Skin Grafts following the Application of DC Electrical Fields," *Plastic and Reconstructive Surgery* 84(2) (August 1989): 267–272.

Weiss, D.S., R. Kirsner, and W. Eaglstein, "Electrical Stimulation and Wound Healing," *Archives of Dermatology* 126 (February 1990): 222–225.

Varicose Veins and Spider Veins

Pittler, Max, and E. Ernst, "Horse-Chestnut Seed Extract for Chronic Venous Insufficiency," *Archives of Dermatology* 134 (November 1998): 1356–1360.

Vitiligo

Capitanio, M., E. Cappelletti, and R. Filippini, "Traditional Antileukodermic Herbal Remedies in the Mediterranean Area," *Journal of Ethnopharmacology* 27 (1–2) (November 1989): 193–211.

Montes, L.F., M.L. Diaz, J. Lajous, and N.J. Garcia, "Folic Acid and Vitamin B_{12} in Vitiligo: A Nutritional Approach," *Cutis* 59(1) (July 1992): 39–42.

Warts

Kainz, J., G. Kozel, M. Haidvogl, and J. Smolle, "Homeopathic Versus Placebo Therapy of Children with Warts on the Hands: A Randomized, Double-Blind Clinical Trial," *Dermatology* 193(4) (1996): 318–320.

Xu, Y., "Treatment of Facial Skin Diseases with Acupuncture—A Report of 129 Cases," *Journal of Traditional Chinese Medicine* 10(1) (March 1990): 22–25.

Wrinkles

Schnitzler, L., and A. Adrien, "Cutaneous Electric Stimulation in Aging. Electroacupuncture of Wrinkles following the Procedure of Ph. Simonin," *Revue Française de Gynecologie et d'Obstetrique (French Review of Gynecology and Obstetrics)* 86(6) (1991): 461–466 (French).

PART THREE: SKIN-CARE TREATMENTS AND TECHNIQUES

Bodywork

Kurz W., R. Kurz, Y.I. Litmanovitch, H. Romanoff, Y. Pfeifer, and F.G. Sulman, "Effect of Manual Lymphdrainage Massage on Blood Components and Urinary Neurohormones in Chronic Lymphedema," *Angiology* 32(2) (February 1981): 119–127.

Norman, Laura, *Feet First: A Guide to Foot Reflexology* (New York, NY: Fireside Books, 1988).

Shapiro, Debbie, *Your Body Speaks Your Mind* (Freedom, CA.: The Crossing Press, 1997).

Guided Imagery Techniques

Epstein, Gerald. *Healing Visualizations: Creating Health Through Imagery* (New York, NY: Bantam New Age Books, 1989).

Light Therapy

Corvo, Joseph, and Lilian Verner-Bonds, *Healing With Color Zone Therapy* (Freedom, CA: The Crossing Press, 1998).

Liberman, Jacob, *Light: Medicine of the Future* (Santa Fe, NM: Bear & Co. Publishing, 1992).

Sound and Music Therapy

Lingerman, Hal A., *The Healing Energies of Music* (Wheaton, IL: Quest Books, 1995).

Resources

Baar Products
P.O. Box 60
Downingtown, PA 19335
800-269-2502 or 610-873-4591
Fax: 610-873-7945
http://www.baar.com
Manufacturer of Glyco-Thymoline.

Caleel-Hayden International
518 17th Street, Suite 1800
Denver, CO 80202
800-348-3078
Fax: 303-573-5400
http://www.cellex-c.com
Manufacturer of Cellex-C skin-care products.

Covermark Cosmetics
157 Veterans Drive, Suite D
Northvale, NJ 07647
800-524-1120
http://www.covermark.com
Manufacturer of Covermark concealing cosmetics.

Dermablend
1135 Pleasant View Terrace West
Ridgefield, NJ 07657
877-900-6700 or 201-313-8823
Fax 201-313-8828
http://www.dermablend.com
Manufacturer of Dermablend corrective cosmetic system.

Dermatologic Cosmetic
Laboratories, Ltd.
20 Commerce Street
East Haven, CT 06512
203-467-1570
Fax: 203-467-1573
Manufacturer of C Scape Serum.

Fallene, Ltd.
677 West DeKalb Pike
King of Prussia, PA 19406
800-332-5536
http://www.fallene.com
Manufacturer of Total Block sunblock.

HonTech Foundation for Medical
Technology
P.O. Box 400956
Cambridge, MA 02140
800-881-2933
Fax: 781-322-4527
http://www.itchstopper.com
Manufacturer of ItchStopper.

Merz Pharmaceuticals
4215 Tudor Lane
Greensboro, NC 27410
800-334-0514 or 336-856-2003
Fax: 336-856-0107
http://www.merzusa.com
Manufacturer of Mederma.

Neostrata Company, Inc.
4 Research Way

Princeton, NJ 08540
800-225-9411
http://www.neostrata.com
*Manufacturer of Exuviance skin-care
products.*

Aesthetics, Inc.
800-934-7455
*Manufacturer of the Rejuvenique facial
electroacupressure device.*

ReJuveness Pharmaceuticals
100 Saratoga Village Boulevard
Ballston Spa, NY 12020
518-899-8115
http://www.rejuveness.com
Manufacturer of ReJuveness.

Sun Precautions
2815 Wetmore Avenue
Everett, WA 98201
888-SOLUMBRA
800-882-7860
http://www.sunprecautions.com
*Manufacturer of Solumbra sun-
protective clothing and accessories.*

ORGANIZATIONS

Conventional Dermatology

American Academy of
Dermatology
980 North Meacham Road
Schaumburg, IL 60173-4965
847-330-0230
Fax: 847-330-0050
http://www.aad.org

American Skin Association
150 East 58th Street, 33rd floor
New York, NY. 10155-0002
800-499-SKIN
Fax: 212-688-6547

American Society of Dermatologic
Surgery
930 North Meacham Road
Schaumburg, IL 60173-6016
708-330-9830

Plastic Surgery Research
Foundation
P.O. Box 2586
La Jolla, CA 92038
619-454-3212

Alternative Medicine (General)

American Association of
Naturopathic Physicians
601 Valley Street, Suite 105
Seattle, WA 98109
206-298-0125
http://www.naturopathic.org

American Chiropractic Association
1701 Clarendon Boulevard
Arlington, VA 22209
Tel. 703-276-8800
http://www.amerchiro.org

American College of Advancement
in Medicine
P.O. Box 3427
Laguna Hills, CA 92654
800-532-3688

American Holistic Health
   Association
P.O. Box 17400
Anaheim, CA 92817-7400
714-779-6152
http://www.ahha.org

American Osteopathic Association
142 East Ontario Street
Chicago, IL 60611-2864
800-621-1773 or 312-202-8061
http://www.am-osteo-assn.org

American Self-Help Clearinghouse
Saint Clare's Health Services
25 Pocono Road
Denville, NJ 07834
973-625-9565
http://www.cmhc.com/selfhelp

Bastyr University of Naturopathic
   Medicine
144 NE 54th Street
Seattle, WA 98103
425-823-1300
http://www.bastyr.edu

Foundation for the Advancement
   of Innovative Medicine
100 Airport Executive Park,
   No. 105
Nanuet, NY 10954
914-371-3246
Fax: 914-371-4790
http://www.faim.org

Institute of Noetic Sciences
475 Gate Five Road, Suite 300

Sausalito, CA 94965
415-331-5650
http://www.noetic.org

National Center for Complementary and Alternative Medicine
P.O. Box 8218
Silver Spring, MD 20907-8218
888-644-6226
Fax: 301-495-4957
http://www.altmed.od.nih.gov

Diet and Nutrition

California Certified Organic
   Farmers
1115 Mission Street
Santa Cruz, CA 95060
831-423-2263
http://www. ccof.org

Florida Certified Organic Growers
   and Consumers, Inc.
P.O. Box 12311
Gainesville, FL 32604
352-377-6343
http://www.floridaplant.com/FOG

Food Allergy Network
10400 Eaton Place, Suite 107
Fairfax, VA 20030
703-691-3179
http://www.foodallergy.org

Food and Water, Inc.
389 Vermont Route 215
Walden, VT 05873
800-EAT-SAFE

Mothers and Others for Pesticide
  Limits
40 West 20th Street
New York, NY 10011
212-242-0010
e-mail: mothers@mothers.org

Water Quality Association
4151 Naperville Road
Lisle, IL 60532
630-505-0160
http://www.wqa.org

Herbal Medicine

American Botanical Council
P.O. Box 144345
Austin, TX 78714-4345
512-331-8868
http://www.herbalgram.org

American Herbalists Guild
P.O. Box 70
Roosevelt, UT 84066
http://www.healthy.net.herbalists

Herb Research Foundation
1007 Pearl Street, Suite 200
Boulder, CO 80302
303-449-2265
http://www.herbs.org

Aromatherapy

American Alliance of
  Aromatherapy
P.O. Box 750428
Petaluma, CA 94975-0428
707-778-6762

American Society for Phytotherapy
  and Aromatherapy
P.O. Box 3679
South Pasadena, CA 91031
818-457-1742

National Association for Holistic
  Aromatherapy
P.O. Box 17622
Boulder, CO 80308
303-258-3791

Homeopathy

American Foundation for
  Homeopathy
1508 South Garfield
Alhambra, CA 91801

American Institute of Homeopathy
703-246-9501

American Association of
  Homeopathic Pharmacists
P.O. Box 61067
Los Angeles, CA 90061

Foundation for Homeopathic
  Education and Research and
  Homeopathic Educational
  Services
2124 Kittredge Street
Berkeley, CA 94704
510-649-8930
http://www.homeopathic.com

Homeopathic Academy of
  Naturopathic Physicians

12132 SE Foster Place
Portland, OR 97266
503-761-3298
http://www.healthworld.com/
associations/pa/Homeopathic/
hanp/index.html

Homeopathic Pharmacopoeia of
the United States
P.O. Box 40360
4974 Quebec Street NW
Washington, DC 20016

International Foundation for
Homeopathy
206-776-3172

National Center for
Homeopathy
801 North Fairfax Street, Suite 306
Alexandria, VA 22314
703-548-7790
http://www.homeopathic.org

North American Society of
Homeopaths
10700 Old Country Road 15
Minneapolis, MN 55441
541-345-9815

Acupuncture and Acupressure

Acupressure Institute
1533 Shattuck Avenue
Berkeley, CA 94709
800-442-2232 or 510-845-1059
Fax: 510-845-1496
http://www.acupressure.com

American Association of
Acupuncture and Oriental
Medicine
4101 Lake Boone Trail,
Suite 201
Raleigh, NC 27607
919-787-5181

American Association of Oriental
Medicine
433 Front Street
Catasauqua, PA 18032
610-266-1433
Fax: 610-264-2768
http://www.aaom.org

National Acupuncture and
Oriental Medicine Alliance
14637 Starr Road, SE
Olalla, WA 98359
253-851-6896
http://www.acuall.org

National Certification Commission
for Acupuncture and Oriental
Medicine
P.O. Box 97075
Washington, DC 20090-7075
703-548-9004
http://www.nccaom.org

Mind-Body Medicine

American Psychiatric Association
1400 K Street NW
Washington, DC 20005
202-682-6000
http://www.psych.org

American Psychological Association
750 First Street NE
Washington, DC 20002-4242
800-964-2000
http://www.apa.org

Hypnosis

American Board of Hypnotherapy
16842 Von Karman Avenue, Suite
   475
Irvine, CA 92606
800-634-9766
Fax: 714-251-4632
http://www.hypnosis.com

American Society of Clinical
   Hypnosis
33 West Grand Avenue, No. 402
Chicago, IL 60610
847-297-3317
http://www.asch.net

Society for Clinical and
   Experimental Hypnosis
2201 Haeder Road
Pullman, WA 99163
509-332-7555
Fax: 509-332-5907
http://sunsite.utk.edu/JCEH/
   scehframe.htm

Guided Imagery

Academy for Guided Imagery
P.O. Box 2070
Mill Valley, CA 94942
800-726-2070
http://www.healthy.net/agi

Biofeedback

Association for Applied
   Psychophysiology and
   Biofeedback
10200 West 44th Avenue, Suite
   304
Wheat Ridge, CO 80033-2840
800-477-8892 or 303-422-8436
Fax: 303-422-8894
http://www.aapb.org

Biofeedback Certification Institute
   of America
10200 West 44th Avenue, Suite
   310
Wheat Ridge, CO 80033
303-420-2902
E-mail: bcia@resourcenter.com

Bodywork

American Massage Therapy
   Association
820 Davis Street, Suite 100
Evanston, IL 60201-4444
847-864-0123
http://www.amtamassage.org

American Physical Therapy
   Association
1111 North Fairfax Street
Alexandria, VA 22314
800-999-2782
http://www.apta.org

American Society for the
   Alexander Technique
P.O. Box 60008

Florence, MA 01062
800-473-0620 or 413-584-2359
http://www.alexandertech.org

The Feldenkrais Guild of North
    America
3611 SW Hood Avenue, Suite 100
Portland, OR 97201
800-775-2118 or 503-221-6612
Fax: 503-221-6616
http://www.feldenkrais.com

Reflexology Association of
    America
4012 Rainbow, Suite K-PMB#585
Las Vegas, NV 89103-2059
http://www.reflexology-usa.org

The Rolf Institute of Structural
    Integration
205 Canyon Boulevard
Boulder, CO 80302
800-530-8875 or 303-449-5903
Fax: 303-449-5978
http://www.rolf.org

Pain Management

American Academy of Pain
    Management
13947 Mono Way # 4
Sonora, CA 95370
209-533-9744
http://www.aapainmanage.org

American Chronic Pain
    Association
P.O. Box 850

Rocklin, CA 95677
916-632-0922
http://www.theacpa.org

American Pain Society
4700 West Lake Avenue
Glenview, IL 60025
847-375-4715
http://www.ampainsoc.org

National Chronic Pain Outreach
    Association
7979 Old Georgetown Road, Suite
    100
Bethesda, MD 20814-2429
301-652-4948
http://neurosurgery.mgh.harvard.
    edu/ncpainoa.htm

Therapeutic Humor

American Association for
    Therapeutic Humor
222 South Meramec, Suite 303
St. Louis, MO 63105
314-863-6232
http://www.aath.org

Humor and Health Institute
P.O. Box 16814
Jackson, MS 39236-6814
601-957-0075
http://www.intop.net-jrdunn

Specific Disorders

American Cancer Society
1599 Clifton Road, NE

Atlanta, GA 30329
800-227-2345
Fax: 404-325-2217

American College of Mohs
  Micrographic Surgery and
  Cutaneous Oncology
930 North Meacham Road
Schaumburg, IL 60173-6016
708-330-9830
Fax: 708-330-0050

American Lupus Society
3914 Del Amo Boulevard, Suite
  922
Torrance, CA 90503
800-331-1802

American Melanoma
  Foundation
USC/Norris Cancer Center
2025 Zonal Avenue
GH-10–442
Los Angeles, CA 90033-1034
213-226-6352
Fax: 213-224-6925

Herpes Resource Center
P.O. Box 13827
Research Triangle Park, NC 27709
919-361-8488
http://www.ashastd.org

Lupus Foundation of America
1300 Piccard Drive, Suite 200
Rockville, MD 20850-4303
800-558-0121
http://www.lupus.org

National Alopecia Areata
  Foundation
P.O. Box 150760
San Rafael, CA 94915
415-456-4644
http://www.alopeciareata.com

National Cancer Institute
National Institutes of Health
9000 Rockville Pike
Building 31, Room 10A31
Bethesda, MD 20892
800-4-CANCER or 301-496-
  6631
Fax: 301-402-4945

National Eczema Association
1221 SW Yamhill, Suite 303
Portland, OR 90035
503-228-4430
Fax: 503-228-4430

National Foundation for Vitiligo
  and Pigment Disorders
9032 South Normandy Drive
Centerville, OH 45459
513-885-5739

National Herpes Hotline
919-361-8488

National Institute of Arthritis and
  Musculoskeletal and Skin
  Diseases
Box AMS
9000 Rockville Pike
Bethesda, MD 20892
301-495-4484

National Pediculosis Association
P.O. Box 149
Newton, MA 02161
617-449-6487

National Psoriasis Foundation
6000 SW 92nd Street, Suite 300
Portland, OR 97223
800-723-9166
Fax: 503-245-0626
http://www.psoriasis.org

National Rosacea Society
220 South Cook Street,
   Suite 201
Barrington, IL 60010
708-382-8971
Fax: 708-382-5567

National Vitiligo Foundation, Inc.
Box 6337
305 South Broadway, Suite 403
Tyler, TX 75711
903-534-2925
Fax: 903-534-8075
http://www.nvfi.com

Scleroderma Federation
Peabody Office Building
One Newbury Street
Peabody, MA 01960
800-422-1113 or 508-535-6600
Fax: 508-535-6696
http://www.sclerofed.org

Scleroderma Foundation
89 Newbury Street
Danvers, MA 01923
800-722-HOPE
http://www.scleroderma.org

Scleroderma Info Exchange, Inc.
150 Hines Farm Road
Cranston, RI 02921
401-943-3909

Scleroderma Research Foundation
Pueblo Medical Commons
2320 Bath Street, Suite 307
Santa Barbara, CA 93105
805-563-9133
Fax: 805-563-2402

Scleroderma Society
1725 York Avenue, Suite 29–F
New York, NY 10128
212-427-7040

Skin Cancer Foundation
245 Fifth Avenue, Suite 2402
New York, NY 10016
212-725-5176
Fax: 212-725-5751

VZV Research Foundation
   (Shingles/Varicella Zoster)
36 East 72nd Street
New York, NY 10021
212-472-3181

Other

Cosmetic Ingredient Review
1101 17th Street NW, Suite 310
Washington, DC 20036-4702
202-331-0651

Cosmetic Toiletry Fragrance
  Association
1101 17th Street NW, Suite 300
Washington, DC 20036-4792

Office of Cosmetics and Colors
The Food and Drug
  Administration
200 C Street, SW
Washington, DC 20204
202-205-4094

Index

Siegers, C.P., Dr., 64
Skin bacteria, 107
Skin biopsy, 21
Skin cancer, 283–293
Skin care. *See also* Individual conditions
   acupuncture/acupressure for, 80–85
   aromatherapy for, 65–71
   conventional approaches, 18–39,
      23–31
   daily regimens for, 357–359
   diet and nutrition for, 40–51
   herbal medicine for, 52–64
   homeopathy for, 72–79
   other therapies for, 86–96
Skin Deep (Grossbart), 91
Skin examination, 20
Skin lesions, 9–10
   primary, 10, *11* tab.
   secondary, 10, *11–12* tab.
   special, 10, *12–13* tab.
Skin self-examination, 360–361
Skin structure, 7–9
Skin ulcers, 294–299
Smith, Captain John, 63
Sollner, W., Dr., 285
Sound therapy, 362–364
Specialist referrals, 37
Spider bites. *See* Bites and stings
Spider veins, 311–316
Spirituality, 92
Squamous cell carcinomas, 283, 286–287
Squamous cells, 8
Staphylococcus aureus, 102, 141
Stasis dermatitis, 174
Stefanovska, A., 129
Stings. *See* Bites and stings
Stress, 86
   reduction of, 86–87
Strickland, F.M., Dr., 59
Subacute cutaneous lupus erythematosus
   (SCLE), 217–218
Subcutaneous layer, 7
Successing, 73
Sullican, Dr., 89
Sunburn, 300–305
Superficial chemical peels, 32
Supplements. *See* Nutritional supplements

Surgery, 306–309
Susskind, W., Dr., 86
Sweat glands, 9, 14–15
Systemic lupus erythematosus (SLE),
   217–218

Tazarotene (Tazorac), 109–110
Tea tree oil, 63, 70
Telogen phase, 10
TENS (transcutaneous electric nerve
   stimulation), 36–37, 198, 215,
   363
Terminal hairs, 10
Therapeutic diet, 41–42
Therapeutic touch, 343
Third-degree burns, 150
Thomsen, R.J., Dr., 92
Ticks, 130
Tinctures, 58, 348–349
Tinea, 253–256
Tinea pedis, 120
Topical antibiotics, 109
Topical application, 67–68
Topical preparations, *23–27* tab.
Toxins, 248
Traditional Chinese medicine (TCM),
   81–83
Transcendental meditation, 353
Treatments
   acupuncture/acupressure, 80–85
   aromatherapy, 65–71
   conventional, 21–38, *23–31* tab.
   diet and nutrition, 40–51
   herbal medicine, 52–64
   homeopathy, 72–79
   other therapies, 86–96
Tretinoin (Retin-A), 44, 109
Troubleshooting guide, 100–101

Ullman, M., Dr., 91
Ultraviolet light therapy, 35, 189–190,
   298
Ultraviolet (UV) rays, 284
Urticaria, 207–211
Urtica urens, 79
UVA light, 189–190, 251, 300, 318
UVB light, 189–190, 251, 300